Springer Biographies

The books published in the Springer Biographies tell of the life and work of scholars, innovators, and pioneers in all fields of learning and throughout the ages. Prominent scientists and philosophers will feature, but so too will lesser known personalities whose significant contributions deserve greater recognition and whose remarkable life stories will stir and motivate readers. Authored by historians and other academic writers, the volumes describe and analyse the main achievements of their subjects in manner accessible to nonspecialists, interweaving these with salient aspects of the protagonists' personal lives. Autobiographies and memoirs also fall into the scope of the series.

Bernadette Bensaude-Vincent • Francis Duck

Paul Langevin: Physicist and Social Activist

First Edition

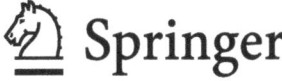 Springer

Bernadette Bensaude-Vincent
CETCOPRA
Univ of Paris 1-Panthéon-Sorbonne
Paris, France

Francis Duck
Bath, UK

ISSN 2365-0613   ISSN 2365-0621 (electronic)
Springer Biographies
ISBN 978-3-031-95259-3   ISBN 978-3-031-95260-9 (eBook)
https://doi.org/10.1007/978-3-031-95260-9

Translation from the French language edition: "Langevin, 1872-1946: Science et vigilance" by Bernadette Bensaude-Vincent © Belin 1987. Published by Belin, Paris. All Rights Reserved.

© The Editor(s) (if applicable) and The Author(s), under exclusive license to Springer Nature Switzerland AG 2025

This work is subject to copyright. All rights are solely and exclusively licensed by the Publisher, whether the whole or part of the material is concerned, specifically the rights of reprinting, reuse of illustrations, recitation, broadcasting, reproduction on microfilms or in any other physical way, and transmission or information storage and retrieval, electronic adaptation, computer software, or by similar or dissimilar methodology now known or hereafter developed.
The use of general descriptive names, registered names, trademarks, service marks, etc. in this publication does not imply, even in the absence of a specific statement, that such names are exempt from the relevant protective laws and regulations and therefore free for general use.
The publisher, the authors and the editors are safe to assume that the advice and information in this book are believed to be true and accurate at the date of publication. Neither the publisher nor the authors or the editors give a warranty, expressed or implied, with respect to the material contained herein or for any errors or omissions that may have been made. The publisher remains neutral with regard to jurisdictional claims in published maps and institutional affiliations.

This Springer imprint is published by the registered company Springer Nature Switzerland AG
The registered company address is: Gewerbestrasse 11, 6330 Cham, Switzerland

If disposing of this product, please recycle the paper.

Preface to the English Revision of *Langevin, science et vigilance*

Langevin, science et vigilance was written in the 1980s. When it was published in 1987, it was the most recent of five full biographies of Paul Langevin published since he had died in 1946: three of them were in French and two in Russian. Another brief volume had also been published in German. Most of these books were testaments to the high regard in which Langevin was held in some quarters during this era. *Langevin, science et vigilance* was the first true biography to be written by a professional historian on the basis of primary sources, thanks to the archives opened to the public by the Langevin family. Since 1987, many of them have been digitized and are now freely available online through *Université PSL* Explore. This facility has enabled deeper research into Langevin's papers. Further archived records have also been accessed, including the Einstein papers published in digital format by Caltech, British Government papers from the UK National Archives, Kew, the British Newspaper archive and French police records from World War II.

Langevin's dual profile as a scientist of high reputation and an intellectual committed to the public arena still retains relevance in the 2020s. Even so, no full account of his life and work has been available to English-speaking readers, apart from the recent translation and publication of André Langevin's descriptive biography of his father.

Our primary purpose in preparing this English revision of *Langevin, science et vigilance* is to move beyond a purely archive-based narrative. We now can provide a more critical evaluation of Langevin's role in science and society during the first half of the twentieth century, in the light of the recent historiographical scholarship. During the time since *Langevin, science et vigilance* appeared, there have been a number of developments that make it appropriate to revisit the narrative. Most recently, 2022 marked the 150th anniversary of the birth of Paul Langevin on January 23, 1872. This anniversary was the occasion for several meetings, talks and presentations, both in France and elsewhere, that served as a reminder of the breadth of Langevin's contributions, to society as much as to science. In particular, medical ultrasound has grown into a multi-billion-dollar industry, and there are few who have never benefitted from this technology. For this reason, the narrative on Langevin's place as the originator of ultrasonics has been expanded, including a number of aspects that have rarely or never appeared in other accounts. It also served to emphasize the continuing scholarship into various aspects of Langevin's private life and views about science and society, which was not available when the biography was originally composed.

In carrying out this translation we have therefore taken the opportunity to revise, enrich and update the original text, taking account of the recent historiography. In particular, the chapters on his private life, on ultrasonics, on the Solvay councils and on his relations with communism and Marxism have been significantly expanded. We have also added 30 new images to enhance the selection of 78 that now illustrate the revised text.

We want to express our gratitude to Catherine Kounelis, head of the Historical Resources Centre of the *Ecole supérieure de physique et de chimie industrielles*, where the Archives of Paul Langevin are kept, and her predecessor Monique Monnerie. They both have been encouraging and extremely helpful throughout this biographical enterprise.

We are also grateful to Martha Cecilia Bustamante for sharing the manuscript of her volume on Jacques Solomon and her views on quantum mechanics.

This biographical account also benefited from the memories of late members of the Langevin family or friends whom one of us interviewed in the 1980s: Luce Langevin, Jean Langevin, Hélène Solomon, Noémie Koechlin and Marie-Élisa Nordmann-Cohen.

Finally, thanks are due to those who have read drafts of this manuscript: Diana Buchwald, Jean-Marc Lévy-Leblond as well as Catherine Kounelis and Martha-Cecilia Bustamante.

Paris, France   Bernadette Bensaude-Vincent
Bath, UK   Francis Duck

References

Bensaude-Vincent B (1987) Langevin, science et vigilance. Belin, Paris
Biquard P (1969) Langevin scientifique, éducateur, citoyen. Éditions Seghers, Paris
Ghimezan I (1964) Paul Langevin. Youth Publishing House, Bucharest
Gross É (2005) La physique de Paul Langevin. Un savoir partagé. ESPCI, Paris
Langevin A (1971) Paul Langevin mon père. Éditeurs Français Réunis, Paris. English edition:
    Duck F (2022) Paul Langevin, my father. EDP Sciences, Paris
Nicolle J (1952) Paul Langevin de grosse französische Physiker und Patriot (1872-1946).
    Aufbau, Berlin
Staroselskaya-Nikitina O (1962) Paul Langevin. State Publishing House for Physical-Mathematical
    Literature, Moscow

A note on the textual citations References to Langevin's works are not included at the end of each chapter, and reference is made as (Langevin 19xx) to the bibliography at the end of the book. Documents from the Langevin digital archive are identified as (Archives) with a reference number (https://bibnum.explore.psl.eu/s/psl/item-set/249135).

A note on the images The sources of some images used in this book are identified in the captions as follows: ESPCI, for *ESPCI Centre for Historical Resources*; PSL University, for *Université (Paris Sciences et Lettres)*; Science et Vigilance for *Bernadette Bensaude-Vincent (1987) Langevin, science et vigilance*, Paris, Belin, for which this book is the authorized English revision. Sources for widely available portraits are not given. Cover images (front) Hebrew University of Jerusalem: (back) *ESPCI Centre for Historical Resources*.

Contents

1 **A "Secular Saint"** 1
   1.1 A Public Icon 1
   1.2 Profile of a Third Republic *Notable* 2
   1.3 Science and Action 4
   1.4 A Dispersed Scholar 6
   References 8

2 **The Road to Glory** 9
   2.1 Child of the *Butte* 9
   2.2 An Effervescent Scientific Community 13
   2.3 A Dazzling Early Career 18
   2.4 A Theory of Magnetism 20
   References 22

3 **A Turbulent Private Life** 23
   3.1 A Circle of Friends 24
   3.2 A Vibrant Social Life 26
   3.3 Troubles in Married Life 28
   3.4 Shame and Scandal 30
   3.5 Drama and Farce 33
   References 36

4 **Atoms in Science Education** 37
   4.1 Debates About Science Education 37
   4.2 Culture Versus Technology 39
   4.3 Historical Versus Dogmatic 40
   4.4 Atomism Versus Mechanics 41
   4.5 Atomism Versus Energetics 43
   4.6 Science Is Life 45
   References 47

5	**The Physics of Electrons, a New World**...........................	49
	5.1 The Triumph of Electromagnetism	52
	5.2 "Thinking in Ether".......................................	54
	5.3 Langevin's $E = mc^2$	56
	References...	59

6	**Promoting the Theory of Relativity**............................	61
	6.1 Breaking with Heroic Historical Narratives..................	62
	6.2 Langevin's Personal Version of the Principle of Relativity.......	64
	6.3 Relativity as Adaptation...................................	67
	6.4 Langevin's Traveller in a Rocket	68
	References...	72

7	**War Service: Underwater Echoes**	75
	7.1 Collapse of a Dream World	76
	7.2 The Creation of Ultrasonics................................	77
	7.3 Forming an Expert Team	80
	7.4 The Chilowsky/Langevin Patent	83
	7.5 The First Echoes	85
	References...	86

8	**The Genesis of Piezoelectric Technology**........................	89
	8.1 A Legacy of Pierre Curie	89
	8.2 A *Quartz Piézoélectrique* Is Sent to London..................	91
	8.3 From Discovery to Prototype...............................	92
	8.4 The Marvel of Quartz Resonance	95
	8.5 The Quartz Sandwich Transducer	97
	8.6 Interallied Conference on Supersonics (19–22 October 1918)....	100
	References...	100

9	**Restoring Science and Peace**	103
	9.1 A Scholar in the Public Arena	105
	9.2 "The Internationale of the Mind"...........................	106
	9.3 Promoting Cultural Internationalism	107
	9.4 Challenging the Boycott of German Science..................	110
	References...	112

10	**Einstein in Paris**	113
	10.1 A Major Media Event	113
	10.2 A Busy Week of Lectures	115
	10.3 A Memorable Session at the *Société française de philosophie*...	118
	10.4 Dialogue and Misunderstandings..........................	119
	10.5 Impacts of Einstein's Visit	121
	References...	123

11	**Ultrasonics in Peacetime**.....................................	125
	11.1 International Patent Competition..........................	126
	11.2 Langevin's 1918 Patent	128

	11.3 Ultrasonics Survives	131
	11.4 Chilowsky Reappears	132
	11.5 Back to Basics	136
	11.6 Claims and Counterclaims	139
	References	142
12	**Figures of Science and Rationalism**	**143**
	12.1 The Prostitution of Science	144
	12.2 "Science, Mother and Daughter of Democracy"	145
	12.3 "Science, Elder Sister of Justice"	148
	12.4 Rationalism or Scientism?	150
	12.5 A Religion of Reason	152
	References	153
13	**Career Profile**	**155**
	13.1 Intensifying Activism for Peace	157
	13.2 Declining Scientific Productivity?	163
	13.3 "Scientific Consultant"	167
	13.4 The "Boss"	168
	References	170
14	**Langevin and the Solvay Physics Councils**	**171**
	14.1 1911: A "Witches' Sabbath"	173
	14.2 A Modest Participation	177
	14.3 President of the Scientific Board	180
	14.4 Mission Impossible, Given the Circumstances	182
	References	183
15	**Sharing Knowledge as a Duty**	**185**
	15.1 Public Outreach	186
	15.2 Three Big Cultural Enterprises in the 1930s	187
	15.3 Actor in Cross-Disciplinary Exchanges	192
	15.4 At the *Centre international de synthèse*	194
	References	195
16	**Langevin in the Debates on Quantum Mechanics**	**197**
	16.1 The First Quantum Theory	197
	16.2 Louis de Broglie "Lifted a Corner of the Great Veil"	198
	16.3 The Crisis of Determinism	201
	16.4 It's a Crisis in the Theory of Mechanics	204
	16.5 Langevin in the Bohr-Einstein Controversy	206
	References	209
17	**Langevin Marxist?**	**211**
	17.1 Quantum Physics as a Prompt Towards Marxism	212
	17.2 Marxist Initiation Through the *Cercle de la Russie neuve*	217
	17.3 Marxist "à la française"	219
	References	222

18	**Langevin and the French Communist Party**	223
	18.1 A Vignette	223
	18.2 The PCF and the Intellectuals	225
	18.3 A Fellow Traveller	226
	18.4 One Step Forward…	229
	18.5 …One Step Backward	232
	References	234
19	**Through the Hardships of World War Two**	235
	19.1 Humiliated, Honoured	236
	19.2 Mandatory Vacation	240
	19.3 The Time of Tributes	245
	19.4 The Flash of Hiroshima	246
	References	251
20	**Changing Society Through Educational Reforms**	253
	20.1 Knowledge-Based Methods of Teaching	254
	20.2 *L'école unique*	257
	20.3 Modern Humanities	258
	20.4 The Langevin-Wallon Plan	259
	20.5 A Dormant Reform?	262
	References	265
21	**Postscript**	267
	References	270
	Bibliography	270
	Chronology	281
	Index	289

About the Authors

Bernadette Bensaude-Vincent philosopher and historian of science, is Emeritus Professor at the University of Paris 1 Pantheon-Sorbonne, and a member of the French Academy of technology. She has authored or edited more than 20 books and 200 articles and essays on the history of chemical sciences and techno-sciences as well as on the issue of science and the public. In 2021 she received the George Sarton Medal, the highest distinction of the History of Science Society and in 2024 the Franklin-Lavoisier prize from the History of Science Institute and the *Fondation de la Maison de la chimie*.

Francis Duck is a retired medical physicist who, until 2018, was visiting professor at the University of Bath, UK. He has degrees from the Universities of Nottingham (BSc in Physics) and London (PhD, DSc). He spent time in research in medical ultrasound in the UK, Canada and the USA, and then made his career as a medical physicist in the UK National Health Service. He has published widely, largely in topics on medical ultrasonics. Since retirement, he has focused on the history of physics applied to medicine, and most recently has edited a history of medical ultrasound with the International Organisation for Medical Physics. In 2007 he was made MBE for services to health care.

Chapter 1
A "Secular Saint"

Abstract The name Paul Langevin, inscribed on the walls of many French cities, is a figure of French heritage. He is neither quite legendary, like his illustrious friends Albert Einstein and Marie Curie, nor completely obscure like so many other activist scientists of his generation. He is just famous enough to be unknown. He was depicted as "the most human of scientists" and "a man of deep kindness, constantly putting his devotion at the service of those who suffered". Langevin combined ethical with intellectual qualities, courage with patience, and reason with generosity and intelligence with humanity. He had all the qualities of a "secular saint". He was also a "dispersed scholar", who crossed boundaries and refused to confine himself to a single research area, but who, as a counterbalance, developed a strong aspiration to unification, to the synthesis of knowledge.

1.1 A Public Icon

Langevin belongs to that uncertain fringe of the past situated between memory and history. The story of his life has been told by relatives, friends and collaborators. These recollections have the qualities of testimony and the flavour of memories. But they tend to create a stereotype, capturing the character into a frozen vignette. They have composed a three-faceted portrait of Langevin: the scientist, the educator and the citizen. All three faces are unified under the banner: a man of progress. Langevin the scientist was a pioneer of the atomic era, always supporting new theories that had shaken the foundations of physics by the beginning of the twentieth century. Langevin the educator was a fierce opponent of tradition and denounced the routine and sclerosis of French education. Finally, as a political activist, Langevin fought tirelessly for justice and to build a world of peace. The image of a man of progress is so powerful that it seems to encapsulate his entire work. Georges Cogniot, who

© The Author(s), under exclusive license to Springer Nature
Switzerland AG 2025
B. Bensaude-Vincent, F. Duck, *Paul Langevin: Physicist and Social Activist*,
Springer Biographies, https://doi.org/10.1007/978-3-031-95260-9_1

fought many political and educational battles with Langevin,[1] selected this trait to depict the character in his obituary.

> The mystery of Paul Langevin was his perpetual youthful spirit. He pushed forward, into battle and to victory, until the end. He renewed himself with an inexhaustible curiosity and ardour at an age when, usually, his peers enjoy, in stillness, a consecrated glory. His intellectual and practical life was, for fifty years, a drama, a progression, a conquest. As we knew him, as this book would like to revive him, in motion. [5, p. 14]

The physicist Pierre Biquard[2] did not hesitate to attribute this progressive inclination to some instinct:

> Faced with the problems of scientific knowledge, Paul Langevin adopted instinctively an attitude oriented towards progress. Far from being frightened, the boldest innovations led to his adherence and active participation. He understood, enriched, taught, spread the truth. Faced with the problems of man and society, his behaviour was exactly the same ... [1, p. 78]

The intellectual portrait of Langevin immortalized by his disciples was enriched with moral features when his death was announced by the press. He was depicted as "the most human of scientists" in *Les Lettres françaises* (27 December 1946); "This genius physicist was also a man of deep kindness, constantly putting his devotion at the service of those who suffered" in the protestant weekly *Réforme* (5 January 1947). Langevin combined ethical with intellectual qualities, courage with patience, reason with generosity, intelligence with humanity. He had all the qualities of a "secular saint".

1.2 Profile of a Third Republic *Notable*

It would not be difficult to denounce the hagiographic, ideological and political components of these heroic portraits. Patiently deconstructing the myth to substitute a more realistic portrait is a relatively easy task, with the hindsight of history. But it would be at the risk of maintaining the mirage of historians as impartial observers of the past. It seems to us more appropriate to take the popular icon seriously in

---

[1] Georges Cogniot (1902–1978), a professor of literature and an activist, collaborated with Langevin on several occasions notably in peace and antifascist movements in the 1930s as well as in the Commission for Educational Reform in 1944–1946. A member of the Central Committee of the French Communist Party (PCF) for about 30 years, in 1938 he co-founded *La Pensée* with Langevin, a journal that was supported by the PCF to spread Marxist thought among intellectuals.

[2] Pierre Biquard (1901–1992), started his career in the General Electricity Laboratory headed by Langevin at the *École municipale de physique et de chimie industrielles* (EPCI), then worked with Frédéric Joliot Curie. During the war, he joined the French Resistance. One of the founders of the French Atomic Energy Commission (CEA) in 1945, he was chief of staff to Frédéric Joliot, the CEA's high commissioner from 1946 to 1950.

1.2 Profile of a Third Republic *Notable*

order to grasp its meaning and thereby shed light on the mentalities of an age when scientists enjoyed a high prestige in Western societies.

The oxymoron "secular saint" was in vogue in the early twentieth century to refer to an exemplary person respected for his or her contributions to a noble cause.[3] In France, the phrase "saint laïc", often applied to scholars like Emile Littré or Louis Pasteur, testifies to the fascination for great intellectuals and political figures during the Third Republic. It suggests that Langevin embodied the values that prevailed in the French society of that time.

And indeed, Langevin's profile and career have been deeply marked by the values and aspirations of the Third Republic, a regime that covers all his lifetime, since he was born in 1872 (2 years after the proclamation of the Third Republic) and died in 1946, at the dawn of the Fourth Republic. Frock coat and stiff collar, small moustache and brushed hair, Langevin has the look typical of the honourable professors of the Third Republic (Fig. 1.1). He belongs to a long lineage of French intellectuals who coupled intellectual achievements with engagement in the public sphere. Dating back to the eighteenth century with figures like Voltaire and Diderot, brilliantly pursued in the nineteenth century with Victor Hugo, this tradition was rejuvenated by the Dreyfus Affair which prompted famous writers such as Emile Zola,[4] scientists such as Emile Duclaux,[5] and many others to accuse the government of lies and injustice [10].

Langevin was by no means a marginal. Let's not imagine an eccentric scientist, away from official science, a kind of "terrible child of the university", a label occasionally used for Einstein. Even when he was a scientist in rebellion against governmental measures, Langevin remained a "notable", a prominent member of the regime, so respected that his ashes were transferred to the Pantheon in 1948 together with the remains of his friend Jean Perrin.

Furthermore, Langevin is an example of the mechanism of social ascent through education typical of the Third Republic. Thanks to the non-clerical system of public education implemented by Prime Minister Jules Ferry it was possible for a youth of modest origin, like Langevin, to be able to become an international star in the physics community. As a student, he bravely climbed all the rungs of the education ladder from compulsory primary school to the elitist Ecole normale Supérieure. He subsequently remained in the educational system for all his life, becoming a

---

[3] According to Google Books NGram viewer, the phrase "secular saint" first used in English language in 1885 reached a peak in 1890 and a second lower peak in 1940–1945. In French literature, "saint laïc", hardly used until 1900, became more and more popular in the first half of the twentieth century with a first peak in 1930–1935 and a second higher one in 1945.

[4] Emile Zola (1840–1902), a French writer, critic, and political activist was the most prominent French novelist of the late nineteenth century. Zola fully committed himself in defending Alfred Dreyfus, a Jewish officer in the French army who was accused of treason by the government.

[5] Emile Duclaux (1840–1904), chemist and biologist was a close collaborator of Louis Pasteur whom he succeeded as director of the Pasteur Institute. He was also fully committed in defence of Captain Dreyfus.

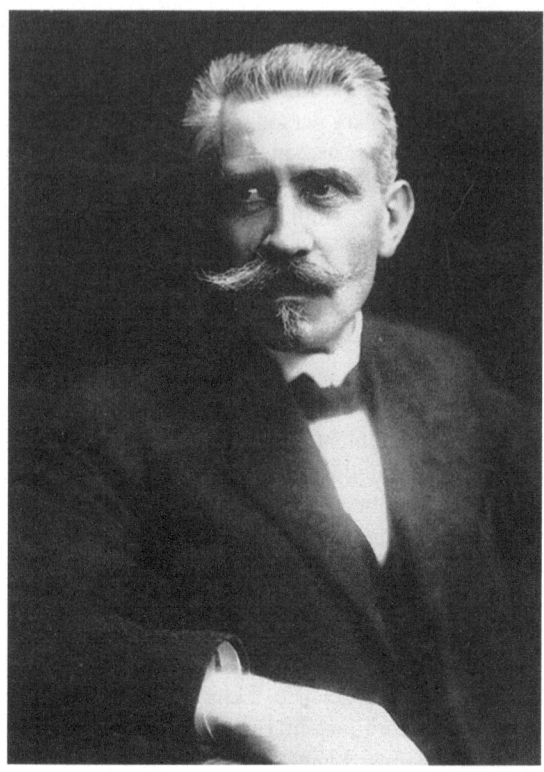

Fig. 1.1 Photograph of Langevin by Genia Reinberg. (ESPCI)

professor at the *Collège de France*[6] and the Director of the Paris *Ecole municipale de physique et de chimie industrielles* (EPCI). Finally, it is in the reorganization of public education that he attempted to materialize his ideal of social justice when he chaired the big reform project of the French educational system set up at the Liberation in 1944, known as the Langevin-Wallon plan.

1.3 Science and Action

How did Langevin manage to become so famous? What did he achieve in his scientific, educational, or political career to become such an icon of progress? Is he the author of a groundbreaking scientific discovery, the founder of a new discipline or theory? Did he invent a new pedagogy? Was he the leader of a revolutionary movement? None of these labels really suits him. Such is the paradox that makes the interest and complexity of this biography. Langevin never became a political leader,

---

[6] The *Collège de France*, created in the sixteenth century, is a prestigious public institution teaching cutting edge research.

1.3 Science and Action

nor a party man; and the reform project that bears his name has never been implemented.

In physics, he had already established for himself a high international reputation by his 30s, through important research on ionized gases and the theory of magnetism. Many of his colleagues also commented on his experimental skills, presumably acquired in his laboratory training under the supervision of Pierre Curie at EPCI. His later work on ultrasound and piezoelectricity added the accolade of engineer to the fame of the theoretical and experimental physicist. However, Langevin was neither a discoverer nor a Nobel Prize winner, although he was nominated 15 times. Sometimes, he didn't even bother to publish his results and was content to present them, mixed with those of others, during his courses at the *Collège de France*, according to his colleagues and students.[7] In 1905, he was exploring the implications of relativity but he was content to disseminate Einstein's ideas. Einstein himself emphasized this effacement in his obituary:

> The burden of duties always undertaken of his own free will however hindered his own research, which is why the fruit of his work appeared more in the publications of others than in his own. It seems certain to me that he would have developed the special theory of relativity if it had not been done elsewhere; for he had clearly recognized the essential points. [4, p. 13]

Like many intellectuals of his generation, Langevin was affected by the shock of the First World War that deeply undermined faith in the progress of civilization and society. Seeking to overcome the shock he found remedies through public engagement. In the 1920s, he joined various world movements with the hope that through campaigns targeting young people and through scientific cooperation, it would still be possible to restore peace. Later, in the face of rising international tensions in the 1930s, he embarked into vibrant activism, restlessly fighting against fascism. Thus, Langevin increasingly spread his activities in multiple directions. He ran from congress to committees, from meetings to commissions, multiplying commitments. Was this at the risk of dissipating his energy in vain? Certainly, one can observe a fairly rapid decline in his scientific production at this time, in stark contrast to the pre-war, extremely fruitful, years. A glance at his list of publications shows that Langevin produced about as many results in the 15 years before the war as during the 30 years that follow.

---

[7] "Three quarters of Langevin's work has not been published" estimates Léon Brillouin, physicist who graduated under Langevin's supervision and collaborated with him. He emigrated to the United States during the First World War and founded information theory. The estimate may be exaggerated but all the testimonies of Langevin's colleagues and those who attended his courses at the *Collège de France* point in the same direction [1, p. 69]. Langevin himself speaks of his "reluctance to publish his work" in a letter dated 13 January 1925, addressed to Albert Einstein [8, p. 23].

1.4 A Dispersed Scholar

While praising the courage, modesty and self-sacrifice of Langevin, one can nevertheless worry about the consequences of his choice. Did he not miss a brilliant scientific career? Did he not waste his talents through his activism? "Dispersed scholar": is this the label that should be substituted for that of "secular saint"? Yes, the young Langevin was dissipated in many senses. The young Langevin was a dandy who led a dissolute life and had love affairs. The mature scientist and activist always opted for dispersion in his scientific works as well as in his social activism. Regardless of his strong pacifist or social convictions, he never identified with any party or movement. He rather diversified his commitments in dozens of organizations. As a young researcher, he decided to work on several subjects at the same time. From the start, Langevin crossed boundaries and refused to confine himself to a single research area. In the single year 1905, he published on electrons, on ionized gases, on the kinetic theory, on magnetism, on the impossibility of demonstrating the translational motion of the earth, on the inertia of energy. Later, in the 1930s, he remained apart from the competition that was taking place in atomic physics as he chose to devote the largest part of his scientific activity to communication and dissemination. Dissipation is, for Langevin, an intellectual strategy, a good practice based on his conviction that disseminating and sharing scientific knowledge matters as much as producing it.

Even in his ways of spreading the most recent developments in physics, Langevin inclined towards maximum dispersion. His work is made of a mosaic of scattered pieces: articles, lectures, talks, pamphlets. He never wrote a big treatise, a textbook, nor a popular science book. Instead, he delivered talks at a variety of institutions and at events all over the world.[8] His preference for oral communication largely shaped his style of thought. Langevin liked to display brilliant synoptic reviews on a topic rather than delivering patient and meticulous analyses. He was fond of images and metaphors and he was able to talk to all kinds of audiences, from colleagues and experts to the lay public. This scientist was a good performer. He used the technical skills that he acquired during his training at the EPCI to accompany his lectures with spectacular experiments on electricity. For example, he used a quadrant electrometer to project a light spot onto a screen, displaying to a large audience the quantities of electricity measured by this device. He fully participated in the new culture of sensitivity that the "fairy electricity" and radiations developed around 1900 with a taste for spectacular demonstrations shrouded in mystery [9].

As a counterbalance to his dispersive inclinations and the spread of his research interests, Langevin developed a strong aspiration to unification, to the synthesis of

---

[8] Langevin's main scientific papers published in scientific journals have been collected in a volume published by the *Centre national de la recherche scientifique* after his death [6]. Twelve of his talks delivered between 1894 and 1946, published in obscure and hardly accessible brochures or journals, have been selected and published by Vuibert in 2007 [7].

knowledge. He developed broad panoramas of the evolution of mankind in his public talks. As Louis de Broglie noted in his portrait of Langevin:

> A lover of general ideas, he was keen to consider the philosophical aspects of advances in physics and, coming at a time when the outlook for science was constantly changing, he enjoyed looking at the ever-changing panorama of our knowledge as a whole and drawing out its broad outlines. [3, p. 237]

Indeed, Langevin was never a professional philosopher. As we will see, his considerations on scientific progress, society and civilization were far from original or innovative. However, his philosophical convictions shaped under the pressure of circumstances, sometimes under the shock of events, deserves the attention of historians. By virtue of their very banality, they open a window on the mentalities of a generation. Moreover, they also provide a key to grasp what makes the unity of Langevin's dispersed life and the coherence of his work. Finally, they afford clues to better understand the meaning of the public icon of Langevin as a secular saint. For this icon may express his unabated attempts to save his faith in progress despite his own doubts and anxieties, and the external threats of barbarism. A human voice trying to drown out the noise of weapons.

So the strong public image of Langevin is not built on the basis of a specific aspect of his work. It rather proceeds from the conjunction of the various and multiple facets of his life. Here was a leading figure of science, an expert in abstract physics who was capable of communicating and interacting with people from all walks of life. A son of the working class who rose to the level of the Collège de France, he remained a friend of the people. Romain Rolland,[9] who long rubbed shoulders with Langevin in peace movements, depicted him in 1934 as "a master of science who leads the popular classes". The same terms are found in the press articles announcing Langevin's death: "A great Frenchman who put his intelligence at the service of the people" (*France nouvelle*, 21 December 1946); "The scientist never ceased to share the aspirations of the people" (*Ce soir*); "The ardent life of a child of the people who became one of the greatest scientists in the universe"; and as a subtitle "An example for the youth of France" (*L'Avant-garde*, 25–31 December 1946). Even those who disapproved of Langevin's project, like Étienne Gilson for instance, considered he was moral authority above the parties (*L'Aube*, 7 August 1947).

Obituaries published in the British press represented the dispersion of his talents. The *Illustrated London News* emphasized his work on magnetism. John D. Bernal, writing in *Nature*, emphasized the importance of Sonar, and of quartz-controlled oscillators, both arising from Langevin's work in the First World War. *The Times* noted that Langevin had long been interested in politics and was "known for his advanced ideas". The British physicist James Crowther remembered "his influence over persons arose from his selflessness; his attention was always directed outside

---

[9] Romain Rolland (1866–1944) was a French essayist and novelist who was awarded the Nobel Prize for Literature in 1915. He put his fame in the service of peace especially in his early membership in the World Committee against War and Fascism.

himself. He was a wonderful listener and friend; young men of talent always felt he was genuinely devoted to them" [2, p. 268].

Bernal recalled that Langevin said: "The scientific work which I can do, can be done and will be done by others, possibly soon, possibly not for some years; but unless the political work is done there will be no science at all". Throughout his career Langevin might have faced the ethical dilemma since he noted at the end of his life:

> Allow me, an old man, to evoke my personal experience, to retrace the path along which circumstances led me to reconcile various tasks as best I could, and along which I was able to verify how much easier it is to fulfil one's duty than to know it. In this way, I was led to an at least apparent dispersion that, before the war and the recent occupation, some of my best friends reproached me for, not so much in the interest of Science, which could do without me, but in my own personal interest. (Langevin 1946a, p. 13)

How to write the biography of such an emblematic character, now that the speeches that held students or the public spellbound are frozen words printed on yellowing paper? Rather than attempting to provide a complete overview of all his achievements we will focus on a few key moments in his life and works. There will therefore inevitably be gaps, differences in tone and breaks in style through the chapters. We will strive, as much as possible, to provide the background of Langevin's claims and actions in order to contextualize them and to better discover how, as a scientist and an activist, he achieved such high social prestige in mid-twentieth-century France.

References

1. Biquard P (1969) Paul Langevin, scientifique, éducateur, citoyen. Seghers, Paris
2. Crowther JG (1970) Fifty years with science. Barrie & Jenkins, London, p 268
3. De Broglie L (1951) La vie et l'œuvre de Paul Langevin. In: Savants et découvertes. Albin Michel, Paris, pp 233–269
4. Einstein A (1947) Paul Langevin. La Pensée 12:13–14
5. Labérenne P (1964) La Pensée et l'action. éditions sociales, Paris
6. Langevin P (1950) Œuvres scientifiques de Paul Langevin. éditions CNRS, Paris
7. Langevin P (2007) Propos d'un physicien engagé (ed: Bensaude-Vincent B). Vuibert, Paris
8. La Pensée (1972) Langevin L. Paul Langevin et Albert Einstein d'après une correspondance et des documents inédits. p 161
9. Sibum O (2008) Experience – experiments: the changing experiential basis of physics. In: Beretta M, Grandin K, Lindqvist S (eds) Aurora Torealis. Studies in the history of science and ideas. Watson Publishing International, Sagamore Beach, pp 181–191
10. Winock M (2015) Le Siècle des intellectuels. Points-Seuil, Paris

Chapter 2
The Road to Glory

Abstract Langevin grew up in the Montmartre district in the aftermath of the violence of the Paris Commune. His background hardly predestined him for a brilliant career as a physicist, but he benefited from the educational system introduced by the French Third Republic. Langevin graduated top of his year at the *École municipale de physique et de chimie industrielles de Paris* (EPCI) in 1891. Continuing his education at the prestigious *École normale supérieure* he was ranked first in the *agrégation* of physics in 1897, in addition to making many life-long friends. The world of physics was febrile, with X-rays, radioactivity and ether, challenging experimentalists and theoreticians who were conflicted in their approaches. A year's scholarship with J.J. Thompson in Cambridge, the basis for his PhD in gas ionization in 1904, gave him a springboard for a dazzling career. His 12 publications that year included topics as disparate as gas ionization, the inertia of energy, the ether and kinetic theory, followed the next year by seminal contributions to Brownian motion and magnetism.

Langevin could serve as a model for graduate students and young researchers because he is a self-made scientist. His background hardly predestined him for a brilliant career as a physicist. But he benefited from the educational system introduced by the French Republic and succeeded thanks to hard, intense work, and a social network of friends.

2.1 Child of the *Butte*

Paul Langevin's grandfather was a locksmith and his father Victor left school to enlist in the army at the age of 18. From 1854 to 1868, he travelled in Algeria with the imperial troops. When Victor Langevin returned to Paris in 1870, he married Marie-Adèle Pinel, great-niece of the famous psychiatrist Philippe Pinel. The couple settled on the Butte Montmartre, a working-class hilltop suburb annexed to the city of Paris in 1860. This neighbourhood was the crucible where the Paris Commune ignited on 18 March 1871. The Langevins thus found themselves on the front line during the revolt that ended up in the "bloody week" at the end of May 1871, while they were expecting their second child. Paul, this second son, was born shortly afterwards, on 23 January 1872, in a family still traumatized by the repression of the riots. He was born on rue Ravignan, which remains famous because, at the turn of the century, many years after the departure of the Langevins, it hosted a group of painters and poets at the *Bateau-lavoir*. André Langevin described the Langevin's apartment during the first year of Paul's life, as "beautiful and very simple", with a "bulls-eye" window above the door, and large-paned windows "each surmounted by an elegant and very sober coat of arms". These architectural details remain.

Paul Langevin is therefore a "child of the Butte", like Gavroche the fictional character in Victor Hugo's novel *Les Misérables*. He could run in the narrow streets of a Montmartre, in complete upheaval because, at the top of the hill, the Sacré Coeur Basilica was under construction. The decision to build this massive basilica at the height of the popular revolt was part of the establishment of a bourgeois "moral order" following the events of the Paris Commune. This did not arouse many religious feelings in the young Paul Langevin who seems to have been much more imbued with the republican past of Montmartre:

> I grew up, in the aftermath of the war of 1870, between a republican father and a mother devoted to sacrifice. Eyewitnesses of the siege of Paris and the bloody repression of the Commune, they instilled in me, through their stories, the horror of violence and the passionate desire for justice. (Langevin 1945d, p. 45)

In 1880, the family moved to another neighbourhood. Paul went to a "communal" primary school in the 15th arrondissement, and passed the primary school certificate in 1883 (Fig. 2.1). Since he was a brilliant pupil this diploma did not mark the end of his educational journey, as was the case for the majority of pupils. Langevin was admitted to the Ecole primaire supérieure Lavoisier . This was a new type of public institution officially created in the 1880s and nicknamed *collège du peuple* (the people's high school), because it was attended by children from the working class whereas the *lycées* which delivered the *baccalauréat* were reserved for the bourgeoisie [2]. Following the course of study at the Superior Primary School, Langevin obtained the highest score at the entrance exam of the *École municipale de physique et de chimie industrielles de Paris* (EPCI) in 1888. The EPCI had been founded in 1882 by the Alsatian chemists Paul Schutzenberger and Charles Lauth on the model of the Mulhouse school [13]. Its aim was to train competent engineers for the industrial sector, and to give them a high level of theoretical background in physics and chemistry as well as experimental skills, thanks to practical classes in the laboratory or the workshop. The municipality of Paris offered scholarships for able students. Langevin attended Pierre Curie's classes here, graduating top of his year in 1891 (Fig. 2.2). He remained part of the school for the rest of his life, becoming director of studies and then director in 1926.

By the end of this 3-year course of study at EPCI, Langevin seemed more attracted to teaching than to industry. Having acquired some teaching skills out of necessity through giving fee-paying maths or physics lessons to make ends meet, he

2.1 Child of the *Butte*

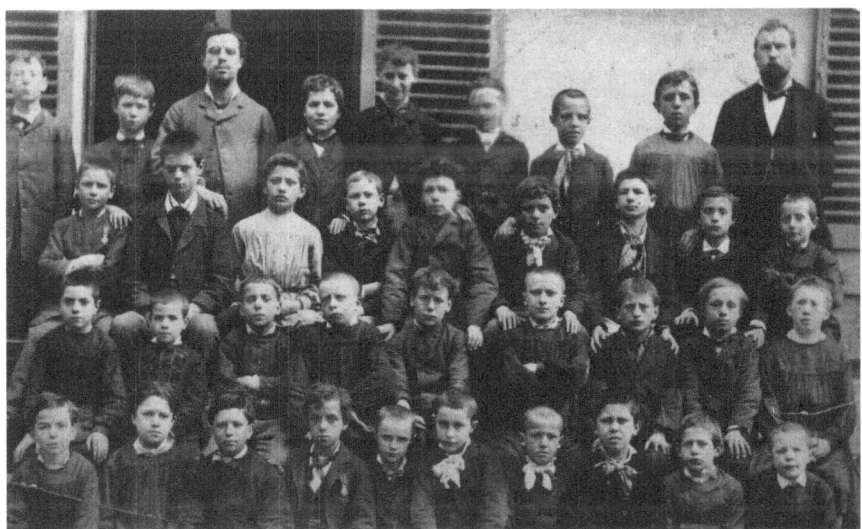

Fig. 2.1 At the "communale" about 1880: Langevin is the third student from the right, bottom row. (ESPCI)

Fig. 2.2 Seventh graduation of the EPCI: Langevin is the second on the left. (ESPCI)

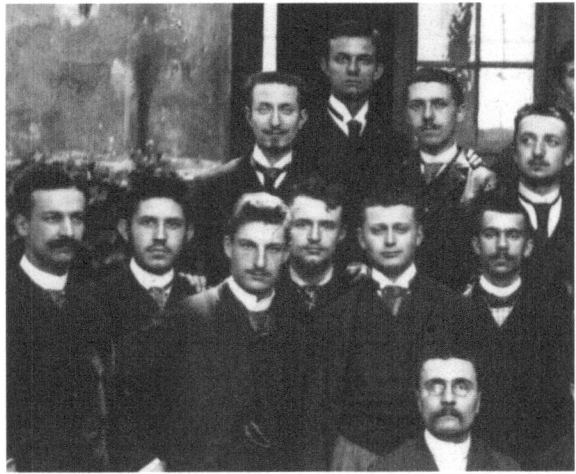

chose to pursue a career in education. Following the BA (*licence*) of physics that he obtained at the University of Paris in 1892, he prepared for the highly competitive entrance exam at the *Ecole normale supérieure* (ENS), an elite institution created by the French revolution to train future teachers. The exam required that he learned Latin and classics but he was motivated by the expected salary paid to the *normaliens* (ENS students). He successfully passed the entrance exam in 1893, at the age of 21 (Figure 2.3). For nearly 12 years, Langevin has been a diligent and hardworking student who passed exam after exam. But now he had a break, a rest, his

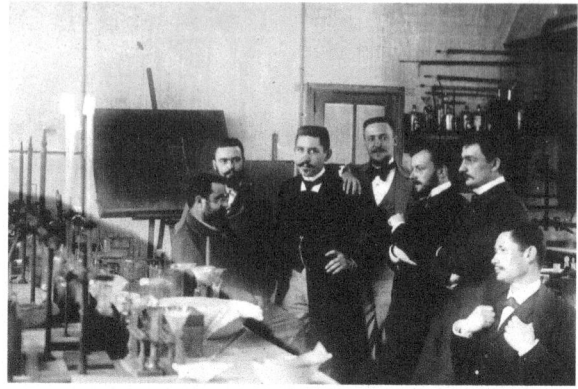

Fig. 2.3 Langevin at the bench at the Ecole normale supérieure, about 1895. (ESPCI)

entrance delayed for a year because of compulsory military service (1893–94). Returning to three years more study, he finally prepared for the additional and final exam, the *agrégation* of physics, that he passed in 1897 and was ranked first.

So remarkable was this achievement that, on Wednesday 10 August 1897, the daily paper *Le Figaro* included a succinct summary of his past and present successes and a prescient observation on his future prospects:

> In the examinations that ended last week for the aggregation in physical sciences, Mr. Paul Langevin achieved a success that deserves to be noted. Having entered the *Ecole normale supérieure* at the top of the class, Mr. Langevin has constantly kept this position and was admitted to the aggregation with the same position, 10 points above the student who followed him. Previously, Mr. Langevin had triumphed in the same way at the *Ecole de physique et de chimie industrielles de la Ville de Paris*. In summary, since 1888, he has not taken any examination without coming out in first place. This is a fine example of perseverance at work and it would be surprising if Mr. Langevin did not, under these circumstances, quickly make progress.

These three years at the ENS proved decisive not only for the excellence of the scientific training but also for the relationships forged with other students from various disciplines who made up a solid network of long-lasting relations for future collaborations.

Langevin was a student at the ENS during a period of political turmoil that was caused by the Dreyfus Affair. When Captain Alfred Dreyfus, a graduate of the *École Polytechnique* and a Jew, was accused of treason and sentenced to life imprisonment, the ENS students, encouraged by the librarian Lucien Herr, supported the petitions against this unfair condemnation [1, 6]. Presumably Langevin was among the students supporting Dreyfus, but he was primarily focused on his studies in physics and was anxious to complete his education with a PhD. Thanks to a scholarship from the city of Paris he was able to commence work for his doctorate in the Cavendish Laboratory, Cambridge, UK. Langevin successfully defended his PhD in 1902 and he immediately got a teaching position as substitute and then supply professor for Eleuthère Mascart at the *Collège de France*.

2.2 An Effervescent Scientific Community

What was the state of physics, in 1900, when Langevin entered this international scientific community? He was immersed into an effervescent research community shaken by a series of major recent discoveries. Roentgen's discovery of X-rays at the end of 1895 attracted considerable public and medical attention. This invisible short-wavelength electromagnetic radiation created astonishment in the popular mind by making the inside of a human body visible without the body being cut open. The boundary between matter and radiation, between the theories of mechanics and electromagnetics was becoming increasingly uncertain. When he arrived in Cambridge as the first foreign research student to be permitted to study there, Langevin found himself immersed in the eye of a tornado. In 1897, John J. Thomson, head of the Cavendish Laboratory, demonstrated that cathode rays were negatively charged particles smaller than atoms and with a negligible mass.[1] In 1898, at the EPCI, Pierre and Marie Curie extracted and isolated from the uranium mineral pitchblende a substance that emits radiation that they named "'radium". Electrons and radioactivity marked the end of an era dating back to antiquity. And, to complete the revolution, in 1900 Max Planck predicted that electromagnetic radiation should be considered, theoretically, to consist of quanta, or packets, of energy. The stable "Victorian era" of the indivisible atom [12, p. 79], and the fundamental pillar of the conservation of matter, was giving way to a wonderful world, populated with mysterious particles and powerful rays.

When considering possible theories to explain these observations, the climate was tense because of the conflict between mechanics and electromagnetism. It crystallized around the problem of the speed of light, because light waves were believed to propagate through an all-pervasive imponderable material, known as the ether. This concept raised the question of the mutual influence between matter and ether and of the relative motion of bodies. On the one hand, a number of physicists, Hendrik Lorentz in particular, assumed that the ether was motionless and that light propagates in this stationary environment, as a transverse wave. On the other hand, George G. Stokes claimed in 1845 that ether is dragged along by matter. In this case, it should be possible to demonstrate the translational motion of the Earth relative to the ether. In 1881, Albert Michelson tried to measure this movement with an interferometer. Morley repeated the experiment in 1887 but they both got negative results. The repeated failure of these experiments challenged the physics community. George Fitzgerald, Hendrick Lorentz and Henri Poincaré all suggested various hypotheses to account for these negative results. Finally, in 1905, Einstein, showed how to get physics out of this impasse, thanks to the two hypotheses of the relativity of space and time and the constancy of the speed of light relative to any inertial

---

[1] J.J. Thomson (1856–1940) is a pioneer of atomic physics. His work led him to consider electrons as the universal constituents of the atom, in vibratory motion that Lorentz mathematically described. Thomson also conceived a model of the atom, sometimes called the "plum pudding model" with positive and negative charges distributed throughout the sphere of the atom.

frame of reference. Between 1900 and 1905, the tension was at its peak. It is therefore a period that could be briefly characterized by an ambivalent climate of crisis and rebirth.

Langevin was a young student in the 1890s, when atomic physics emerged. However, during these crucial years, these challenges were barely being discussed in French universities. In most teaching institutions, physics courses remained focused on rational mechanics with hardly any mention of electromagnetic theory and atoms. The emphasis remained on experimental physics, with theoretical physics assigned to be taught by mathematicians. The divorce between the two approaches to physics inhibited progress [10]. But it was at the core of Langevin's thoughts when he commenced his career in physics.

During these formative years, Langevin managed to overcome this institutional divorce because he was fortunate enough to meet with the few scholars who were exceptions to the rule. They were all in Paris and taught in the Latin Quarter. Langevin acquired an excellent basic training in both mathematical and theoretical fields at the ENS,[2] as well as both experimental and technical skills at the EPCI. In this school, where a famous shed housed the discovery of radium in December 1898, Pierre Curie introduced the student Langevin to research by offering him a modest collaboration on his work in the electricity laboratory (Langevin 1906a). At the Sorbonne, Langevin attended courses given by Henri Poincaré, one of the few professors who taught electromagnetism as well as molecular kinetic theory and the statistical interpretation of Carnot's principle (Langevin 1913f). At the ENS, Langevin attended the courses of two professors who were open to theoretical and new ideas. Eleuthère Mascart, who was also the fifth holder of the chair of General and Experimental Physics at the *Collège de France* gave the course on electricity and magnetism, at the time he was publishing his 2-volume Treatise On *Electricity and Magnetism*, which covered both theory and "Methods of Measurement and Application". Langevin replaced him in 1902 at the *Collège de France* and later became the sixth holder of chair of General and Experimental Physics. In his obituary, Langevin described Mascart as someone who cared for theoretical knowledge:

> When the extraordinary development of the electrical industry led him from science to applications, he saw his role clearly, and tenaciously upheld the rights of even the highest science as the surest guide for the emerging industry. (Langevin 1908a)

Langevin also attended Marcel Brillouin's course on kinetic and molecular theories at the ENS. Holder of two doctorates in mathematics and physics (1880 and 1882), he introduced Boltzmann statistical theory in France in his book *Théorie cinétique des gaz* (Langevin 1902). When he was elected Professor of Mathematical Physics at the *Collège de France* in 1900, he was not content with teaching only the official lectures associated with his chair. He introduced the German model of seminars into France, where a few specialists discuss new theories [9]. When Langevin returned from Cambridge, he participated in one of these elite seminars, where the thermodynamics of radiation was discussed, based on the work of August Kirchoff,

---

[2] His mathematical expertise would later be recognized by the French Mathematical Society, which wanted to count him among its members (H. Lebesgue, 20 Nov 1919. Archives L075/039).

2.2 An Effervescent Scientific Community

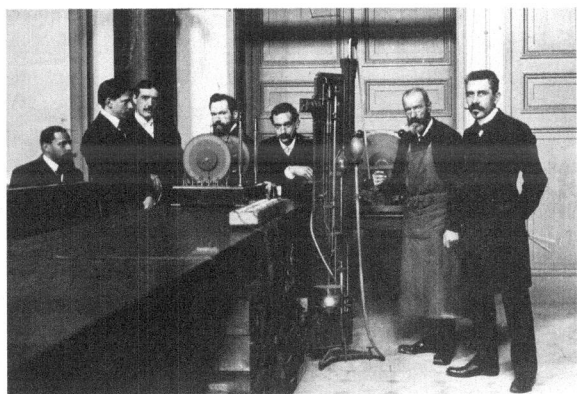

Fig. 2.4 Langevin in his laboratory at the *Collège de France*, surrounded by his main collaborators: Edmond Bauer, his assistant and relativity theorist; Marcel Moulin, who developed with Langevin an electrometer for recording atmospheric ions used in meteorology; finally Maurice de Broglie, elder brother of Louis de Broglie. (ESPCI)

Adolfo Bartoli, Wilhelm Wien and Max Planck. Langevin presented Wien's memoir on the thermal radiation displacement law [3]. Langevin thus became, with Brillouin, one of the few French physicists familiar with statistical mechanics and radiation thermodynamics.

At the ENS, he also collaborated with Jean Perrin, who was then a young teaching assistant (*préparateur*) for the *agrégation*. During the period 1894–1897 Perrin was studying cathode rays and X-rays for his PhD and in 1895 he demonstrated that cathode rays carried a negative charge (Fig. 2.3).

In 1897, Langevin moved to the Cavendish Laboratory in Cambridge, thanks to a scholarship from the Municipality of Paris, to undertake research on ionized gases. Here, independently of Georges Sagnac, who was working in Paris, he discovered that secondary rays were emitted by solids when exposed to X-rays. Langevin's studentship in this dynamic laboratory, which had been founded in 1874, as renowned for its experimental tradition as for the bold theoretical speculations of its members, was a critical moment in his development [8]. A new laboratory had been opened the year before, and the Cambridge regulations had only recently been changed to accept students with degrees from other universities. Not only was he immersed in the cradle of atomic physics—he was there when J.J. Thomson measured the speed of electrons—but also because he made friends with other young researchers, destined for fame, like Charles Wilson, John Townsend and especially Ernest Rutherford.[3] Appointed replacement professor at the *Collège de France*, in 1902, Langevin took the chair of experimental physics in 1909 (Fig. 2.4).

---

[3] Ernest Rutherford (1871–1937), a New Zealander, commenced a brilliant career at the Cavendish Laboratory that he continued at McGill University in Montreal. He then succeeded Arthur Schuster at Manchester before returning to direct the Cavendish Laboratory in Cambridge. He developed a theoretical interpretation of radioactivity, and analysed the structure of the atomic nucleus.

At the same time, Paris was not left behind, since at the same time Marie and Pierre Curie were conducting their research on radioactivity. Langevin who was also friend of the Curies might have participated in their adventure at EPCI by associating with their physical-chemical research. But he followed a parallel, more theoretical, research pathway.

Rutherford had arrived at Cambridge two years before Langevin, initially to work on a wireless detector of his own design. (Fig. 2.5) But Röntgen's discovery of X-rays later that same year had redirected all the experimental work at the Cavendish Laboratory. So, by the time Langevin arrived, he was faced with fundamental questions raised by the investigations being conducted on cathode rays, on their nature, their charge and their speed. What are the relationships between matter and electricity? How to reconcile the concepts of theoretical mechanics and electromagnetic theory? At the turn of the century, these questions were also being tackled by others, notably by Lorentz and Poincaré. Thus, paradoxically, the studentship in Cambridge brought Langevin closer to Poincaré and led him towards a global approach driven by a concern with the coherence of the theories of physics.

Langevin was so concerned with the unification of physics that this question underlies all his research between 1900 and 1905. Research on ionized gases (Langevin 1902d), the choice of subject for his PhD thesis, was directly linked to the work of J.J. Thomson on the conductivity and the formation of ions in gases under the action of X-rays. Langevin's project seems modest, at first glance: to provide an experimental confirmation of Thomson's views on the mobility and recombination of ions. But Langevin does not think only of his work in relation to that of Thomson. He introduces the problem as emerging at the crossroads of two independent but simultaneous research pathways: on one side, Thomson's experimental research; on the other, the evolution of electromagnetic theory from Faraday and Maxwell to Lorentz and Larmor. This theoretical development that, Langevin noted, allows the prediction and explanation of the Zeeman effect, the separation and polarization of the spectral lines emitted by an atom subjected to a magnetic field, leads to the reversal of the traditional considerations on the relationships between matter and the electromagnetic ether. It invites a view of the electron as a link between them, and subsequently a redefinition of matter as a special form of the "universal substratum" of the ether. In 1902, Langevin addresses the question of unification with the help of kinetic theory. His doctoral dissertation also contributes to experimental physics by developing a new method to measure the recombination of ions and their mobility (Fig. 2.6). Langevin shows that the combination coefficient varies with pressure and becomes very small in rarefied gases. This result was very strongly endorsed by Marcel Brillouin in his report to the Academy of Sciences. In any case, Langevin's doctoral dissertation raised widespread interest as shown by the correspondence that he received from all over the world, and it firmly established Langevin's international reputation.

2.2 An Effervescent Scientific Community

Fig. 2.5 Langevin at Cambridge, sitting next to J.J. Thomson and in front of Ernest Rutherford: 1898. (ESPCI)

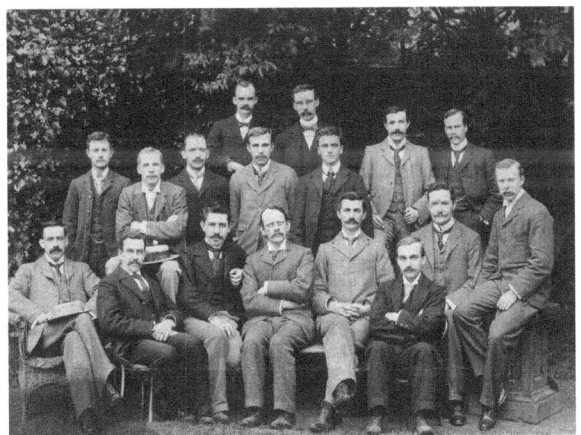

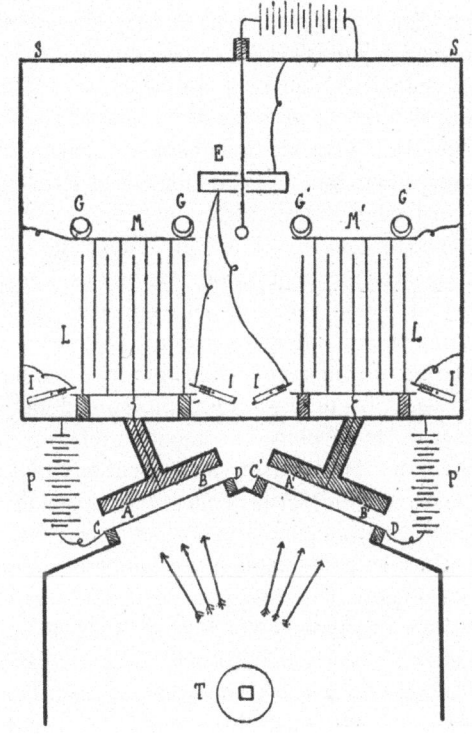

Fig. 2.6 Langevin's apparatus for his PhD studies into ionized gasses. T: Crookes' tube to generate X-rays: ABCD, A'B'C'D', ionization chambers, exposed simultaneously: ILGM, I'L'G'M', adjustable air capacitors: E, electrometer. (ESPCI, PSL University L165-05-04, Langevin 1902b, c, d)

2.3 A Dazzling Early Career

Back in Paris from Cambridge, Langevin conducted research on atmospheric ions in the laboratory located on top of the Eiffel Tower, in accordance with Gustave Eiffel's intention to use the Tower as a laboratory for scientific measurements and experiments (Langevin 1904d). There, Langevin applies to the atmosphere the methods he has developed in his dissertation on the ionization of gases. He identifies two categories of distinctly different ions: ordinary ions produced by the action of radiation and ions a thousand times heavier, which he simply calls "large ions". Langevin gives a theoretical discussion on the mode of evaporation of water droplets. He shows that, for thermodynamic reasons, there can be no stable droplets of intermediate size and that these "large ions" are produced by the fixation of ordinary ions on the particles suspended in the air (Langevin 1905d, e). The results of this research have repercussions in several fields, notably for the explanation of meteorological phenomena, such as the different types of clouds and their electrical conductivity, which will be studied by Langevin's students at the *Collège de France*. This research is also an opportunity for Langevin to try out new electrometric techniques and to propose, in collaboration with Moulin, a recorder of atmospheric ions (Langevin 1905e, 1907).

Langevin published 12 articles during 1905. Only five of them result from his research on ions. Langevin also addresses the inertia of energy (Langevin 1905h), questions the negative result of the Michelson-Morley experiment (Langevin 1905m). He also tackles kinetic theory, undertaking a difficult and very skilful analysis that allows him to specify the law of action of one molecule on another, leading to the tracing of trajectories in certain cases (Langevin 1905g). This work is undoubtedly one of the first in France that shows the importance of statistical mechanics and its application possibilities. Langevin himself developed the kinetic theory of osmotic pressure, of magnetism and later, of the electric and magnetic birefringence of colloidal solutions.

Perhaps the most innovative, intuitive and far-reaching of Langevin's scientific advances at this time was his exploration of the fundamental concept of the inertia of energy. He developed an equation relating energy to mass at the same time as Einstein did, but by using a different and more general approach (Chap. 5). He went on to use the inertia of energy to explain the nuclear mass deficit, the observed difference between the masses of atoms and integer multiples of the mass of hydrogen. Thus, he could explain the source of radium's apparently inexhaustible creation of energy. This discovery opened a path to a future in which the vast reserves of nuclear energy would be released for both creative and destructive purposes.

Langevin's early publications made a breakthrough on the international stage. Unlike Einstein, who had some obscure years before success, Langevin gained early visibility. In 1904, when he was only 32 years old, he was invited to represent French physics at the International Congress in St Louis along with the senior scientist Henri Poincaré,[4] acting as the rapporteur on the topic of the "Physics of Electrons".

---

[4] Mathematician and theoretical physicist, Henri Poincaré (1854–1912), excelled in mathematical physics and pioneered new research fields such as topology, chaos theory and relativity theory. He was also influential as a philosopher of science.

2.3 A Dazzling Early Career

This huge multifaceted congress, organised in conjunction with the Louisiana Purchase Exposition, lasted from April to December and attracted a total of nearly 20 million visitors. It was during the peaceful days on board his returning voyage that he formulated the foundation for his theory of diamagnetism. Later in his life, he would travel widely, but this was the only occasion that he ever visited the USA.

He started to accrue distinctions. In 1897 he was elected associate member of the Cambridge Philosophical Society; in 1907, he was awarded a prize from the Academy of Sciences; in 1915 the Hughes Medal from the Royal Society of London for his work on electrical science, followed by the Guthrie lecture and medal from the Physical Society of London in 1917. Other countries seem decidedly quicker than France to officially recognize the merits of the young physicist, in spite of joining the French contingent at the first Solvay conference in 1911: as early as 1921, he was invited to become a foreign member of the Royal Institution of London, soon followed by membership of academic institutes in Rome, Prague, Moscow, Bologna, Buenos Aires and Copenhagen. He will have to wait until 1934 to be elected at the French *Académie des sciences*.

Around 1905, Langevin tackled the question of Brownian motion, which also occupied his friends Jean Perrin and Albert Einstein. In a study of colloids, Perrin showed that a liquid at equilibrium is in fact agitated by the incessant internal motion of its molecules. He used this invisible motion as an argument in support of the reality of molecules and the determination of Avogadro's number. In 1905, Einstein published a paper that sought to establish the size of molecules and determined the diffusion coefficient as a function of temperature and solvent concentration, assuming spherical colloids. In 1908 Langevin published a short note in the *Comptes rendus de l'Académie des sciences* (Langevin 1908a) where he found Einstein's formula in a simpler way, and derived a mathematical formula stating that the average force of molecules does not depend solely on viscosity, but also depend on another complementary force. This force, later named "Langevin's noise", maintains particle agitation despite the viscous resistance that would eventually halt motion. Langevin's formula, which marks a milestone in the interpretation of Brownian motion, has inspired and continues to inspire research in many fields. In the 1920s, it occupied the mathematical community because this noise appeared as a mathematical monster subverting classical differential calculus and opened the way to stochastic calculus. Langevin's formula is still used today to model events as diverse as random biophysical and climate phenomena and financial movements on the stock market.

At the same time, to increase his income, Langevin, like Marie Curie, accepted in 1904 a position as a lecturer at the *Ecole normale supérieure de jeunes filles de Sèvres*. For decades, in this capacity, he taught the female students for the Physics aggregation (Fig. 2.7).

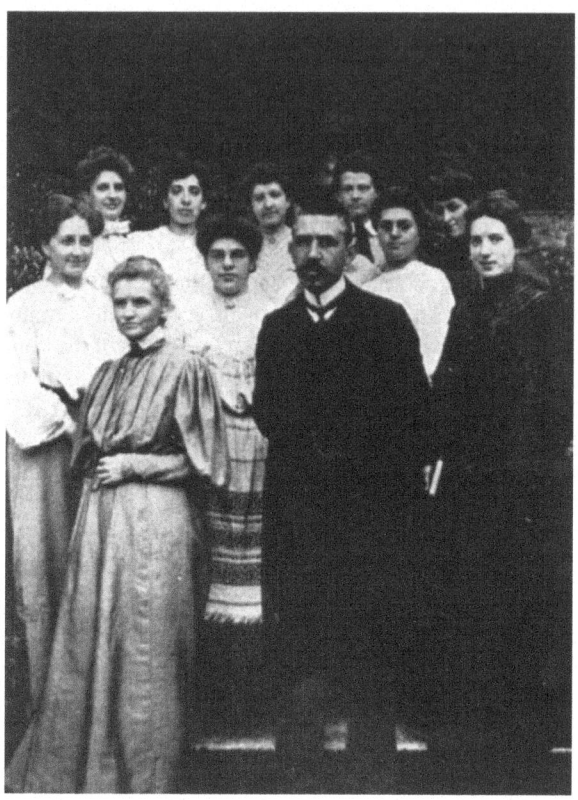

Fig. 2.7 Langevin at Sèvres in 1906. (ESPCI)

2.4 A Theory of Magnetism

Of all Langevin's scientific works, it is the theory of magnetism that is considered today as his major contribution to the advancement of physics (Langevin 1905i, j, k). It is all the more memorable because Langevin established illuminating and clear formulae in a mysterious field that had generated theories of suspect validity and practices such as Mesmerism. In any case, Langevin's approach demonstrates the unity of his work and the continuity of his thought. As in 1902, he approaches this new subject by placing himself at the crossroads of two streams of thinking. On one side, he relies on the electronic theory of Lorentz and, on the other, on the work of his former mentor, Pierre Curie.

In 1895, Curie had distinguished three types of magnetic substances, diamagnetic, weakly magnetic and ferromagnetic, and stated an experimental law according to which the specific magnetization coefficient of weakly magnetic substances varies in inverse proportion to the absolute temperature [4]. Langevin describes diamagnetic phenomena in terms of Jean Perrin's orbiting electrons. In other terms, he treats diamagnetism as a general property of matter, independent of temperature. Given the uncertainties about the electronic structure of atoms in the early 1900s, it

2.4 A Theory of Magnetism

was a very bold hypothesis. In fact, Langevin drew his inspiration from the history of physics, more precisely from André-Marie Ampère's identification of electricity with magnetism. He treats the movement of electrons as closed circuits forming small magnets, to which he applies Faraday's laws of induction. The application of a magnetic field on a molecular structure produces a molecular orientation and a resulting "magnetic moment" in the opposite direction of the field. Langevin also uses the recent kinetic theory to provide a theoretical explanation. Both paramagnetic and ferromagnetic behaviours proceed from a reorientation of the molecules endowed with the same magnetic moment under the effect of two opposing forces: the action of the magnetic field which tends to orient all the molecular moments parallel to the field and the thermal agitation which tends to create a uniform distribution in all directions. A statistical equilibrium results from this struggle between the forces of order and disorder. Langevin gives a formula that allows the calculation of paramagnetic susceptibility as a function of the field intensity and inversely proportional to the absolute temperature. Thus, Langevin confirms the experimental results of his former professor and also determines, by calculation, an estimate of the radius of the electron orbit. His results were exploited, as early as 1906, by Pierre Weiss, a physicist at the Polytechnic School in Zurich, who proposed an explanation of the main aspects of ferromagnetism by representing the magnetic interactions from the hypothesis of a "molecular field", a fictitious magnetic field, and by introducing the concept of "spontaneous magnetization" [11].

What remains today of Langevin's theory of magnetism? Langevin and Weiss can be seen as the distant founders of a "French school" of magnetism, which develops throughout the century until the Nobel Prize of Louis Néel in 1970. Langevin's formula on diamagnetism is retained with all its value because quantum mechanics leads to the same result, while his formulae for paramagnetism have been modified and completed by assuming discrete orientations for atomic moments. However, Langevin's formula remains valid in the case of supermagnetic bodies composed of ferromagnetic grains. In a sense, the notion of a permanent magnetic moment, which Langevin intuitively put at the base of his theory of paramagnetism, was already a quantum notion.

Beyond the explanation of magnetism, Langevin's interpretation had a broader impact on twentieth-century physics. Debye applied the methods he used in the study of para-magnetism to electric polarization and Langevin himself generalized his explanation by applying it to electric birefringence [5, pp. 251–253]. Finally, Langevin's theory of magnetism served as a springboard for investigations into the electronic structure of the atom. Langevin had suggested that the properties of a molecule, unlike those underpinning diamagnetism, were caused by a few electrons only, undoubtedly by the electrons of the *outermost shell* that determine the valence of atoms. It seems that this remark strongly influenced Niels Bohr when he designed a quantum model of the atom in 1913 [7].

This too brief survey of the works published between 1900 and 1905 clearly shows that it was an extremely creative period, a brilliant and promising start in a scientific career. It also reveals Langevin's characteristic style of research practice. From the outset, he was not inclined to walk on a single untrodden research pathway. He did not try to be recognized as the authoritative expert on a small specialty. Instead, he developed a distinctive way of thinking outside traditional boundaries. In place of pursuing a single method when he addressed any problem of physics, Langevin criss-crossed several pathways and took inspiration from a variety of fields of physics. In thus creating interferences between various domains, he invented radically new results. This characteristic and fruitful style of thought proceeded from his concern with the consistency of physics theory raised by the conflict between electromagnetism and mechanics. For the young Langevin, the unification of physics theories was a goal as much as a research strategy. In each subject that he tackled, he constantly tried to make bridges, thus creating underlying links between all his scientific contributions on seemingly very disparate themes.

References

1. Andler C (1932) Vie de Lucien Herr. Bibliothèque La civilisation française, Paris
2. Briand J-P, Chapoulie J-M (1992) Les Collèges du peuple: L'enseignement primaire supérieur et le développement de la scolarisation prolongée sous la Troisième République. CNRS, Paris
3. Bustamante C (2011) Paul Langevin et le conseil Solvay de 1911: Au cœur de l'histoire de la physique du XXe siècle. Images de la Physique:3–9
4. Curie P (1895) Sur les propriétés magnétiques des corps à diverses températures. Annales de Chimie et de Physique 5:289–405
5. De Broglie L d (1951) "Vie et œuvre de Paul Langevin" Address given at the *Académie des Sciences*, 15 Dec 1947. In: Savants et découvertes. Albin, Paris, pp 231–269
6. Duclert V (1999) L'engagement scientifique et l'intellectuel démocratique. Le sens de l'affaire Dreyfus. Politix 48(4):71–94. https://doi.org/10.3406/polix.1999.1808
7. Heilbron JL, Kuhn TS (1969) The genesis of Bohr Atom. Historical Studies in Physical Sciences 1:211–290
8. Longair M (2016) Maxwell's enduring legacy: a scientific history of the Cavendish Laboratory. Cambridge University Press, Cambridge
9. Olesko K (1991) Physics as a calling: discipline and practice in the Königsberg seminar for physics. Cornell University Press, Cornell
10. Pestre D (1984) Physique et physiciens en France, 1918-1940. Archives contemporaines, Paris.
11. Quédec P (1986) Le Magnétisme de Weiss: péché d'orgueil ou fraude vénielle. Revue du Palais de la Découverte 14(137):36–45
12. Rusk RD (1937) Atoms, men and stars: a survey of the latest developments of physical science and their relations to life. Ayer, London
13. Shinn T (1980) From 'corps' to 'profession': the emergence and definition of industrial engineering in modern France (ed: Fox R, Weisz). Cambridge University Press, Cambridge, pp 183–208

Chapter 3
A Turbulent Private Life

Abstract Langevin married Jeanne Desfosses in 1898, on his return from Cambridge. By 1904 the family had grown to include two sons, Jean and André, and a daughter Madeleine. Hélène followed in 1909. Langevin was part of an intimate circle of friends, known as the "Arcouest group" from the location of their family holidays, which included the Curies, the Perrins and the Borels. As parents they also combined their efforts in educational support for their children. The Langevin marriage was stormy. A few years after the premature death of Pierre Curie, Langevin developed an intimate relationship with Marie Curie. When their love affair became public in 1911, salacious press reports vibrated through the international scientific community. Langevin challenged the journalist Téry to a duel. The scandal caused huge distress and led to Langevin living separately from his family. His return to the marital home after the war did not prevent him having another liaison.

Langevin's early professional successes were somewhat overshadowed by the difficulties in his private life. In 1898, he married Emma Jeanne Desfosses, the daughter of an artisan in ceramics and a primary school-teacher (Fig. 3.1). She was 22, he was 26. During the next decade, four children were born: Jean (in 1899), André (in 1901), Madeleine (in 1903) and Hélène (in 1909). The family rented a house with garden close to Fontenay-aux-Roses, a suburb south of Paris. Although after his graduation in 1902, the young Dr Langevin got the enviable position of substitute professor in the Chair of General and Experimental Physics at the *Collège de France*, his income did not suffice to cover the expenses of the growing family. Langevin took an additional teaching load with the course on electricity at the *Ecole Normale Supérieure* for women in Sèvres, replacing Marie Curie. In a letter to his wife in April 1904, we see Langevin anxious that he was not being able to make ends meet, due to a simple delay in the payment of his fees.

The financial situation of his household at this time depended on the professional appointments of the Curies. Langevin was vying for Pierre Curie's position at EPCI. But the situation of this famous couple of scientists was no less precarious. Pierre Curie had no certainty of obtaining the chair of physics at the Sorbonne and, in 1900, he was considering taking a position in Geneva. Marie Curie had a modest

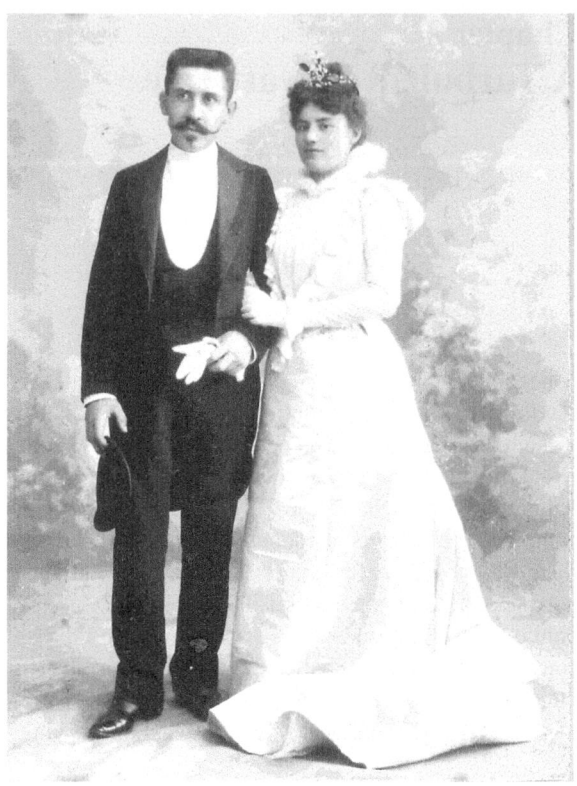

Fig. 3.1 In 1898, Langevin married Jeanne Desfosses. (ESPCI)

position of lecturer in physics at the Ecole normale supérieure de jeunes filles de Sèvres. In short, the daily life of these brilliant researchers was not always easy or calm.

3.1 A Circle of Friends

Fortunately, Langevin had a number of close friends whom he met in his student's years. At EPCI he developed a strong friendship with his supervisor Pierre Curie who soon recognized the talent of his student. They shared wide scientific interests and were so puzzled by the interactions between energy and matter that they seriously considered paranormal phenomena that caused a stir in Europe by the turn of the century. In 1905, Pierre Curie took part in the scientific experiments conducted at the Sorbonne around the medium Eusapia Palladino and Langevin continued this kind of experiments in the early 1920s [1].

3.1 A Circle of Friends

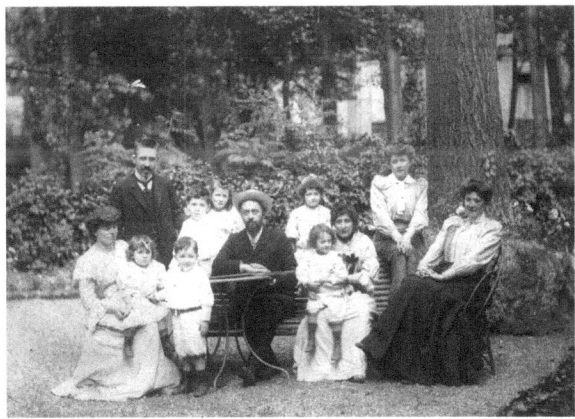

Fig. 3.2 Jean Perrin's family, with Langevin and his family c 1910. (ESPCI)

As a student at ENS, Langevin developed a close friendship with Jean Perrin who became his confidant.[1] Through the ENS network, he later became a friend of the mathematician Emile Borel and his wife Camille Appel.[2] Langevin was part of a typical network of friends in intellectual Parisian circles, a network formed in the course of studies in the *grandes écoles* of the Republic.

The Curies married in 1895 and their two daughters, together with the Langevins and their four children, the Perrins (married in 1897) with their two children, and the childless Borels (married in 1901), had social gatherings and loved to enjoy relaxing Sundays together (Figs. 3.2 and 3.3). They used to meet at each other's homes for impromptu dinners or more formal evenings. For many years they shared the joys and sorrows of everyday family life. As a novelist writing under the pen name Camille Marbo, Marguerite Borel recalls these evenings with fondness:

> Jean Perrin loved to host dinner. He had an exuberant childlike joy. The Langevins opened up to us, between Sceaux and Fontenay, a house with a fairly large garden, under the trees in which we freely wandered on summer evenings. I walked there a lot with Jean Perrin; I still breathe in the fresh smell of grass and foliage. Meanwhile, Émile Borel and Paul Langevin were discussing mathematical physics. [6, p. 85]

---

[1] Jean Perrin (1870–1942) was one of Langevin's closest friends. Like him he had a dazzling early career, but mostly in physical chemistry. In 1895, he demonstrated that cathode rays are of corpuscular nature: in short, that they are electrons. In 1908, he deduced a precise value of Avogadro's number, N, from his research on colloidal solutions and Brownian motion. He then proved the existence of atoms from the remarkable concordance of his results with the determinations of N by chemists [7]. Later, after the harsh blow dealt to scientific research by the human losses of the First World War, Perrin devoted himself to what is now called "the politics of science": he led in the 1930s a "campaign for science" which resulted in the creation of the C.N.R.S. and the Secretary of State for Research under the *Front populaire* [10].

[2] Émile Borel (1871–1956), mathematician, distinguished himself by his research on probability. He was married to Marguerite Appel (daughter of Paul Appel, rector of the University of Paris), novelist under the pseudonym of Camille Marbo. Her memoirs, *Through Two Centuries, Memories and Meetings* (1883–1967), provide a rich source of information about this circle of intellectuals and scientists.

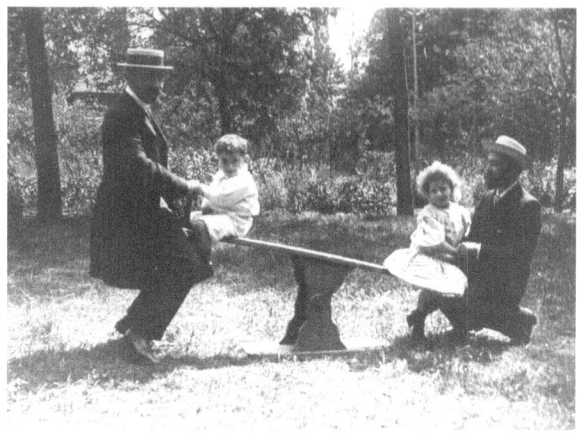

Fig. 3.3 Sunday in the Langevins' garden at Fontenay-aux-Roses. Jean Perrin with his daughter Aline and Paul Langevin with his son André. (ESPCI)

After the death of Pierre Curie in 1906, Marie Curie, herself a teacher's daughter, took the initiative to organize a cooperative school at home for the children of this group. They took turns teaching private lessons to their children, Langevin taught mathematics, Jean Perrin physics in his small laboratory at the Sorbonne, Marie Curie chemistry in Pierre Curie's laboratory at EPCI, Henriette Perrin taught history and French. Notably, Jeanne Langevin is not involved in this initiative. She does not share the culture of this circle of intellectuals. Marie Curie also included in the cooperative school the offsprings of Henri Mouton from the Pasteur Institute who taught natural sciences, and of Edouard Chavannes from the *Collège de France* whose wife taught English, German and geography.

3.2 A Vibrant Social Life

The Perrins, Curies and Langevins also spent holidays together in a small fishing village in Brittany (Fig. 3.4). L'Arcouest, near Paimpol, opposite Bréhat, became a famous location in the history of French science. For years, so many Parisian intellectuals gathered there on vacation that L'Arcouest has been nicknamed Sorbonne-Beach. This fashionable resort was launched by the historian Charles Seignobos, who opened his beautiful granite house to all his friends and colleagues. At L'Arcouest, this honourable professor of the Sorbonne was "the Captain", wearing a faded hat, always with a song on his lips. He took his guests aboard his sailing boat, *l'Églantine*. Baths and walks, songs and laughter, this warm and unconstrained life was so pleasant that soon the Perrins, then Marie Curie, built their own houses there. Today, the descendants of Irène and Frédéric Joliot-Curie still own their house in L'Arcouest.[3] Unsurprisingly as the children of the Langevins, Perrins, Curies and

---

[3] See the documentary film *L'esprit de l'Arcouest* by Florence Riou 2024. https://www.dailymotion.com/video/x9bngfe

3.2 A Vibrant Social Life

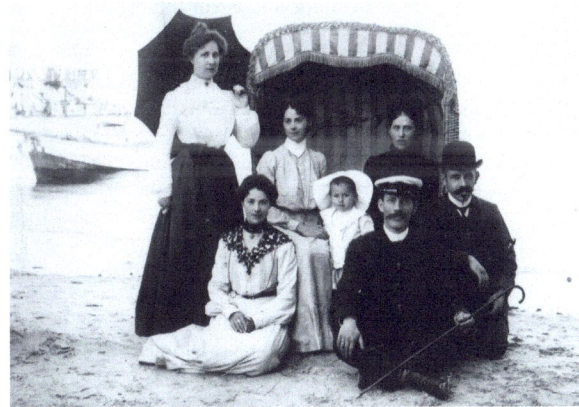

Fig. 3.4 Langevin and family on the beach, a favourite holiday destination for Parisian intellectuals at the beginning of the century. (ESPCI)

Augers spent their holidays together, some of them intermarried. For instance, Hélène Joliot-Curie, born in 1927 married Michel Langevin, Paul's grandson.

At the turn of the twentieth century, this small circle of friends became visible on the stage of Parisian Belle époque social life by the foundation of a monthly journal: *La Revue du mois*. The initiative came from the Borels, with Camille Marbo assuming the role of editor-in-chief. The editorial board included Langevin, Perrin, and other famous intellectuals. Launched on 1 January 1906, *La Revue du Mois* aimed to cover a wide spectrum of fields including science, literature, theatre, law, medicine, and politics. The philosopher Henri Bergson Paul Painlevé, mathematician and politician, and Edouard Herriot and Léon Blum, both politicians, all contributed to the journal. The 120 issues published between 1906 and 1915 highlight the life and activities of a Parisian network of left-leaning intellectuals.

Remarkably, despite his working-class roots, Langevin easily moved in this circle of intellectuals. He rubbed shoulders with the poet Paul Valéry, the writer J.H. Rosny the elder, and felt comfortable in the Parisian salon of Aline Ménard-Dorian.[4] This rich cultural milieu was formed in the 1890s among the group of Dreyfusards at the ENS. Langevin, raised by his parents with the memory of the Commune, shared their political ideals and their admiration for the socialist leader Jean Jaurès. Nevertheless, before the First World War, his political opinions were mostly expressed by his immersion in this social network. He was not yet involved in any political activity, apart from his participation in the big demonstration caused by the murder of Jean Jaurès in 1913. Like Perrin, Langevin was at this time primarily dedicated to his scientific research.

The accidental death of Pierre Curie on 19 April 1906 fell like a bombshell into this intimate group. In his eulogy for his mentor and friend, Langevin tried to

---

[4] In her Parisian salon, Aline Ménard *née* Dorian (1850–1929) welcomed leading figures from the worlds of literature, art and politics and inspired Marcel Proust in his painting of the Verdurins' salon. She diligently campaigned for Captain Dreyfus, and became vice-president of the *Ligue des droits de l'Homme* in 1922 and general secretary of the International Federation of Human Rights.

express the feelings of them all, set in the conflicting events that were beginning to challenge his own life:

> It is this constant need for truth and clarity, extended to all activities, which made him, in a natural and simple way, always keep his thoughts directed towards the most important issues, which gave so much nobility and strength of example to a life of courage and free examination, in an invigorating and healthy atmosphere that he created around him.
>
> It is the same discipline, applied by him throughout his mental life, which gives us the key to all his personality, which always kept so far away from the hustle and bustle, in the serenity of an existence entirely devoted to science and the people he loved, in the quiet of the laboratory where glory came to seek him to disturb for a moment the admirable unity of his life.
>
> [...] For no one has known better how to intimately mix work and enjoyment, to associate his affections and his thoughts more harmoniously. As work companions, he had first his brother and then his wife, and these two collaborations, which in a way mark out the history of his life and his output, have created around him the atmosphere he loved and where his ideas have matured. (Langevin 1906a)

3.3 Troubles in Married Life

Exciting research, close friends, and a rich social life: Seen from afar, the pre-war years appear idyllic. Yet the correspondence housed in various archives reveals a darker, sadder face. Unlike Perrin's, Langevin's marriage had never been peaceful. There were "terrible scenes" even before their first son was born. Camille Marbo recalls:

> Under the pretext of distracting Paul Langevin, we would sometimes take him out, my husband and I, with Jean Perrin, to some show or some meeting (…) One evening, coming out of a club, Jean Perrin exclaimed: "We must wash ourselves of this stupid and depressed atmosphere!". He hailed a cab and drove us to the front of the Arc de Triomphe "to salute Rude's bas-relief at sunrise". After which, Paul Langevin took us to *les Halles*, at Baratte's, to eat onion soup. All these men, who became famous, were making discoveries at this time that would carry their names to the four corners of the learned world. But they seemed to the young woman I was, like big, often clumsy, children. [6, p. 94]

From the very beginning Paul confided his worries to Jean Perrin. It seems that Jeanne could barely tolerate the financial hardship and pressed her husband to leave teaching for a more lucrative career in industry. Langevin complained about the interference of his in-laws. He suspected the "three women who tormented his life" (including his mother-in-law and sister-in-law) of stealing money from him [8]. He even asked Perrin to look after 800 francs because he thought that this money was not safe at home. On the other side Jeanne, taking Henriette Perrin into her confidence, complained about her husband's harshness and insults and reported violent arguments between them that upset the 8-year-old Jean.

For about 10 years, tensions and fights between the couple alternated with reconciliations, sometimes followed by the birth of another baby. The periods of depression undermined Langevin's health: stomach pains, more or less acute, more or less chronic, but serious enough to raise worries among his friends and colleagues.

3.3 Troubles in Married Life

While taking Paul Langevin's side, they deplored his weakness and lack of firm will. For instance, Charles-Edouard Guillaume, a Swiss physicist friend of Pierre Curie, describes Langevin as:

> a delicate being of high mentality. Unfortunately for him, his will is wavering, and has shown this on many occasions. His marriage was not a happy one. His wife, who came to his parents as a seamstress, succeeded, with her mother's help, in circumventing him and dragging him into a situation that was always painful. I've heard it for myself: he didn't have a single year of happiness. (Letter 5 December 1911 quoted in Blanc [2, p. 127])

The tensions in Langevin's marriage reached a climax in 1907 when Marie Curie organized the cooperative school. Paul left home and took refuge with the Perrins. But he came back "for the children", as he said. Henriette Perrin frequently came to the Langevins' house where she witnessed a number of terrible scenes. She shared her concerns with Marie Curie. In turn, she became a confidant for Paul Langevin who increasingly talked to her about his marital difficulties (Fig. 3.5).

It is not clear when or how Marie's and Paul's friendship turned into love. Their children later took the view that it was inevitable. Ève Curie wrote:

> Marie, who had exercised a man's profession, had chosen her friends and confidants among men. And this exceptional creature exercised upon her intimates, upon one of them in particular, a profound influence. No more was needed. [3, p. 279]

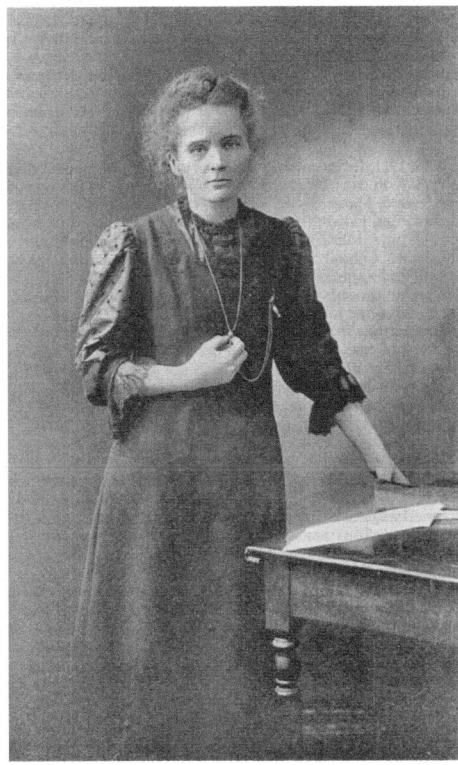

Fig. 3.5 Marie Curie: Photograph taken for her unsuccessful election to the *Académie des sciences*. (Science et Vigilance)

André Langevin was equally non-judgmental:

> How could it be considered abnormal, when Paul Langevin considered it his duty to encourage and help Marie Curie in her misfortune, and when he continued to discuss with her the new physics that radioactivity had brought about and which fascinated them both [...]. Is it not quite natural that this friendship, together with mutual admiration, gradually turned into a love and an affair, several years after Pierre Curie's death? [5, p. 55]

The circle of friends noted that in spring 1909, Marie Curie, the widow now overworked and saddened by the death of her father-in-law Dr Eugène Curie, appeared cheerful wearing new bright clothes instead of her usual black dress. It seems that in 1910, Langevin and Marie used to meet in a small apartment rented in the Latin Quarter and exchanged letters through their friend Henriette. A long letter that Marie wrote to Paul, presumably in the summer of 1910, sheds light on their mutual feelings (transcribed by Karin Blanc [2, pp. 63–69]). She was certainly sexually attracted by him but she above all expresses tenderness and care, an almost motherly care. She was quite directive with him: she urges him to break with his wife for good; she suggests that a separation would not deprive him from his children and that his wife and her family are toxic and constitute a major obstacle to his scientific creativity:

> Finally, my Paul, it's not just your children to consider. There's you, your scientific future, your moral and intellectual life. All this has been in great danger for years. (…) Your family is an environment of irresistible destructive power, and I believe, quite exceptional. You can't live in this family without being digested by it for its own use … (ibid., p. 65)

She worries that Jeanne Langevin might hire someone to follow her husband and that his children might be used to spy on him. She warns him that she will not bear it if Jeanne became pregnant again and, if so, it would mean "a definitive separation between us…because I can risk my life and my position for you, but I couldn't accept this dishonour in the face of myself, of you and of people I hold in esteem" (ibid., p. 67).

Their liaison took place at a time when Marie Curie, who had succeeded Pierre as a professor at the Sorbonne, took the lead in the management of the research laboratory. In 1910, she applied for nomination at the *Académie des sciences* with the strong support of a number of leading scientists who knew her scientific merits. The candidacy of a woman in this venerable institution attracted the public attention. Over the months before the election, there were comments in the daily press mocking her and denouncing the threat to future harmony. She strongly resented her defeat by the catholic physicist Edouard Branly, but she was definitely a woman under public scrutiny.

3.4 Shame and Scandal

In 1911, Langevin's torments culminated with the revelation of their liaison, on 4 November by *Le Journal*, a widely circulated newspaper in Paris. A two-column article on the first page with a photo of Marie Curie was titled *Une histoire d'amour: Mme (et pourquoi pas le professeur) Curie et le professeur Langevin.*

3.4 Shame and Scandal

It turns out that, in spring 1911, Jeanne Langevin had effectively hired someone to steal letters in their pied à terre. Immediately afterwards, Henri Bourgeois, her brother-in-law and editor of the newspaper *Le Petit Parisien,* visited Marie Curie with threats that a scandal was imminent, and blackmailed her. She alerted Perrin and the Borels who invited Marie and her daughters to come with them to Genoa where they would travel for a conference. Marguerite Borel remembers that Marie insisted that she wanted to save Paul from himself because he is a genius but he is weak. Marie went back at work and travelled to Poland with her daughters during the summer.

Meanwhile Langevin, who had fled to the Perrins to protest against the stolen letters, returned home "for the children". But the arguments and insults became so violent that on 26 July he gathered up his two young sons and took the ferry to Newhaven, England, where they stayed for a month in lodgings in Meeching Road, above the harbour. He also borrowed a lot of money, presumably to pay the blackmail, whereas Jeanne obtained alimony from him after requesting an official separation. Paul's lawyer, Raymond Poincaré, attempted conciliation, and failed.

Blackmail prevented the publication of the letters for only a few months. In late October, Langevin and Curie travelled to Brussels to attend the first Solvay Conference in physics. The official photograph shows Marie Curie surrounded, protected, by the rest of the French contingent, Ernest Rutherford behind her, while Langevin stands away to one side, next to Albert Einstein. This professional meeting exacerbated Jeanne's jealousy and she decided to publish the letters anyway. *Le Journal* reported Fernand Hauser's visit to Fontenay-aux-Roses where he met Langevin's mother-in-law, who pretended that Paul and Marie had fled together to an unknown destination.

Marie Curie bravely counter-attacked from Brussels, responding to the lies in *Le Temps* the next day. She clearly proved that everyone in her entourage knew where she was. She managed to get apologies from Hauser, the author of the article (*Le Temps*, 8 November 1911). *Le Temps* added the denials of Marie Curie's collaborators and concluded that the whole story was "folie pure" (a pure invention).

But it did not stop the press. On the same day she received a telegram from Stockholm to inform her that she was the recipient of the Nobel Prize for Chemistry. This was the supreme reward for the years of work since the Pierre Curie's death. The news that should have delighted Marie Curie and her friends was met with anxiety. It was impossible now to escape the publicity that the newspapers had unleashed. In *L'Action française*, Léon Daudet, a writer, and active monarchist, published an article titled *Science and Virtue* stating that "We find here, in concrete form, one of the superstitions most cherished in a democracy ... Science (with a capital S) confers virtue ... Today the republican Dreyfusism needs the dogma of the virtue of scientists" (L'Action française, 17 November 1911). This affair was more than a private drama that tore two families apart; it became a political affair because the right-wing press launched a xenophobic and anti-science campaign. *L'Action Française* tries to revive the climate of the Dreyfus affair.

Marie Curie was an easy prey for the media. In *L'Œuvre*, on 23 November, Gustave Téry, a former classmate of Langevin at ENS, published a lengthy article titled *The Scandals of the Sorbonne* quoting large excerpts from the stolen letters of Marie to Paul. Téry posed as the noble defender of a mother of four children abandoned by an irresponsible husband, ironically nicknamed the "Chopin of the Polonaise", manipulated by the seductive and malevolent power of the "Vestal of radium". Téry's article, titled *Pour une Mère*, addressed towards Langevin, starts thus:

> No sir, Curie's wife should not be suspected.
> Why is this?
> Why ask? Madame Curie is the honour of the University, she is all of French science.
> So much! We shudder to think that, if this fatal student had not come from Poland expressly to witness the discovery of radium, there would no longer be French science ... And there are still patriots obtuse enough to consider the invasion of foreigners as a national scourge!
> Do not joke on such a subject.
> You speak of it, in fact, with terrible seriousness. It really seems that the Dreyfus affair has been turned around. You, the former Dreyfusard, you invoke "the honour of the university" in the same tone that your adversaries once pronounced "the honour of the army." And for you, anticlerical savage, Science with a capital S has become the New Idol, whose Grandfathers and Vestals are infallible and taboo!

The prestige of the academic world was under threat and Raymond Poincaré asked the newspapers to self-censor. Faced with such a scandal, Marie Curie did not collapse. On 22 November she wrote to Svante Arrhenius chair of the Nobel Committee to "talk to him about a delicate affair" and ask him to prevent its disclosure in the Swedish press. But excerpts of the letters had already spread to the foreign press, especially in the widely circulated *Berliner Tageblatt*. Arrhenius, initially in favour of Marie Curie's visit to Stockholm for the official ceremony, changed his mind. On 1 December he wrote to her:

> Honour and esteem for our Academy as well as for science and for your country seem to me to demand that in such circumstances you withdraw from coming here to accept the prize. [2, p. 114]

Marie responded on 5 December 1911:

> The approach you suggest would be a serious mistake on my part. The prize was awarded to me for the discovery of radium and polonium. I believe that there is no connection between my scientific work and the facts of my private life, which are being invoked against me in cheap publications, and which are, moreover, completely misrepresented.
> I cannot accept the principle that the appreciation of a scientific work can be influenced by slander and libel concerning private life. I am convinced that this opinion will be shared by many people. I'm very sorry that you don't share it yourself. (Ibid., p. 116)

Actually many French scientists, including Georges Urbain[5] and Guillaume, wrote to Arrhenius to convince him that she should come for the ceremony on 10 December. What she finally did attend, she was acclaimed by the king and queen of

---

[5] George Urbain (1872–1938), a French chemist who specialized in the isolation and separation of rare earth elements, was a professor at the Sorbonne and the founder of the *Institut de Biologie Physique* in Paris. A former student of the EPCI like Langevin, he was also a composer, a sculptor and a regular visitor on holiday at L'Arcouest.

Sweden and by a crowd of feminists, according to the Swedish press. But there was no report on the Nobel ceremonies in the French press. Marie Curie was treated with silence at home.

3.5 Drama and Farce

How did Langevin face this scandal? Like a number of French colleagues he wrote to Arrhenius to defend Marie Curie's reputation to the Nobel Committee:

> It is impossible for me to hide the cruel pain that I felt when I noticed, by your letter to Mr. Urbain, the impression produced on yourself and on some of your colleagues by the abominable publication directed against Madame Curie. One cannot judge, if indeed anyone has the right to, the correspondence that is reproduced there in a distorted form by text alterations and cuts, one cannot judge Madame Curie's attitude in this whole affair, if one does not know under what conditions I have lived for thirteen years nor from whom these attacks have come.
>
> First of all, a life of relentless labour entirely devoted to the highest concerns with the success that you know and that you have recently contributed to reward as it deserved, should it not be the best defense against baselessly injurious suspicions? One cannot be aware of the moral height of Madame Curie, the beauty of her existence from all points of view, her constant concern for dignity and pride in herself and in those to whom she attaches some value, and misunderstand her intentions and the motives that have guided her.
>
> Remember, to justly appreciate her moral value, the dignified and firm manner in which she knew how to decline the honours that were offered to her from all sides to remain the tireless and disinterested worker she wanted to be.
>
> I suffer from needing to shout with all my strength that such a woman has not done all that she is accused of, that her work and affectionate relationships are irreproachable, that everyone, especially those who can best appreciate her value, must trust her in the name of her past life.
>
> All my friends, all those who know the difficulties I have endured for thirteen years, all those who are interested in my scientific future, are ready, and have spontaneously told me when they knew them, to sign with both hands the advice that Madame Curie decided to give me in a period of anguish for her, after having been threatened with death for several months, more than a year ago, by a jealous, violent woman capable of anything.
>
> I absolutely did not follow the advice, which was no longer discussed between Madame Curie and me, and I tried with complete sincerity to stay in my family. It took their mother to insult me in a particularly serious way in front of them for me to seek to withdraw, during the holiday period, two of my children from the suffering they are experiencing and from the harmful influence of the environment in which they were living.
>
> I cannot give you more precise details about what this environment was: let it suffice for you to know that my wife's brother-in-law and her advisor in this whole affair, did not hesitate, a year ago, at the time of Madame Curie's candidacy for the Academy of Sciences, long before the published correspondence was stolen, to himself write ignoble anonymous letters to smear Madame Curie—I have absolute proof of this; that this man, a low-level journalist, took the stolen correspondence to his newspaper editor, immediately and without asking for any explanation from those who had written it; finally that this man is currently denying with the utmost effrontery a loan of several thousand francs that I made to him without demanding a receipt. I neither can nor should tell you anything about my wife, but you will understand the atrocious alternative in which she put me, either to let an irreproachable woman be smeared, who is today crucified for having tried to save, in the name

of the friendship that I was asking her for, what she saw in me of a scientific future or to say, to defend her in a public trial all that has been my life and all that my children could reproach me later for having said.

I am currently trying, at the cost of painful sacrifices, to ensure this trial does not take place, allowing Madame Curie, whom I admire with all my power, the possibility of pursuing those who dared to throw her to the wild beasts because they hated her glory and greatness.

The sincere sympathy that I felt for you when I saw you here makes me hope that you trust my word and that you will not let yourself be led to a deeply unfair judgment. [2, pp. 120–122]

Langevin himself felt humiliated by Téry's portrait of him in *L'Oeuvre* as "a man who allows the woman who carries his name, the woman who remains the mother of his four children, to be dragged into the mud by all his friends, this man, if he is a professor at the *Collège de France*, is nothing but a boor and a coward" [8, p. 323]. Adopting an attitude he would like to be noble and generous, Langevin responded to the insult by challenging Téry in a duel. This old medieval practice seems to have been revived in the late nineteenth century among politicians, journalists and writers, the last defence against the press in the absence of any French laws of libel. But Langevin's chivalrous gesture turned into a "farce". He managed to convince the mathematician and future minister, Paul Painlevé, and Albin Haller the director of EPCI, to act as his seconds. He then shared lunch with Marguerite Borel in a bistro and went to buy a weapon on a shop where he tried his hand at discharging the pistol in the firing range. On the morning of 26 November, he and Téry convened with their seconds in the Bois de Vincennes, east of Paris. A few reporters were there but no one heard a gunshot. According to the reports in the daily newspapers, Langevin lifted his arm half way up as though to discharge his gun but Téry kept his pistol barrel pointed to the ground. Langevin then also lowered his gun. Téry later reported that he did not want to shoot because he wouldn't have done a service to Madame Langevin by killing her husband nor to French science by depriving it of a brain [4, 9]: a happy outcome for this honourable scientist.

Langevin subsequently lived separately from his wife in an apartment on rue Larrey, meeting his children for walks on Sundays. His youngest daughter Hélène hardly knew her father. But a few years later, at the request of his wife, he returned to the household. This reconciliation did not put an end to the fights between them. Marie-Elisa Cohen,[6] a close friend of their daughter Madeleine, who often had dinner at the Langevins in their apartment at EPCI in the late 1930s, reported that:

Madame Langevin was always arguing with "le père Langevin" … Her husband addressed her formally, and she replied informally. They had a relationship like that. I remember a

---

[6] Marie-Elisa Nordmann-Cohen (1910–1993) was a chemist who obtained a PhD in George Urbain's laboratory. She joined the *Comité de Vigilance des Intellectuals Antifascistes* in 1934 and the *Comité Mondial des Femmes contre la Guerre et le Fascisme* where she collaborated with Madeleine Langevin. As a member of the Resistance, she was deported to Auschwitz in 1943. After the war, she was president of the *Amicale des anciens déportés d'Auschwitz*. She was Frédéric Joliot-Curie's assistant at the Atomic Energy Committee (CEA) and a member of its scientific council.

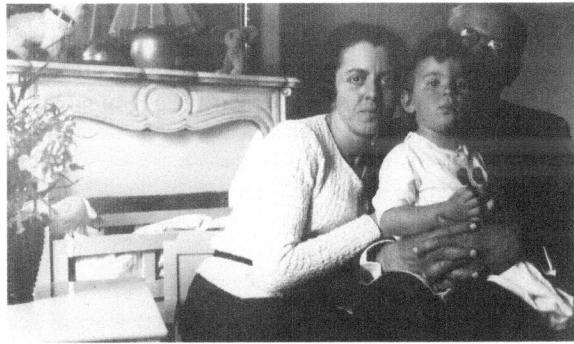

Fig. 3.6 Eliane Montel, with Paul-Gilbert and Paul Langevin c. 1934. (Paul-Éric Langevin)

dinner in the spring of 1939. She had brought a melon ("le père Langevin" was very, very fond of good food). He tasted it, gave it back to his wife saying: it's a turnip. She sent back for another melon. It's a turnip three times. It wasn't pleasant. (Cohen, 1985, Bernadette Bensaude-Vincent, "personal communication")

Marie-Elisa Cohen added that Jeanne Langevin "was considered as nothing by everyone … she was stupid and so no-one could forgive her for the way she had behaved in 1911".

Langevin's return to the marital home did not prevent him from having another liaison.[7] He had a love affair with the physicist Eliane Montel (1898–1993), who had graduated from the female *Ecole normale supérieure* in Sèvres in 1920. In 1929 and 1930, she worked in Marie Curie's laboratory and published a paper in the *Journal de physique*. In 1931, she was hired as "attachée de recherche" at EPCI in Langevin's laboratory. On 5 July 1933 she gave birth to a son Paul-Gilbert Langevin who regularly visited his father until his death in 1946. After a university training in physics, Paul-Gilbert became a musicologist and died in 1986 (Fig. 3.6).

By contrast to the aftermath for Langevin, the Langevin-Curie scandal really undermined Marie Curie's health and completely shattered her emotional life. For months she was depressed and her work was affected, whereas Langevin conscientiously pursued his research, his courses, his lectures and his publications. Perhaps stimulated by the uncertainties of his private life, encouraged by his friends, he threw himself passionately into physical theory and mobilized all his energy in the service of a scientific revolution. In fighting for the triumph of electron physics, in campaigning for relativity, Langevin would learn the language of the activist. This is how he forged the weapons for his future educational, pacifist, or political battles.

Clearly, as Marie Curie's biographer Susan Quinn remarks, the scandal about the Langevin-Curie affair reflects the social conventions of the *Belle Epoque*. It was perfectly acceptable for bourgeois males to have off-marriage relations and to keep

---

[7] According to Marie-Elisa Cohen, extra-marital relationships were common among male scientists. She mentioned Urbain's affair with a Russian woman working in Marie Curie's lab at the *Institut du radium*. After the death of his wife Henriette in 1938, Perrin had an affair with Nine Choucroun, a biochemist who developed the technique of electrophoresis. She fled with him to the United States when Paris was occupied by the Nazi troops in 1941.

a mistress provided the elected partner did not show up in public and let the official wife assume the conventional role of a married woman in polite society [8, p. 295]. Langevin, however, could not fit in to this bourgeois model because not only was Marie Curie too famous to stay in the background but also because his wife was not integrated into the society he inhabited.

References

1. Bensaude-Vincent B, Blondel C (eds) (2002) Des savants face à l'occulte, 1870–1940. éditions de la découverte, Paris
2. Blanc K (1999) Marie Curie et le Nobel. Uppsala Studies in the History of Science, Uppsala, p 26
3. Curie È (1938) Madame Curie. Tr. Vincent Sheen. Doubleday, Doran, New York
4. Giroud F (1981) Une femme honorable. Hachette, Paris
5. Langevin A (2022) Paul Langevin, my father. EDP Sciences, Paris. English edition: Duck F
6. Marbo C (1967) Souvenirs et rencontres (1883–1967). Grasset, Paris
7. Perrin J (1913) Les atomes. Félix Alcan, Paris
8. Quinn S (1995) Marie Curie. A life. Simon & Schuster, New York
9. Reid R (1979) Marie Curie derrière la légende. Seuil, Paris
10. Weart S (1979) Scientists in power. Harvard University Press, Cambridge

Chapter 4
Atoms in Science Education

Abstract The 1902 French educational reform opened up a debate about ways of teaching science. In 1904 Langevin gave a lecture at the *Musée pédagogique* entitled *The Spirit of Scientific Education*. Starting with a fierce critique of physics courses and textbooks used in secondary education, he rejected the separation between culture and technology and proposed a historical approach as an alternative to the dogmatic teaching of physics. Langevin valued the historical method to serve the promotion of atomism. He used history to legitimize atomism as a theoretical synthesis as powerful as rational mechanics. Sceptical chemists challenged his argument that atoms are no longer a hypothesis. Langevin also had to defeat a second opposition to atomism that came from the energeticists, who attempted to explain all phenomena in terms of energy relations and to dispense with the hypothesis of atoms. According to Langevin, energetics and mechanics were, despite their divergent positions, in the same camp. His historical insights are woven with a host of biological metaphors suggestion that science grows like a living organism.

As early as 1904, Langevin combines his research and teaching activities with a passionate interest in education. Shortly after his PhD defence, he is involved in the debates surrounding a national project of reform of secondary education [10]. A brief sketch of the debates going on in the French educational system at the turn of twentieth century will help understand this facet of Langevin's actions.

4.1 Debates About Science Education

Science became an important subject in the education system set up in the aftermath of the French Revolution with the implementation of courses of mathematics, physics and chemistry, and natural sciences in secondary schools. Science had been given more prominence in the *lycées* following the 1852 reform, which introduced a "bifurcation" between two routes, the science and the classics curricula—leading to two different baccalaureates. The contents to be taught each year and the teaching methods were (and still are) strictly defined by the government in the syllabus.

A further reform was prompted in 1902 by continuing debates on education during the Third Republic. The controversy set the advocates of classical education, which included Latin and Greek, against the advocates of modern education, who wanted to strengthen and enhance science teaching. The latter claimed that the sciences are an integral part of education because they contribute through their methods to the formation of the man and the citizen.

The 1902 reform changed both the curriculum and the syllabus [10]. It reunified secondary education by introducing a single baccalaureate, which was arranged in four sections: A (Latin-Greek), B (Latin-Languages), C (Latin-Sciences) and D (Languages-Sciences). It introduced an innovative way of teaching science through practical exercises, which would be subject to assessment. The overall aim, as outlined by Louis Liard, vice-rector of the *Académie de Paris*, was to transform the spirit of teaching the sciences. "Until now, they had been treated mainly as subjects for examinations and competitions. From now on, they will be instruments of culture" [11, p. 247].

The 1902 reform opened up another debate about the ways of teaching science. Before 1902, physics and chemistry teaching was mainly theoretical. The course was dictated by the teacher and then repeated, in written or oral form, by the student. The 1902 reform aimed to put an end to such dogmatism with the introduction of practical classes, in which students performed bench-top experiments without expensive apparatus. The ministry recommended the use of the inductive method, inviting students to carefully consider their experimental observations, then to explain them.

In support of the reform, a series of lectures on mathematics and physics was organized in early 1904 at the Musee pédagogique in Paris. They attracted a large audience of leading scholars as well as secondary school teachers. These lectures were published in 1904 by the *Imprimerie Nationale* "to be sent free of charge in triplicate to the libraries of all high schools". In other words, they were semi-official explanations of the reform. Nevertheless, the speakers were free to express their own opinions.

In this context, Langevin gave a lecture with the title *The Spirit of Scientific Education* (Langevin 1904a), which caused a lively discussion with the audience at the end of the session.

The lecture begins with a harsh and biting critique of the physics courses and syllabus in secondary education. Then Langevin proposes a historical approach as an alternative to the dogmatism of physics teaching. To support his proposal, he embarks on a long survey of the history of physics that ends in praise of the modern atomic theory. Thus, throughout the pages, the plea for the history of science turns into a plea for atomic physics.

Langevin's distinctive enthusiasm for new theories, which generated for him the icon of "man of progress", thus seems to proceed from a respect for history. How can he reconcile these two attitudes, which could appear to be antagonist at first glance? The revolutionaries, in science, as elsewhere, are rather inclined to proclaim: "Let's wipe the slate clean of the past". Galileo, according to legend, called for the books of Aristotle to be abandoned in order to decipher the great book of nature. And Lavoisier, wanting to re-establish chemistry exclusively on facts, strongly condemned history and asked his reader to forget everything he knew to better listen to nature. Langevin, by contrast, wants both to recall the past and to overthrow tradition. Far from considering, like Lavoisier, that history conveys a jumble of errors and prejudices, he sees it as a remedy against dogmatism and sclerosis. He cultivates history in order to subvert it.

How is this strategy developed? What are the underlying scientific and historical assumptions? Let's follow Langevin's argument carefully in order to characterize his positions in the controversies of the time.

4.2 Culture Versus Technology

The first criticism of the methods of physics teaching is that they are "dogmatic" and "fragmentary". Teachers present isolated, disjointed facts as principles, and ask their students to memorize them. Thus, secondary education that aims at a dual "educational" and "utilitarian" purpose fails miserably on both counts.

This criticism is part of a heated debate on the place of technology in education. Langevin alludes to it in the first lines by presenting the desire to train technicians as a "recent phenomenon", "a new concern". In fact, the concern to train engineers and technicians was nothing new. During the nineteenth century, numerous engineering schools, both general and special, were created in France—among them the *École centrale* and the *École municipale de physique et de chimie*—along with special institutes for training technicians. But the "desire to train technicians" in the universities was new [8]. This project was hotly debated. Overall, the academic world was hostile, especially in Paris. It feared that it would be contaminated by the German model and that the prestige of the university would be undermined by degrading the nobility of pure science through contact with empirical and routine techniques [13].

What is Langevin's position? (Fig. 4.1). He is neither on the side of the knights of pure science, like Emile Picard, academician, mathematician, author of a theory on functions of a variable complex, nor on the side of the apostles of industry, like Henry Le Chatelier, chemist, famous for his contribution to chemical thermodynamics. He dismisses both of them, because he rejects the dichotomy between culture and technology.

> In agreement with this conception that to educate is to prepare to act, I do not believe that there is a need, in scientific matters, to establish *side by side* two distinct teachings, one speculative, the other practical, one giving the spirit, the other giving the letter, one of method, the other of results (…) These two faces of scientific teaching are inseparable like the two sides of an equation, in the way that the question posed deductively by theory is inseparable from the answer provided by experience and from which the law is derived by induction, and how this inner representation that is our science is inseparable from the recorded facts. (Langevin 1904a, p. 26)

Fig. 4.1 Young Langevin.
(Photograph Henri Manuel.
All rights reserved)
(ESPCI)

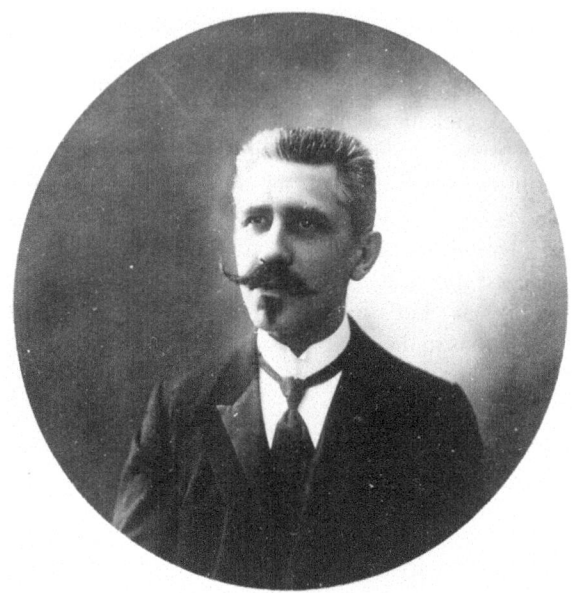

Thus, Langevin condemns "side by side" as a pathway to dogmatism. To separate, isolate and juxtapose different subjects never brings good results in education. It is as absurd to juxtapose two types of teaching as it is to juxtapose facts and laws in science teaching.

4.3 Historical Versus Dogmatic

Langevin is especially robust in his criticism of physics textbooks. He found them dogmatic in two respects: sometimes it is "the statement of a law that falls from who knows where"; sometimes it is "the statement placed above all verification" (Langevin 1904a, p. 75). In both cases, the word dogmatism suggests a transcendent authority; almost divine in the first, and metaphysical, in the second. Physics textbooks are "admirable catechisms of experimental science", exposing a dead and frozen science, a science that Langevin describes as senile and deeply objectionable.

He envisages a unique remedy. He suggests that a historical approach that reveals the efforts of the human mind to adapt to reality is the way to make science more attractive, young and vigorous. In addition, history is good at conveying a "confident and thoughtful" trust in the laws of physics. In emphasizing the limits of their validity, the historical presentation of science avoids arguments of authority and prevents the illegitimate extensions of the laws outside their domain of application. In short, history is a panacea. It brings life back to the most rigid discussions and rejuvenates science; it transmutes science teaching into true scientific education of the mind.

Yet is this plea for a historical approach to science truly innovative? The opposition between the historical and the dogmatic, which structures Langevin's argument, is reminiscent of a major distinction made by Auguste Comte in the *Cours de philosophie positive*. In the Second Lesson, Comte clearly stated that the historical approach to science was the best way to understand it. However he also acknowledged that "As science progresses, the historical sequence of explanation becomes more and more impracticable [...] while the dogmatic sequence becomes more and more possible, as well as necessary" [5, pp. 50–51].

Moreover, a glance at the official recommendations of the Ministry of Education, or at the science textbooks of the late nineteenth century, shows that the historical method was already widely implemented in teaching [9]. In sciences, as in literature, the courses included extensive retrospective reviews: general histories were published, the classics were reissued, and attempts were made to organize the teaching of the history of sciences [6]. Langevin himself benefited from this insertion of history in science teaching, since he had to read the original memoirs of past scientists to prepare the lessons for the *agrégation* examination in physical sciences (Langevin 1926c, p. 23). So why does he passionately advocate a cause that seems to have been won already? Why does he criticize the "spirit of scientific teaching" when he seems to be in agreement with the conventional methods?

This mix of conformism and revolt is an indication that there are other stakes in this plea for the historical approach. Langevin is in fact challenging the Comtean heritage. Indeed, physics textbooks were full of names and dates of past discoveries. But they were content with providing an accumulation of experimental demonstrations along with an endless sequence of laws and principles. For Langevin, that is dogmatic history, dead science. He firmly rejects the historical method used in textbooks. Two conceptions of history confront each other and behind them two conceptions of science itself. The historical approach used in science textbooks was based on an empiricist vision of scientific knowledge: its major aim was to convey the view that scientific statements are based on experiment. Through the lens of history, Langevin hopes to deliver a quite different message. He puts the emphasis on the role of hypotheses and theory in knowledge production (Langevin 1904a, p. 76). For him the educational virtue of the historical method is to develop the spirit of synthesis in science.

4.4 Atomism Versus Mechanics

Langevin values the historical method because it serves the promotion of atomism. He uses history to legitimise atomism as a theoretical synthesis as powerful as rational mechanics.

Let us remember that the atomic hypothesis, formulated in 1805 by the English chemist John Dalton, had sparked many disputes in the nineteenth century [3, 16]. Thanks to its experimental support and to its explanatory power of chemical combinations, it ended up being adopted by most of the chemists who gathered at the first

Congress of Chemistry at Karlsruhe in 1860. However, in the chemistry community, it remained a mere hypothesis, that could be accepted without assuming the existence of atoms and molecules [1]. In the physics community, by contrast, the kinetic theory of gases that related the mechanical and thermal properties of gases to the independent motion of molecules presupposed the physical reality of molecules. Then, on the basis of his experiments on Brownian motion in colloids, Perrin developed a demonstration of the molecular reality in *Les Atomes* [14]. His demonstration relies on the convergence of the values of Avogadro's number, N, calculated by a dozen methods taken from independent disciplines. Such a remarkable convergence of independent results would be a miracle without the existence of unobservable molecules. This proof of molecular reality, based on probability, also implies the real existence of the atomic components of molecules, and consequently electrons as components of atoms. Ironically, atoms became an indisputable reality only when they ceased to be a-tomic, that is to say indivisible.

Yet, in the early twentieth century, the game was not won because there were two strong opponents to atomic theory. First, a number of chemists remained sceptical about molecular reality. Marcellin Berthelot is the most famous of these and, as he was still powerful at the turn of the century, he maintained the censorship on atomism that Jean-Baptiste Dumas had imposed before him in French education. Certainly, atoms were not totally banned from chemistry courses in 1904, because chemists couldn't work without them. But they could use them as instrumental fictions, as convenient images without assuming their real existence.

Unsurprisingly, the audience at the *Musée pédagogique* disagreed with Langevin when he argued that atoms are no longer a hypothesis, but a strong theory which embraces several branches of physics. Émile Borel, for example, agrees to talk about atoms in secondary education: it's necessary in chemistry and useful in physics, he says. But he immediately adds:

> There is a big difference between illustrating Mariotte's law,[1] for example, using the atomic hypothesis, and deducing it as a particular consequence of this *a priori* hypothesis. In this latter case, we would really have an atomic synthesis; I believe we agree on the inconveniences of this mode of presentation. (Langevin 1904a, p. 105)

An even more sceptical teacher at the Fénelon high school, Marie Mourgues, informs us about the nature of the alleged difficulties:

> Our students are only 18 years old. Is it reasonable to give as the goal of their research the intimate constitution of matter? Isn't there a great danger in making them see life beyond our senses, even armed with a powerful microscope? Do they have enough physical and moral health to withstand, better than Pascal, being face-to-face with the unknown? And this eagerness on their part to catch the expressions of molecules and atoms, which we are given as an argument in favour of the use of the theory, isn't this rather proof that they make the image a reality? (Ibid., p. 48)

---

[1] This law, also known as Boyle's Law or Boyle-Mariotte law, describes the relationship between pressure and volume of a confined gas. The absolute pressure exerted by a given mass of an ideal gas is inversely proportional to the volume it occupies if the temperature and amount of gas remain unchanged within a closed system.

4.5 Atomism Versus Energetics

Here we see the extent of the resistance that Langevin must face. But how does he hope that history can overcome it?

History provides Langevin with a powerful critique of mechanistic theories. Critique in the almost Kantian sense, because it is indeed about defining the conditions of possibility and the success of Newton's mechanics, but, this time, to awaken physicists from their mechanistic slumber. Thus begins the trial of mechanics, in the court of history. Langevin gives a contrasting historical survey of mechanics and of atomism.

In his historical survey of the theory of mechanics, Langevin often refers to Ernst Mach. A French translation of his *Mechanics* appeared around the time of this conference [12]. Mach developed a critique of classical mechanics, arguing that Newton's absolute space and time are metaphysical notions and claiming that only relative motion between bodies makes sense. In its form as well as in its contents, Langevin's critique of theoretical mechanics is relying heavily on this non-Comtean positivist tradition. He emphasizes both the obscurities that envelop the origins of mechanics—Descartes and Maupertuis are accused of having tainted it with metaphysics—and the difficult notion of absolute movement.

His genealogy of atomism aims to highlight that this theory is independent from the theory of mechanics. Langevin mentions the laws of chemical combination and Faraday's laws of electrolysis, and when he later encounters mechanical models, he suggests that the interference of mechanical notions with atomism has been the source of anti-atomism. He acknowledges that, in the nineteenth century, thermodynamics and electromagnetism could do without atoms, although there is no contradiction between the Carnot principle and atomism. But atomism rests on more recent results from physics: recent experiments on conduction in gases allow us to "count" atoms; and above all, the discovery of electrons or "atoms of electricity" transforms the atomic hypothesis into a real principle.

Langevin firmly concludes that mechanics can no longer hold the monopoly in theoretical physics. It must share the sovereignty with atomism. "Each in its place", says Langevin (ibid., p. 95). Thus, his critical historical glimpse leads to a new geography of physics. The venerable mechanics must limit itself to the visible, "to the movement of matter taken *en masse*". Atomism is tasked with synthesizing everything else. The two rivals have to coexist in a single domain, the kinetics of gases. A new map of knowledge emerges from his lecture that diminishes the territory of mechanics and confines it to the surface of things.

4.5 Atomism Versus Energetics

In addition to sceptical chemists, Langevin had to defeat a second opposition to atomism which came from a vigorous contemporary movement: energetics. Energeticists attempted to explain all phenomena in terms of energy relations and to dispense with the hypothesis of atoms. In 1895, Wilhelm Ostwald, professor at the University of Leipzig, presented his project at a conference in Lübeck which stirred strong reactions in both Germany and France [2]. In his lecture, Ostwald began by stressing the inadequacy of theoretical classical mechanics: he denounced its abusive extensions to electricity and energy, and criticized its ontological assumptions of a reversible nature, whereas the phenomena we observe are irreversible. Then, in a second step, he argued that energetics opens up a safe—albeit long and arduous—theoretical pathway. The two principles of thermodynamics are necessary and sufficient to describe and explain all physical phenomena using the concept of energy. This lecture outlining his project of energetics aroused strong reactions in Austria and Germany from Ludwig Boltzmann and Max Planck. In France, Pierre Duhem, professor of physical sciences at the University of Bordeaux, was also on the side of energetics. He emphasized the contrast between the simplicity of the principles of classical mechanics and the multiplicity of complex assumptions required to extend them to thermodynamics. He described a "counter-revolution", a physics of qualities, reviving Aristotelian physics without renouncing the use of mathematical formulas.

The controversy mainly rested on antagonist philosophical choices. Energeticists claimed that we transgress the limits of science by trying to explain everything by a single hypothesis. Reality is beyond physics, which must be content to classify, describe and predict phenomena. As we can very well achieve this with the concept of energy and the two principles of thermodynamics, there is no need for an atom. The atomists wanted to explain physical and chemical phenomena with the help of atoms and they tried to figure out its structure using models. It is about "explaining the complex visible by the simple invisible" as Perrin put it, by providing an account of a variety of independent phenomena with a single hypothesis [14].

Such were, roughly speaking, the terms of the dispute. It is easy to guess which side Langevin was on. After following Mach's historical critique to weaken the empire of theoretical mechanics, Langevin parted from him because Mach shared the phenomenological epistemology of energeticists. He considered the laws of physics as summaries of experiments, constructed for the purpose of making sense of experimental data. These mathematical, idealized expressions of phenomena do not describe the reality beyond sensations. Thus Langevin used Mach's history of mechanics to free a territory of theoretical physics and find a place for atoms. But because of his epistemological choices, Mach was no longer a good guide to establish that atoms have a right to exist in the liberated territory.

Langevin does not however fully side with the atomist party in the on-going controversy over energetics. He adopts a unique position. In the standard accounts of this controversy we find, facing the energeticists, the mechanists and the atomists. This alliance is based on historical evidence because the atomists have often resorted to mechanical models, plum pudding, nuclear or planetary for example, to describe the structure of the atom. The alliance between mechanics and atomism is also based on philosophical considerations: both theories aim to provide explanations rather than just descriptions of phenomena. So strong was this epistemological affinity that Abel Rey, a French philosopher of physics, published a book on this controversy that he called *L'énergétique et le mécanisme* from the point of view of the conditions of knowledge [15].

Langevin's lecture outlines a quite different landscape. Energetics and mechanics find themselves, despite their divergence, in the same camp. Because each, in its own way, seeks to stop history: energetics by imposing the famous *ignorabimus*; mechanics by locking itself in the illusion of a closed, complete, definitive body of knowledge. What kind of argument does Langevin use to make this point? He cannot use history against the energetics camp, because it turns out that history is also the favourite weapon of Langevin's adversaries. The two energeticists that Langevin attacks by name, Wilhem Ostwald and Pierre Duhem, know more about history of science than he does.[2]

4.6 Science Is Life

Since the scientific dispute between energeticists and atomists is settled through the mediation of historical arguments, we should more closely examine the kind of history that Langevin practices and wants to promote in science teaching.

Unlike Pierre Duhem, he is not inclined to dig seriously into the past. One searches in vain in his works for the precise analyses of the history of mechanics that are found in Duhem. Instead, Langevin practices a historical "glance", a vigorous panorama which summarizes in one sentence the main features of the contribution of individual scientists, or even a century of scientific endeavours. He does not care to follow the details of scientific changes through a chronological sequence of events. Instead, he aims to identify a principle that can guide future investigations.

His historical insights are woven with a host of metaphors borrowed mainly from biology. The metaphor of living science guides the argument. Science is viewed as a living organism, a tree whose trunk is formed by the two principles of thermodynamics and the principle of symmetry of Gabriel Lippmann and Pierre Curie. The tree has three major branches: mechanics, electromagnetism and atomism. This metaphorical description is indifferent to the chronology of events. Langevin even notes, considering the principle of conservation of energy, that it is extremely harmful to present it, as is sometimes done, following the second principle, on the pretext that historically it was formulated later. And the Carnot principle itself, formulated in 1824, should be presented in Boltzmann's probabilistic interpretation of entropy, "the only way to give Carnot's principle its true meaning" (Langevin 1904a, p. 40).

Finally, Langevin's major reproach to energetics is that it would stop the growth of the tree of physics. In his plea for atomism, he intends to defeat energetics through

---

[2] Before dedicating an entire work to the history of chemistry, *The Evolution of a Science, Chemistry* (1909, French trans. Paris, 1910), Ostwald had presented chemistry in historical order in the work criticized by Langevin, *Elements of Inorganic Chemistry*, Leipzig, 1900, French trans. Paris, 1904. As for Duhem, he had already published a historical volume on *The Electrical Theories of James Clerk Maxwell* (Paris, Hermann, 1902) and *The Evolution of Mechanics* in 1903. In 1904, he was drafting the beginning of *The Physical Theory*, where history is mobilized to criticize explanatory theories in general, and atomism in particular [4, 7, pp. 42–43].

a few rhetorical appeals to a life "instinct" to protest against the idea of imposing barriers to knowledge. Langevin mobilizes microbiology to emphasize that it is time to move from a superficial, macroscopic description of physical phenomena, to a deep understanding of the atomic structure of matter. He invokes the memory of Louis Pasteur and speaks of "atomic colonies" which he compares to "bacterial colonies" to convince the audience of the reality of atoms (ibid., p. 41). The image of living science is therefore much more than simple rhetoric. As early as 1904, it underlies his view of physics and transforms the rebellion of the young physicist against textbook science into a noble fight of life against death.

Still, once again Langevin shares this way of thinking with his opponents. Duhem also uses a host of arguments borrowed from life sciences. They first provide him with a model: physical theories should be like natural classifications of phenomena [7, pp. 30–40]. They also provide a metaphor—the parasite—for rejecting atomism. The living and powerful syntheses that Langevin wishes for are, for Duhem, "parasites" that weaken the theory and hasten its end because they quickly become outdated (ibid., pp. 42–43).

Thus, the controversy between these two physicists is played out in a battle of biological metaphors. They illuminate the dispute by revealing the tangles from which the disagreement proceeds. Duhem and Langevin are on the same ground: they both agree about the importance of historical considerations in physics teaching and research. They share a view of the history of physics as a slow, gradual and continuous process. They disagree on the function that is assigned to history. For Duhem, the creativity of physicists rests on historical considerations because physics theories are incompletely determined by experiment and logic (ibid., pp. 36–37). For Duhem, history limits the number of possible hypotheses. For Langevin, on the contrary, history is a liberating factor that frees the physicist from the prevailing dogmatism.

To sum up, subversion and emancipation are the major functions assigned to history by Langevin. He wants to promote history in the teaching of physics to achieve the triumph of atomism both in scientific research and in science teaching. This revolutionary purpose leads him to take an original position both in the debates about the reform of secondary education, where he dismisses both the proponents of technical education and the defenders of pure science, and in the current scientific controversy between advocates of mechanics and advocates of energetics, where he dismisses both camps.

His lecture also shows the limits of the revolutionary potential of history. While it may be very relevant to destabilize established doctrines to weaken mechanics, it then becomes an obstacle to the triumph of atomism. Langevin therefore uses an artillery of biological metaphors that allows him to confuse all opponents under the same banner. In the light of living science, the difference between energeticists and mechanists fades away. Both embody sclerosis and death.

Finally, this 1904 lecture will emerge as a founding text. Not only does it announce or foreshadow themes that Langevin develops later, such as thought and action, for example, but above all it forges a personal style of thought that can be labelled as an art of speaking with multiple voices. Langevin manages to conduct multiple battles at once, by linking various pairs of notions covering a variety of subjects.

References

1. Bensaude-Vincent B (1999) Atomism and positivism: a legend about French chemistry. Annals of Science 56:81–94
2. Bensaude-Vincent B (2005) Revisiting the controversy on energetics. In: Görs B, Psarros N, Ziche P (eds) Wilhelm Ostwald at the crossroads between chemistry, philosophy and media culture. Leipziger Univertätsverlag, Leipzig, pp 13–18
3. Brock WH (1967) The atomic debates. Leicester University Press, Leicester
4. Brouzeng P (1987) Pierre Duhem. Belin, Paris
5. Comte A (1830) Cours de philosophie positive, Lesson 2. Cited in the reprint by Hermann, Cours de philosophie positive, vol 1. Paris (1975)
6. Coumet E (1981) Paul Tannery, l'organisation de l'enseignement de l'histoire des sciences. Revue de Synthèse 101–102:87–123
7. Duhem P (1906) La théorie physique, son objet, sa structure. Vrin, Reprint Paris (1981)
8. Fox R, Weisz G (eds) (1980) The Organization of Science and technology in France (1808–1914). Cambridge University Press, Cambridge
9. Hulin N (1984) L'histoire des sciences dans l'ensignement scientifique. Rev Française de Pédagogie 66:15–27
10. Hulin N (ed) (2000) Physique et humanités scientifiques. Autour de la réforme de l'enseignement de 1902. Etudes et documents. Presses universitaires du Septentrion, Lille
11. Liard L (1904) Les sciences dans l'enseignement secondaire. Revue Universitaire 1:185–191. Cited in Hulin 2000, 247
12. Mach E (1904) La Mécanique, exposé historique et critique de son développement. Paris, Vienne
13. Paul HW (1972) The issue of decline in nineteenth-century French science. French Historical Studies 8:416–450
14. Perrin J (1913) Les atomes. Alcan, Paris
15. Rey A (1908) L'Énergétique et le mécanisme au point de vue des conditions de la connaissance. Alcan, Paris
16. Rocke AJ (1984) Chemical atomism in the nineteenth century from Dalton to Cannizzaro. Ohio State University Press, Columbus

Chapter 5
The Physics of Electrons, a New World

Abstract Langevin was invited to the 1904 International Congress in St. Louis, to speak in a session on the "Physics of the Electron". He described these "grains of electricity", as a scientific revolution. The purpose of his presentation was to overcome the conflict between theories of mechanics and electromagnetism by sketching a theoretical synthesis of physics based on electromagnetic concepts. He invited physicists to break away from thinking "in matter" and to think "in ether". He tackled the basic notion of mass and claimed that the inertia of the electron is of electromagnetic origin. While seeking an electromagnetic definition of mass, Langevin went on to predict its consequences, to explain deviations from Prout's Law and the origin of radioactive energy. In 1913, Langevin consolidated the views of his St. Louis lecture, demonstrating how Einstein's relationship $E = mc^2$ emerged from his search for an alternative definition of mass, without recourse to relativistic theory. Thus he reached the same conclusion as Einstein by considering the inertia of energy.

At the turn of the twentieth century, world fairs followed one another every 4 years. After Paris 1900, which marked the triumph of the "Electricity Fairy", Louisiana organized the "World's Greatest Exhibition", titled the *Louisiana Purchase Exposition* in St. Louis in 1904. World exhibitions in general celebrate science and technology. In 1904, however, visitors could discover a department in the physical sciences division devoted to theoretical concepts such as matter, ether and the electron.

International congresses were organized during the World Fairs [7], the first one for physics being held in Paris in 1900. Convened by the committee of the World Fair, these congresses were not intended to be meetings of experts debating their cutting-edge research results. Like the exhibition, they were aimed at a broad audience and to arouse public support and enthusiasm for science. Therefore Langevin did not hesitate to present electron physics as "a new America, where one breathes easily, which solicits all activities and which can teach many things to the Old World" (Langevin 1904b, p. 62) (Figs. 5.1 and 5.2).

Langevin's invitation to speak at the St. Louis Congress was arranged by Ernest Rutherford. He wrote to Langevin on 15 June 1904:

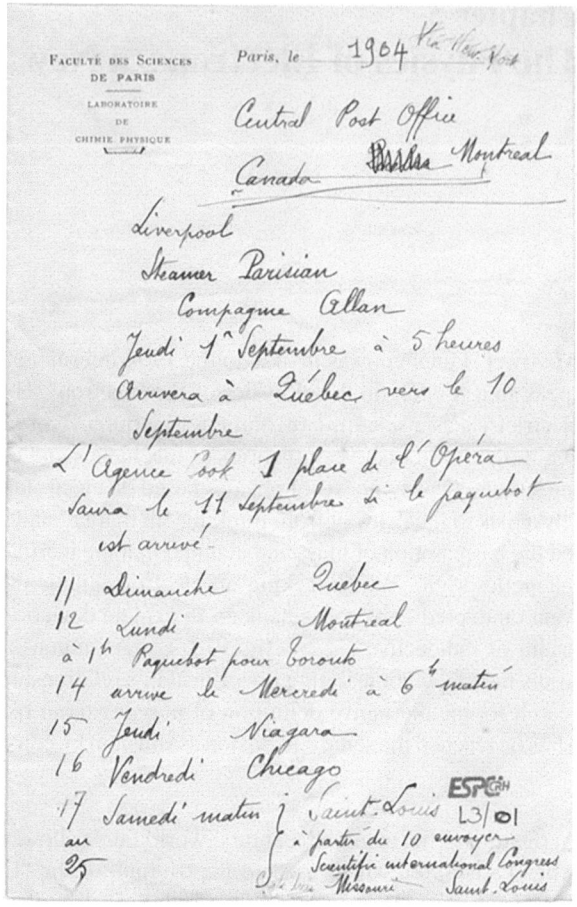

Fig. 5.1 Langevin's notes for his itinerary during the voyage to St. Louis 1–17 September 1904. (ESPCI, PSL University L003/001)

I have just been visited in Montreal by Simon Newcomb who wishes you to come over to St Louis to take part in the discussion with me on the Physics of the Electron. The division of the subject will be left to a mutual arrangement, but I suggested you should take the part dealing with cathode rays and I should confine myself to radioactivity. I hope that you will see your way to come. (Archives L076/014-1)

Newcomb was the chair of the organizing committee. Rutherford's proposed division of topics reveals his priorities. He had just published his seminal work on radioactivity, and his selection of this topic for himself in a session on the electron, presumably on the pretext that he would include β particles, would give him a platform to promote his book.

Langevin was uncomfortable about the topic assigned to him by his friend. When he replied on 28 July, worrying that he had yet to receive a formal invitation from Newcomb, he stated emphatically that "I know absolutely nothing about this subject": that is, he had not studied in depth the specific behaviour of a stream of electrons accelerated in a Crookes' tube. Thinking of the much broader topic of the

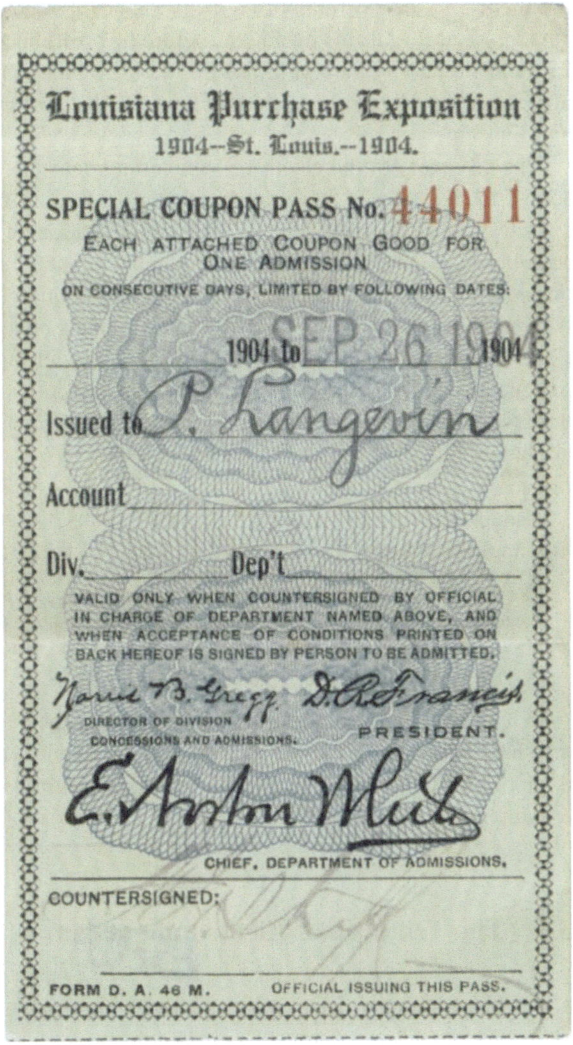

Louisiana Purchase Exposition
1904--St. Louis.--1904.

SPECIAL COUPON PASS No. 44011

EACH ATTACHED COUPON GOOD FOR ONE ADMISSION
ON CONSECUTIVE DAYS, LIMITED BY FOLLOWING DATES:

1904 to SEP 26 1904 1904

Issued to P. Langevin

Account

Div. Dep't

VALID ONLY WHEN COUNTERSIGNED BY OFFICIAL IN CHARGE OF DEPARTMENT NAMED ABOVE, AND WHEN ACCEPTANCE OF CONDITIONS PRINTED ON BACK HEREOF IS SIGNED BY PERSON TO BE ADMITTED.

Norris B. Gregg — DIRECTOR OF DIVISION CONCESSIONS AND ADMISSIONS.

D. R. Francis — PRESIDENT.

CHIEF, DEPARTMENT OF ADMISSIONS.

COUNTERSIGNED:

FORM D. A. 46 M. OFFICIAL ISSUING THIS PASS.

Fig. 5.2 Langevin's pass for the Louisiana Purchase Exposition, St. Louis, 26 September 1904. (ESPCI, PSL University L003/006)

"Physics of the Electron", he expressed his concern that it "will be difficult for me to find much time between now and then to attend to it" (Archives L003/052). He soon received an invitation from Newcomb, who confirmed the arrangement: "You have doubtless heard from Professor Rutherford, who will be your associate, as to the nature of the address which is desired of you" (Archives L003/010). When he attended the British Association meeting in Cambridge later in August, accompanied by his wife Jeanne, Langevin would have had plenty of opportunity to develop the approach he would use, in discussion with his British mentor J.J. Thomson.

The published record of Langevin's lecture is a valuable survey, about 70 pages long, of the state of the art in physics before Einstein's famous 1905 article founding the theory of special relativity. Of all Langevin's lectures, it is perhaps the most personal as it reveals his own ideas before he positions himself as the spokesman of Einstein's relativity theory. It also allows us to grasp Langevin's relationships with contemporary physicists such as Thomson, Rutherford, Lorentz,[1] HenriPoincaré and Einstein.

The discovery of the electron,[2] which historians often simply attribute to Joseph John Thomson, was in fact a process that took 10 years engaging a number of physicists from various countries [4]. The identification of cathode rays, observed by Jean Perrin in 1895, with the universal constituents of the atom was hotly debated during the next years. But Langevin does not mention such hesitation, for his gaze is resolutely turned towards the future. He takes advantage of this conference to sketch out a grand plan. For him, the discovery of electrons represented less a hope of penetrating the architecture of atoms than a hope of reunifying physics under the umbrella of electromagnetism. The existence of "grains of electricity" meant above all that an interface was possible between the physics of matter and the physics of radiation.

Langevin describes the advent of these "grains of electricity" as a scientific revolution, a paradigm shift in the ultimate theme of the paper:

> The notion of the electron (…) has in a few years taken an immense step which makes it break the frameworks of the old physics and overturn the established order of notions and laws to lead to an organization that is foreseen to be simple, harmonious and fruitful. (Langevin 1904b, p. 104)

What does this revolution consist of? For Langevin, it is a reversal of the relationships between electromagnetism and mechanics, the end of a centuries-long reign of mechanics, and the promise of a new synthesis. The major goal of his presentation is to sketch a synthesis that replaces and, if possible, extends mechanics.

5.1 The Triumph of Electromagnetism

To begin with, Langevin argues that the whole of physics can be understood using only electromagnetic notions. He proceeds in two steps: first, he breaks the historical connections between atomism and mechanics, to put an end to what he describes as a historical compromise. Therefore, in the historical introduction to the paper, he claims that modern atomism emerged from Maxwell and Lorentz theories alone, leaving classical mechanics aside. In the second section, Langevin tries to deduce mechanics from electromagnetism:

---

[1] The Dutch physicist Hendrik Lorentz (1853–1928) shared the 1902 Nobel Prize in Physics with Pieter Zeeman for the discovery and explanation of the Zeeman Effect, and derived the Lorenz transformation that underpinned the theory of special relativity. He was described by the Nobel Foundation as "the world's leading spirit, who completed what was left unfinished by his predecessors and prepared the ground for the fruitful reception of new ideas based on the quantum theory".

[2] The term "electron" was coined by the Irish physicist George Johnstone Stoney in 1891.

5.1 The Triumph of Electromagnetism

> To what extent can the known properties of matter be deduced from these two notions of the electron and the ether, and what must we introduce beyond these to build a synthesis? (Ibid., p. 71)

To meet this challenge, Langevin tackles the basic notion of all mechanics, mass. He assumes that the inertia of the electron is of electromagnetic origin; and as he admits that matter is composed of "electrons of both signs", he boldly concludes that the inertia of matter is of electromagnetic origin. But this attempt to absorb classical mechanics encounters an irreducible obstacle: gravitation stubbornly refuses to fit into an electromagnetic synthesis. Newton resists! Langevin admits it and submits, but he thinks he can quietly translate all other domains of physics into electromagnetic terms.

This quick overview of Langevin's lecture suggests that, in 1904, he hoped to solve the inner conflict that divided physics theory, using a victory of electromagnetism over mechanics. Although the approach was not entirely original, since Langevin heavily relied on Hendrik Lorentz's recent work,[3] this lecture highlights Langevin's distinctive style. In particular, the historical approach to the notion of electron is a personal trait. A look at Thomson's courses and lectures that Langevin brought back from Cambridge shows that Thomson always proceeded from experiment to theoretical conclusion, without any reference to history (Archives L126/02). Moreover, Langevin is not interested in the questions, that were foremost in Thomson's mind, related to the structure of matter and the model of atom. He only mentions them towards the end, to account for the electrical and magnetic properties of matter.

The key question for Langevin, as for Lorentz, Poincaré and Einstein, is the conflict between electromagnetism and mechanics. However, his approach is not driven by a sense of crisis. So Langevin is not looking for a compromise formula between the two conflicting theories, let alone a rescue solution. The contrast is made clear in the paper delivered by Henri Poincaré in St Louis [11]. His lecture, "The Principles of Mathematical Physics", describes a crisis in physics that puts all fundamental principles—conservation of matter and conservation of energy, equality of action and reaction, and the law of least action—in danger. To deliver a diagnosis and a prudent prognosis, Poincaré chooses a historical approach like Langevin, to show that this is not the first crisis in physics. He nevertheless insists that the current crisis is serious and creates a climate of uncertainty about the future. The negative results of the Michelson-Morley experiments force mathematicians to be ingenious to save the "The Principle of Relativity", according to which the laws of physical phenomena must be the same for a stationary observer as for one carried along in a uniform motion of translation, so that we have a means of knowing whether we are at rest or in motion. To conclude he envisages a new mechanics subverting all principles:

> Perhaps (…) we should construct a whole new mechanics, that we only succeed in catching a glimpse of, where as inertia increases with velocity, the velocity of light would become an insurmountable limit. (Ibid., p. 23)

---

[3] Lorentz hybridized Maxwell's theory with the corpuscular notion of *grains d'électricité*. He interpreted optic and electromagnetic phenomena in terms of interactions between electric particles and a stationary ether [5].

However, he immediately nuanced this revolutionary vision as he states that classical mechanics would remain valid "as a first approximation, since it would be true for velocities that are not too great, so that we would still find the old dynamics within the new". The old principles "are so useful" that they would remain in place. And his advice is that "the surest way in practice would be still to act *as if* we continue to believe in them" (ibid., p. 24).

Langevin, by contrast, seems to be driven by a spirit of conquest and a hunger for a renewal. And this time he is much closer to Einstein than to Poincaré. But he follows a quite different path. In his 1905 paper, *On the Electrodynamics of Moving Bodies*, Einstein began by listing difficulties and contradictions before seeking to solve them by using one or two hypotheses. By contrast, Langevin does not "cut the Gordian knot", as has been said of Einstein. Instead he finds in electromagnetic theory a principle capable of overturning the whole framework of theoretical mechanics. One can say, to underline the difference between these two styles of thought, that Einstein does physics by playwriting, introducing a "deus ex machina" that emerges from the outside to resolve the crisis. Langevin rather thinks of it as an epic where the young hero "electron", the latest in the tradition, disrupts the old order thus reshaping the entire landscape of physics theory. In other words, Langevin indeed describes an "electronic revolution" but not at all as a break. Instead he suggests a reversal of perspective:

> It thus seems more natural to consider the analogy pointed out by Maxwell between the equations of electromagnetism and those of Lagrange's dynamics as justifying much more the possibility of an electromagnetic representation of the principles and notions of ordinary, material mechanics, than the reverse possibility. (Langevin 1904b, p. 82)

This inversion generates a prodigious effect of novelty: a non-mechanical conception of matter. Langevin considers ether as the key concept of all physics and invites physicists to break away from the age-old habit of thinking "in matter" and to get the habit to think "in ether".

> It is unreasonable to try to construct what is simple and singular—that is the ether—from a complicated and diverse medium like matter. I believe that we will have to get used to thinking "in ether" independently of any material representation. (1904b, p. 65)

To us today, this bold attempt at reconstructing the whole of physics around the notion of ether in 1904 may appear outdated because, in the next year, Einstein would abolish this hypothetical mechanical medium from the theory of physics. Thus, paradoxically, this concept of an electromagnetic ether emerged just one year before Einstein seems to demote it to the rank of superfluous hypothesis. But how then can we understand that Langevin welcomes Einstein's article with enthusiasm, a year later?

5.2 "Thinking in Ether"

The question of internal consistency forces us to clarify Langevin's proposal of "thinking in ether". In 1904, the existence of this fluid medium, infinitely light and universal, was considered to be established, and nothing exceptional. This opinion

5.2 "Thinking in Ether"

is shared by the physics community. This hypothetical elastic medium to support the propagation of light waves was widely accepted when James Clerk Maxwell proposed that light is an electromagnetic radiation, and published a mathematical model of its propagation [3]. The idea seemed to be confirmed when, during the 1880s, Heinrich Hertz carried out a series of experiments to demonstrate the existence of electromagnetic waves and revised Maxwell's equations. The ether is even, in the eyes of some physicists like George Fitzgerald, a very positive notion that finally eliminates the mystery surrounding action at distance. It reflects the collective endeavour of dozens of physicists from various countries to solve the puzzle raised by the conflict between mechanics and electromagnetism. Langevin heavily relies on J.J. Thomson's notion of electromagnetic inertia. In 1881, Thomson noted that charged bodies are harder to move than uncharged bodies and hypothesized that an electromagnetic mass was added to the mechanical mass of bodies, giving a mathematical formula for this effect. He went on to confirm that the increase of the mass of bodies varies with its velocity and added that it also depends on its direction. In 1893, he clearly stated that it is impossible to supersede the velocity of light because that would require an infinite amount of energy.

Does this betray the influence of the Cambridge milieu of physics? Although historians of physics often contrast the mechanistic inclinations of English physicists with the primacy of electromagnetism in Germany by the end of the nineteenth century [13], Cambridge physicists were the exception. In his lecture, Langevin never mentions the German physicist Wilhelm who developed an electromagnetic worldview in 1900 [5, 12]. He assumed that all forms of mass, inertial and gravitational, are of electromagnetic origin. Unlike Langevin, he even suggested that if gravitation was of electromagnetic origin there should be a proportionality between the various forms of mass. Lorentz also embraced the view that there exists only electromagnetic mass in 1904. While the rest of the international physics community was focused on the mutual influence between matter and ether, a specific and distinctive ambition of the Cavendish Laboratory was to explain all physical phenomena as resulting from movements of the ether. Joseph Larmor, whose courses Langevin attended in Cambridge, published *Aether and Matter* in 1900, a theoretical physics book, where he outlined a theory of ether that was independent of a theory of mechanics [8]. Thomson was close to the Society for Psychical Research, and Oliver Lodge suggested that matter is ether structured in a special way and that ether could be the instrument of thought [10]. So, speculations about ether were conducive to spiritualism [14].

What did Langevin retain from such ethereal speculations? No certainty, because he admits that all attempts at understanding the structure and functions of the ether were a failure (Langevin 1940b, p. 7). But he keeps a firm intention to exclude mechanistic interpretations of ether. He rejects totally all hypotheses of this kind by noticing a logical contradiction in their assumptions. And he concludes that, instead of stubbornly applying to ether the properties of matter, one must proceed in reverse. In considering ether as the primordial reality, we only give it what it has, electromagnetic properties. Langevin hopes to achieve unity between ordinary matter and ether, thanks to the notion of electron. This "grain of electricity", as he calls it, can bridge the gap between matter and the ether and reconcile the two hitherto irreconcilable theories of physics.

Thus, the call to "think in ether" can be seen as a programme of counter-attack against the mechanistic ambitions of some physicists. It is less about promoting the ether than blocking the path to attempts to extend mechanics into electromagnetism. Nevertheless, in his effort to nibble at the empire of mechanics, Langevin leans towards those scientists who dematerialized matter. But he will not have to be embarrassed for this inclination when he converts to dialectical materialism in the 1930s, since his 1904 lecture received the approval of Lenin.[4] In *Materialism and Empirical Criticism*, Lenin has a chapter titled *Matter Disappears*, where he refers to the Lodge, Righi, Thomson and Langevin. He assumes that their position is not anti-materialist [9, p. 363]. For, to be a materialist, he claims, is to accept an objective reality and not to assume that reality is exclusively material. Lenin even encourages physicists in their attempts at unification.

Anyway, materialist or not, Langevin's project of unification through electrons proved extremely fruitful. His paper in St Louis inspired many of his research projects in the next few years. In particular, it led him to investigate the concept of electromagnetic inertia: in an important article *On the Origin of Radiations and Electromagnetic Inertia* (Langevin 1905h), he establishes a clear distinction between "velocity waves" and "acceleration waves" and how they are generated. The former he described as the electromagnetic "wake" of a moving charged particle and travels with it: the energy in this wave remains local and is not propagated away from the source. By contrast, acceleration waves produce radiation and carry energy away of a magnitude proportional to the square of the acceleration. These concepts were also included in his 1906 course at the *Collège de France*, where Langevin demonstrated that the emission or absorption of radiation by a material system results from a change in its electromagnetic inertia.

5.3 Langevin's $E = mc^2$

According to Edmond Bauer, his assistant at the *Collège de France*, Langevin discovered the formal relationship between energy and mass, equivalent to the famous equation $E = mc^2$, in 1904. Langevin himself later made a similar claim (Langevin 1913c). It is inappropriate to assume, however, that this demonstrates Langevin as a precursor of the principle of relativity (see Chap. 6), although certainly we can at least suggest, as did Einstein himself, that "he had perceived some essential points" [6, p. 14]. In fact, Langevin and Einstein were following quite different creative pathways: Langevin was seeking an electromagnetic definition of mass: Einstein was exploring the consequences of the principle of relativity. At the crossroads, they

---

[4] For further discussion on Langevin's materialism and its connection with Marxism, see Chap. 17.

5.3 Langevin's $E = mc^2$

were bound to meet, and both reached the same conclusion by considering the inertia of energy.[5]

Langevin set out a summary of his non-relativistic development of the equivalence of mass and energy in a lecture at the Society française de physique on 26 March 1913 (Langevin 1913c). This lecture, fortunately published, unlike his earlier lectures at the *Collège de France*, can be seen as the culmination, the drawing together, of all Langevin's "thinking in ether", and of his view of a physics that may be understood using only electromagnetic phenomena. As an integral component of this long lecture, Langevin showed the theoretical equivalence of mass and energy, at least for the specific circumstance he was considering.

He starts with the concept of mass, comparing three mechanical definitions: as a coefficient of inertia, as a capacity for impulse, and as a capacity for kinetic energy. Reviewing these definitions he states:

> Mass is no longer invariable, since its various definitions cease to coincide when the speed of matter ceases to be small compared to that of light and since they all lead, for the same portion of matter, to variable values as a function of speed, according to three different laws. (Ibid., p. 399)

Under these definitions, the concept of the conservation of mass no longer has validity "and becomes mixed with the conservation of energy".

Langevin therefore seeks an alternative, electromagnetic definition of mass. He does not seek electromagnetic characteristics in mechanical mass. Instead, he seeks mass, or at least mass-like phenomena, in the electromagnetic ether. To do this, he considers the inertia of a moving electrically charged sphere. The sphere is surrounded by radial electrical lines of force. When the charged sphere moves, it creates a magnetic field. He cites as evidence the experiments of Rowland. When the velocity is constant, an electromagnetic wave is formed in the surrounding region, local to the sphere. It is this region that carries with it the extra energy that will form the basis for his electromagnetic mass. With his talent for communication using loose metaphors, he describes the lines of force as a mane (chevelure) and the velocity wave as a wake (sillage).[6]

In this 1913 paper he writes:

> Although we are still far from being able to affirm that an electromagnetic synthesis is possible, the effort attempted to constitute it, and the change of view which it implies, have already shown themselves to be very rich in consequences and new insights, some of which I would like to point out. (Ibid., p. 400)

---

[5] Max Born explained Einstein's approach in his book *Atomic Physics* (1935) in a section on the inertia of energy, based on a thought experiment with two opposed light sources in an enclosed box. ([2, p. 54] and Appendix VII, 323).

[6] As noted above, he had used the same approach in *Sur l'origine des radiations et l'inertie électromagnétique* (Langevin 1905k) in order to create a theory for the origin of electromagnetic radiation. In that case, the source of the wave was an accelerating charged sphere, giving rise to the term "acceleration wave".

By considering the energy needed to create the convection current associated with the moving charged sphere, and noting that this is equivalent to the kinetic energy of a moving mass, he derives an expression for an equivalent electromagnetic mass in terms of magnetic permeability μ_0, charge and radius. He then introduces the pressure on the surface of a charged sphere as described by Poincaré, finding an energy minimum for stability between outward electrical pressure and pressure exerted in the ether. This gives the energy in terms of dielectric permittivity ε_0, charge and radius.

Combining these two equations gives electromagnetic mass as the product of energy, permittivity and permeability: $m = \mu_0 \varepsilon_0 E$ (Fig. 5.3).

Langevin's equation and Einstein's equation are simply two sides of the same coin, two mathematically equivalent ways of expressing the same fundamental truth. Using Maxwell's relationship for the speed of light in vacuum, c, in terms of the permeability and permittivity of free space, which can be expressed as $c^2 = 1/(\mu_0\varepsilon_0)$, Langevin's relationship between energy and mass is identical to Einstein's equation $E = mc^2$ and it carries the same profound insight into fundamental physics.

Langevin's derivation does not make any reference to the Lorentz transformation, relative frames of reference or other issues related to relativity. Nevertheless, Langevin also recognized and explored the changed physics that would accompany high velocities, concluding that the same principles would still hold. He worked out that his electromagnetic mass would also be subject to the same relativistic changes at high velocities as would a mechanical mass.

Finally, he extends his analysis to predict the presence of electromagnetic mass inside a body. Following directly from this, Langevin has the priority in the discovery of a consequence of the relationship between energy and mass which is of importance for chemistry. At the beginning of the nineteenth century, the English chemist William Prout hypothesized that all chemical elements were formed from a primordial element, hydrogen. Despite its longstanding success among nineteenth-century chemists who strove to build up a classification of elements, this conjecture encountered obstacles, when it became clear that most atomic mass values were not integer multiples of that of hydrogen. The deviations being of the order of 1%, they could not be considered as mere experimental errors although Prout's hypothesis was criticised by Dmitri Mendeleev, in particular [1]. Langevin had the idea that electromagnetic inertia could account for these deviations.

---

14. Masse et énergie. — La comparaison de cette expression avec celle de la masse électromagnétique initiale m_0 donnée par (4) nous conduit immédiatement à la relation remarquable :

(20) $$m_0 = K_0\mu_0 E_0 = \frac{E_0}{V^2}.$$

La masse initiale électromagnétique d'un électron est égale au quotient de son énergie potentielle totale par le carré de la vitesse de la lumière.

Fig. 5.3 Langevin's expressions for the equivalence of energy and mass. (Langevin 1913c)

It seems to me that the experimental proof of the inertia of the gravity of internal energy is provided by the now certain existence of the deviations from Prout's law, by the fact that atomic weights, although substantially integer multiples of a same quantity, however present small irregularities from this law (…) The explanation I propose results immediately from all the above: the deviations would come from the fact that the formation of atoms from primordial elements (by disintegration, as we see in radioactivity, or through a reverse process not yet observed that would give birth to heavy atoms), would be accompanied by variations in internal energy by emission or absorption of radiation. The sum of the weights of the atoms would differ from that of the transformed atoms by an amount equal to the quotient of the energy variation by the square of the speed of light. (Langevin 1913c, pp. 422–423)

In thus shedding light on the enigma of deviations from Prout's law, Langevin possibly inspired the Rutherford hypothesis of neutrons in his 1920 Bakerian Lecture at the Royal Society on the "Nuclear Constitution of Atoms". This confirms just how heuristic was his approach to the physics of electrons, using electromagnetic inertia as its basis.

References

1. Bensaude-Vincent B, Stengers I (1996) A history of chemistry. Harvard University Press, Cambridge
2. Born M (1935) Atomic physics. Blackie, London
3. Buchwald J (1985) From Maxwell to microphysics. Aspects of the electromagnetic theory in the late nineteenth century. The University of Chicago Press, Chicago
4. Buchwald J, Warwick A (eds) (2002) Histories of the electron. The birth of microphysics. MIT Press, Cambridge
5. Darrigol O (2000) Electrodynamics from Ampère to Einstein. Oxford University Press, Oxford
6. Einstein A (1947) Hommage à Paul Langevin. La Pensée 12:13–14
7. Forest P-G (1986) Montrer pour démontrer. Le Congrès des arts et des sciences de l'exposition universelle de St Louis. Relations internationales 46:131–152
8. Larmor J (1900) Aether and matter. Cambridge University Press, Cambridge
9. Lenin W.I. (1908) Materialism and Empirio-criticism. Critical Remarks about a Reactionary Philosophy. https://www.marxists.org/archive/lenin/works/1908/mec/
10. Lodge O (1907) Ether and reality. Cambridge University Press, Cambridge
11. Poincaré H (1905) The principles of mathematical physics. The Monist 15(1):1–24
12. Seth S (2004) Quantum theory and the electromagnetic worldview. Historical Studies in Physical Sciences 35(1):67–93
13. Wheaton BR (1983) The Tiger and the Shark. Empirical roots of the wave-particle dualism. Cambridge University Press, Cambridge
14. Wynne B (1979) Physics and psychics: science, symbolic action, and social control in late Victorian England. In: Barnes B, Shapin S (eds) Natural order, historical studies. Sage Publications, Beverly Hills, pp 167–187

Chapter 6
Promoting the Theory of Relativity

Abstract Langevin invites a change in the focus of historians of relativity, from the genesis of the theory and priority issues to the multiple ways of exploring and interpreting it. For Langevin, Einstein's paper on the inertia of energy confirmed his own results and increased the strength of the principle of relativity. Langevin did not conclude that the ether was unnecessary, only that it could not be detected, so there was no incompatibility between relativity and electromagnetism using the ether. Langevin was among the first scientists to promote the theory of relativity in France as he understood that Einstein's principle shocked the foundations of physics, and that the shock resonated beyond its boundaries. In an effort to reconceptualize space and time, he presented two lectures on this new physics to a philosophical audience, in 1911. To exemplify the break between the common view of time and the notion of time in relativity physics he emphasized the time shift between a space traveller and a stationary one. Langevin's personal contribution in the history of relativity was to develop a conceptual view of the principle of relativity that interpreted Einstein's conclusions in philosophical terms.

In his obituary of Langevin for the Royal Society of London, Frederic Joliot-Curie devotes as much text to his contributions to relativity as he does for dia- and paramagnetism, and in both cases twice the length of the section on ion transport [6]. Yet the section on relativity is full of generalities, with little evidence for any specific contribution. It is difficult to emphasize Langevin's contribution as long as the attention is focused on the road to the discovery. In most historical studies of the theory of relativity, the name of Langevin is barely mentioned. Or it is only associated with the formulation of a famous thought experiment known as "Langevin's traveller" or "the twins paradox" [15, 21]. To evaluate Langevin's contribution to the history of the physics of relativity it is necessary to critically examine the usual practices of historians of science.

6.1 Breaking with Heroic Historical Narratives

Most historical studies of relativity theory have been conducted by physicists who turned to the history of science. In line with the moral values prevailing in research communities in the twentieth century, they tend to overestimate the role of individuals and downplay the role of research infrastructures [20]. The history of the theory of relativity has been accordingly largely centred on Einstein. The debates between the historians of relativity usually turn around the question: "who discovered relativity?". They follow the genesis of Einstein's papers from Maxwell's integration of light and optics into electromagnetism to Einstein's foundational paper "on the electrodynamics of moving bodies". They scrutinize dozens of papers published on the negative results of Michelson-Morley experiments that discussed the dynamics of moving bodies and they extract from them the major steps leading to the formulation of the theory of special relativity. They finally focus on potential priority disputes between three candidate discoverers Einstein, Lorentz and Poincaré.[1] Lorentz is credited with the notion of a stationary ether in which microparticles circulate and for his mathematical treatment of the negative results of Michelson-Morley experiments: i.e. the Lorentz transformations that Poincaré considered as the "coup de pouce", an ingenious remedy to prevent the collapse of the fundamental principles of physics (see Chap. 5). Poincaré is credited with the formulation of the principle of relativity and for his physical interpretation of the Lorentz transformation. But Einstein alone eliminated the ether and recognized that the principle of relativity demanded that space and time could be determined in any inertial frame of reference. So Einstein remains the sole legitimate discoverer of the theory of relativity.

The debates prompted by the hundredth anniversary of Einstein's foundational paper in 2005 and the intense scholarship encouraged by the project around the collection of Einstein's papers slightly displaced the focus of historical studies. For instance [10], dismisses all priority disputes as tedious and fruitless. He rather focuses on the socio-technical context that favoured the discovery and points to the concern with the synchronization of clocks generated by the extension of the railway networks. Olivier Darrigol [4, 5] emphasizes the collective endeavour of generations of physicists and considers that the contributions of Einstein, Lorentz and Poincaré should be considered as the three final steps in this process. Nevertheless, most historical studies remain focused on the genesis of Einstein's foundational paper, although Darrigol concedes that the construction of the special relativity theory did not end with this paper [5, p. 22].

The case of Langevin is of special interest because it forces historians of science to give up the quest for the founding father of what is considered today as the official theory of relativity. Langevin invites decentring the attention of historians of relativity from the genesis of the theory and the priority issues to the variety of pathways to and interpretations of the theory that Einstein named relativity.

---

[1] See, for instance, the entry https://en.wikipedia.org/wiki/Relativity_priority_dispute

6.1 Breaking with Heroic Historical Narratives

In 1905, Langevin published a paper entitled *Sur l'impossibilité physique de mettre en évidence le mouvement de translation de la terre* (Langevin 1905m). The paper is brief, with two pages only. It considers the Trouton-Nobel experiment, which was based on a suggestion by Fitzgerald that a charged parallel-plate capacitor moving through the ether should orient itself perpendicularly to the motion. Langevin shows simply that the null result may be completely explained by the Lorentz contraction of the charged plate.

Langevin's second engagement with relativity occurred in the same year, 1905, with his investigation into the inertia of energy: although he published his results only in 1913. Langevin studied the inertia of energy in association with a moving spherical charge and uncovered a formal relationship between mass and energy He demonstrated that the constant of proportionality was the product of the permittivity and the permeability of free space.

Langevin's assistant Edmond Bauer brought to his attention that Einstein had derived the same result, on the basis of the principal of relativity: "the laws that govern changes of physical systems do not depend on which one of two coordinate systems moving in uniform parallel relative motion these changed are referred to". The title of Einstein's brief paper *Does the Inertia of a Body Depend on Its Energy Content?* also emphasizes the convergence between Einstein's and Langevin's thinking. In fact, he found in Einstein's theory a confirmation of the grand vision that he had outlined in his paper of the physics of electrons. According to Bauer, he was pleased to discover in Einstein's 1905 papers a number of arguments to substantiate his project of a new synthesis of physics based on electromagnetic dynamics. Michel Paty summarizes the contributions of his reading of Einstein's theory of special relativity:

> Among other things, Einstein's theory gave him what his theory and model of the deformable electron lacked at the time: the principle of relativity and the physically reconstructed concepts of space and time that replaced the absolute concepts of the old mechanics. He saw in Einstein's theory the reformulation he had been waiting for. He himself drew many original results from it as consequences, some linked to his own way of understanding the theory as a "dynamic" (such as his demonstration of the inertia of energy), others due to his own sense of physics as a "thought phenomena" (close to that of Einstein, by the way), such as his analysis of physical distances and durations in systems in relative motion, expressing to its last consequences Minkowski's representation of space-time and its relationship to causality. [17, p. 20]

For Langevin, Einstein's paper on the inertia of energy confirmed his own results. Conversely it established at the outset the strength of the principle of relativity as articulated by Einstein. Langevin did not conclude from reading Einstein's paper that the ether was unnecessary. It may best be assumed to be Poincaré's interpretation, as described in Jeremy Gray's extensive biography [11]. By developing the "Lorentz group", Poincaré made it possible to ignore the ether in relativistic considerations, finding "the perfect invariance of the equations of electrodynamics". Instead, in 1905 Langevin could consider that relativity made the ether undetectable rather than unnecessary. Thus there was no incompatibility for Langevin in accepting relativity while still building a physics of electromagnetism using the ether. As late as 1922 he still retained the ether in his paper on relativity (Langevin 1922e).

We have little evidence for Langevin's view of relativity during the next few years. So Langevin could continue to study electromagnetism, continue to think of an electromagnetic ether, while at the same time accept the new principle of relativity. But, apart from integrating the Lorentz transformations into his work, the principle of special relativity, applied to inertial systems, had no particular impact on his scientific thinking.

It doesn't matter whether or not Langevin clearly revealed the relation between mass and energy summarized in the equation $E = mc^2$ before or at the same time as Einstein. He certainly went on to develop this solution and the further ramifications of electromagnetic inertia during the following years as he notes when he published his results:

> By one of the most beautiful and important applications of the principle of relativity, Einstein was able to generalize the preceding relation (ie $E = mc^2$) to other cases than those of electrostatic equilibrium (that I have) considered so far. I myself developed, independently of him, in 1906, the following considerations and presented them in my teaching at the *Collège de France* in a less elementary and more general form than here. (Langevin 1913c, p. 414)

For Langevin, the inertia of energy, already central in his 1904 paper on the physics of electrons and clearly developed in his 1905 course at the *Collège de France*, was an entrance way to the special relativity, whereas for Einstein it was a consequence that he first mentioned in a letter to a friend in 1905 and considered as "an amusing and fascinating line of thought" (quoted in Darrigol [5, p. 19]). Langevin followed a research pathway that differed from Einstein's. Their paths converged at some point and Langevin adopted the modest position of Einstein's spokesperson, while Einstein considered him as a faithful interpreter of his views [9]. Thus, to break with the heroic historical accounts, it is first and foremost necessary to consider the multiple versions of a theory instead of digging into the roots of the official standard version.

6.2 Langevin's Personal Version of the Principle of Relativity

The case of Langevin also invites historians of the physics of relativity to broaden the scope of their investigations and to consider that communicating science is an integral part of scientific activities [19]. The advancement of science is not limited to the act of discovery, to the enunciation of a new law or principle. It also involves the communication of knowledge. The campaign launched by Langevin to disseminate the theory of relativity in France is a good example of the importance and creative power of knowledge communication.

For Langevin was among the first scientists to defend the theory of relativity in France. As early as 1909–1911, he devoted his course at the *Collège de France* to the theory of relativity and gave two important lectures in 1911, at a time when the community of French physicists ignored, rejected, or contested it. Henri Poincaré, who was best placed to understand it since he had clearly envisaged an entirely new

6.2 Langevin's Personal Version of the Principle of Relativity

mechanics in his St. Louis lecture in 1904, saw in Einstein's theory a convenient convention (Poincaré 1928, pp. 37–54). Until his death in 1912, he developed a conventional view of the principles of physics as initially inspired by experiment and later converted into matters of belief or conventions. This was the philosophical attitude that Langevin describes as "eclectic" in his obituary of Poincaré (Langevin 1913f). Pierre Duhem was downright hostile. He considered all this as a "creation of the mind" that offends common sense.

Langevin played a key role in the history of relativity for two major reasons. First, he developed a personal interpretation of the principle of relativity that emphasized the reconceptualization of space and time. This version of the relativity principle seems more appropriate and accurate to a number of physicists than Einstein's formulation in 1905 [13]. Second, he immediately perceived that Einstein's principle shocked the foundations of physics, and that the shock resonated beyond its boundaries. He managed to turn a new theory in the field of physics into a groundbreaking turning point in the history of Western culture [16, 18]. In 1911 he addressed two lectures on the new physics to a philosophical audience. The first one entitled *The Evolution of Space and Time*, at the International Congress of Philosophy in Bologna (Langevin 1911a); the second one titled Time, Space and Causality at the *Société française de philosophie* (Langevin 1911b). Let us try to identify the major points that he developed in these lectures.

From the outset Langevin presents the principle of relativity as an "experimental fact" established by the negative result of the attempts to discover the translational motion of the earth in the ether.

> The result has been consistently negative and, independently of any interpretation, we can state as an experimental fact the content of the following principle, known as relativity. If various groups of observers are in uniform translation with respect to each other (such as observers linked to the Earth for various positions of the latter in its orbit) all mechanical and physical phenomena will follow the same laws for all these groups of observers. (Langevin 1911a, p. 113)

Nevertheless he seems to distance himself from Einstein's formulation because he speaks of "the principle known as relativity" *(principe suivant, dit de relativité)*. Did Langevin use this cautious phrase because of the lack of clear empirical evidence? The experimental investigation on the speed of light was very difficult. The predicted time-shift was not confirmed before Sagnac's experiment in 1913. However, Langevin fully embraced the principle of relativity. In his obituary of Eleuthère Mascart written in 1908 he argued that Mascart had already grasped this principle when he stated in 1872 that the translational movement of the earth has no appreciable influence on optical phenomena and he concluded "There, written for the first time, in definitive form for optical phenomena, is what we now call the principle of relativity, whose perfect accuracy has been confirmed by all subsequent experiments, in all domains, and whose importance grows ever greater, equal at least to that of the principle of conservation of energy" (Langevin 1909a). Langevin's hesitation concerns the term relativity rather than the empirical status of the principle. His reservation about the term "relativity" seems to proceed from his conviction that what is fundamental in relativity theory is what is invariant. Indeed, the Galilean principle of relativity which states that the same laws of physics apply in any frame of reference that is moving in a straight line at constant speed has been extended to all moving frames of references. But in Langevin's view it means above all that the invariance of the laws of physics is rescued. Einstein himself would later agree with Arnold Sommerfeld who remarked that "relativity" was a misnomer [13, p. 25].

Langevin thus presents an empiricist interpretation of the emerging theory. And, in fact, the first philosophical lesson he draws from relativity is the failure of a priori arguments:

> There is neither space, nor time, *a priori*: at each moment, each degree of perfection in our theories of the world of physics corresponds to a conception of space and time. Mechanics implied the old conception, electromagnetism requires a new one which does not allow definitive statements. (Langevin 1911a, p. 110)

Langevin clearly condemns Kantianism although he does not fully embrace an empiricist interpretation of the relativity principle. Certainly, he admits that experiment is the source of all knowledge and the criterion of its validity, but he also emphasizes the intimate connection between physics theory and the familiar notion of an absolute time. Thus relativity can denounce the illusion that has made us believe, for centuries, that the universal and absolute time of Newtonian physics is "The" natural time. The major message that Langevin wants to convey to the assembly of philosophers at the 1911 International Congress of Philosophy in Bologna is the solid link between the classical notions of space and time and rational mechanics:

> I would like to show that the manner, usually insufficiently analysed, under which these notions were presented until now, was determined, conditioned, by a particular and temporary synthesis of the world, by the mechanistic theory. Our space and our time were those required by rational mechanics. (Ibid., p. 109)

The target of his attacks is, in fact, intuition. He undertakes a sort of genealogy of the classical concepts of space and time in order to prove that two implicit hypotheses underlie them: the absolute notion of simultaneity and, connected to it, the notion of instantaneous causality at a distance (ibid., pp. 116–119).

After the demonstration of the "mutual adaptation" of Newtonian physics and the classical notions of space and time, Langevin emphasizes, by contrast, the solidarity between the new relative conceptions of space and time and the theory of electromagnetism. He presents them as the necessary consequence of the Lorentz transformations that change the coordinates of space and time while keeping the velocity of light constant in all inertial frames of reference. In other terms, he derives the new concepts of space and time from electromagnetism, thus reviving his familiar aspiration for an electromagnetic synthesis of physics. And to establish the superiority of the electromagnetic synthesis over the rival theories of mechanics, Langevin strongly emphasizes that mechanics introduces an asymmetry between space and time: while we have accepted, for centuries, the evidence of relative distances in space, we persist in considering as invariant the time interval for all observers regardless of their relative movement. On the contrary, the principle of relativity restores a perfect symmetry between space and time. Thus the theme of the antagonism between mechanics and electromagnetism still dominates Langevin's interpretation of the principle of relativity. And the most obvious conclusion is that relativity ensures the triumph of electromagnetic synthesis. This may be the reason why Langevin still, in 1911, designates relativity as a "principle" and not as a "theory of relativity". In his view, Einstein supports Lorentz's vision, but he is not viewed as the founder of a new physics.

6.3 Relativity as Adaptation

A second major feature that emerges from Langevin's 1911 talks is the conflation between the principle of relativity and historical relativism. Relativity means above all that space and time have no absolute, eternal, universal character, but are subject to evolution. And this historical perspective is so present in Langevin's mind that he immediately embarks, after the introduction, on a long digression on epoch-making changes in science. At the risk of confusing an audience waiting for insights on relativistic physics, he develops biological comparisons. He likens scientific theories to living beings, endowed with an inner force of expansion that pushes them to conquer new territories. This metaphorical "vital force" of expansion opens two possible outcomes: either there is a mutual adaptation of the rival paradigms in presence, or there is conflict and survival of the fittest (ibid., pp. 109–110).

Thus Langevin resorts to a dubious Darwinist interpretation of the history of science to make sense of what is going on in the field of physics. He uses the notion of *adaptation* extensively. The term occurs on almost every page and features as the essential driving force in the evolution of science. Langevin describes a complex process of adaptation based on three steps—experiments, concepts and theories—that must be adapted to each other. Experiment is the driver: the discovery of new facts either provokes an adaptation of concepts that leads to a weakening of the theory, or to the emergence of new concepts which enrich the theory. The actors, in both cases, are the human mind and reality, that is to say anonymous entities and not creative individuals subject to the whims of genius or chance. Langevin does not speak of the theory of relativity as the invention of Einstein. He is not trying to reconstruct Einstein's creative pathway to the discovery, although he probably knows about Poincaré's psychological descriptions of scientific creativity in *Science and Hypothesis*. For him, science in general and physics in particular are a collective human adventure, which requires painful efforts of adaptation of the human mind to the outside world. This is an intimate conviction based on his own experience of changes in science that occurred throughout his career.

While Langevin will stay with this vitalist vision of science until the end of his life, in 1911, he placed emphasis on the notion of "conflict with survival of the fittest", that he later repudiated. It comes from his attention to the conflict between mechanics and electromagnetism that dominated physics in his formative years. It inspires an epic historical narrative. Mechanics has conquered a significant territory that goes from the infinitely small to the infinitely large. However, the empire of electromagnetism is hardly less powerful, since Maxwell has "assimilated optics without any effort" and "conquered the largest part of physics, invaded chemistry and grouped an immense number of facts that were hitherto formless and without link" (ibid., p. 112). As these territorial evaluations do not make it possible to decide between the opponents, Langevin resorts to direct political language: he grants to classical mechanics the *noblesse* attached to the *ancien régime* and to electromagnetism the dynamism of the rising classes. Langevin mixes the social and biological metaphors and does not care for the boundaries between description and prescription. All languages are good for his purpose: convincing physicists and philosophers to co-operate and forge new concepts, as well adapted to the current state of knowledge as those of our ancestors to their original environment.

6.4 Langevin's Traveller in a Rocket

Forging new concepts of space and time is the third message that Langevin addresses to philosophers as he invites them to cooperate for "the formation of an adequate language" (ibid., p. 110). The task is difficult because it requires thinking about time in the plural. Relativity shatters the uniqueness of time and confronts us with several representations. In Bologna, Langevin insists particularly on the break between the common notion of time and the physicist's time. He introduces the notion of "proper time"; that is the time of a portion of matter measured within a frame of reference. To clearly mark the separation between our familiar representations of space and time and those of relativity, he develops the famous example of the traveller in a rocket launched around the Earth and moving at a speed close to that of light. When after 2 years, the traveller returns to Earth, he finds our globe aged by 200 years. Langevin imagines the type of communication that could establish the traveller and a correspondent on Earth, highlighting the asymmetry of their measurements of duration during the forward trip to the star, which takes the traveller away from the Earth, and the return trip that brings him back. The interval between his departure and return in the proper time of the traveller who has undergone an acceleration will be 2 years while the same interval in the proper time of the one who stayed at home, on earth will be 200 years (ibid., pp. 125–130).

Langevin calls on fiction to rescue science, to convince the audience that the traveller's clock and the clock of the observer on Earth are two physical machines that did not run the same number of cycles because they belong to two distinct frames of reference. In its original context, this fiction, possibly inspired by the British novelist H.G. Wells (Fig. 6.1),[2] is presented as an educational example

---

[2] H.G. Wells published *The Time Machine* in 1895. Although a work of imaginative fiction, it starts with references to science thinking at the time: "Some philosophical people have been asking why three dimensions particularly … and have even tried to construct a Four-Dimensional geometry. Professor Simon Newcomb was expounding this to the New York Mathematical Society only a month or so ago". This book also includes a strong social theme with the two races of the Eloi and the Morlocks, the "haves" and "have-nots".

Fig. 6.1 The French translation of *The Time Machine* by H.G Wells in 1898 remained in print for many decades. Langevin's challenge was to persuade his audiences that the effects of relativity were not science fiction. (F. Duck)

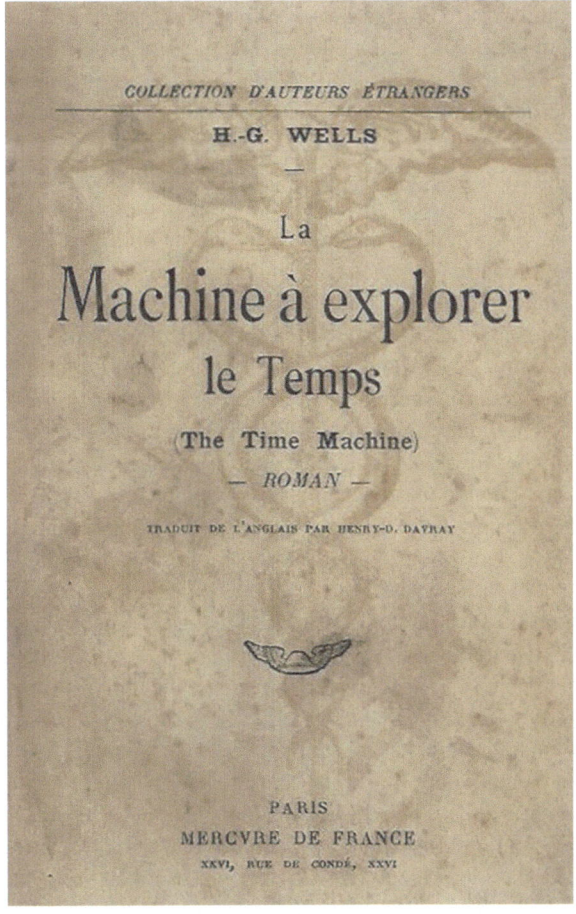

intended to highlight the gap that separates the everyday universe from the physicist's universe. But one could also say that it is science that becomes fiction and see this example as a thought experiment. Isn't it, indeed, an experiment imagined according to theory so as to highlight one of its fundamental consequences, the asymmetry between the proper times of two observers, belonging to two different frames of reference but who compare their respective aging in the same frame? The experiment is not materially feasible—Langevin takes care to highlight the difficulties that it would pose—but it is theoretically possible, that is in accordance with the principles and laws of the theory of relativity. Therefore "Langevin's traveller" has sparked countless comments from amateurs and specialists [17, pp. 528–532]. Elie During argues it has been appropriated by many commentators who portrayed the travellers as twins and reformulated the example as a paradox raised by the principle of relativity [7, 8]. Many physicists consider that the paradox disappears in the context of general relativity. Others continued to seek solutions in various directions. It is indisputable, in any case, that "Langevin's traveller" played a key part in the popularization of the theory of relativity, but at the cost of an ambiguity due to its dual status, of teaching device and thought experiment.

At the *Society française de philosophie*, Langevin insisted on the chasm between the time of philosophers, which he defines as a "succession of states of consciousness of the same individual or events that follow one another in the same portion of matter" (Langevin 1911b, p. 3), and the time of relativity physicists who compare the actual times in the various inertial frames in relative motion to each other. Each one, his own time: there is a time for the philosopher, a time for the psychologist, a time for the physicist ... a multiplicity of times. The discussion at the end of the session reveals that this is what most interested the audience of philosophers. For it seems that they did not care too much about giving up the a priori notions of space and time. They consented to it without pain while they were deeply upset by the prospect of assuming a multiplicity of times, of times intrinsic to physical or biological frames of reference. They strived to think about a plurality of times, presumably because it disrupted the clear divide between subjective and objective notions. Their comments suggest that they would like to bring all this multiplicity back to a single time. Léon Brunschvicg,[3] in particular, bombards Langevin with questions and suggests with humour that physicists, confronted by multiple clocks that are unable to agree with each other, could become the clockmaker (ibid., p. 43). In short, to save the unity of time, he suggests that physicists should take the place of the Great Clockmaker, of God. Langevin declines the generous offer and responds that there is no need to seek to recreate the unity of time. He is confident that the lost unity will reappear at a higher level, in the notion of Universe, of which time is only a relative and variable dimension. This perspective leaves Édouard Le Roy, a mathematician-philosopher[4] unsatisfied. He wittily noted: "if you ask a philosopher 'what is time?' he will begin a long discourse; ask the same question to a physicist, he'll pull out his watch and tell you 'that's it'". To close the discussion, he suggests endorsing the break between the philosophers' and the physicists' use in the language: Philosophers would continue to speak of "time", while physicists should only use the term "hour" (ibid., p. 46). Unsurprisingly this proposal confining physicists to an operational approach to time did not reach a consensus. Ironically, while Langevin invented the "traveller in a rocket" in an effort to engage philosophers and physicists in a collaborative attempt to forge new concepts of space and time, the main idea he conveyed in the audience was that of a divorce. Anyway, we can wonder what kind of collaboration Langevin had in mind, since he himself outlined the philosophical consequences of the principle of relativity.

---

[3] Léon Brunschvicg (1869–1944) was a French philosopher professor at the Sorbonne and active member of the French Society of Philosophy who enjoyed a high reputation. His "critical idealism"—a revised version of Kantianism adapted to the contemporary state of scientific knowledge—has been very influential. He emphasized the role of judgment in scientific activity.

[4] Edouard Le Roy, philosopher and mathematician, succeeded Bergson at the Collège de France and at the French Academy. He contributed by focussing the French community on the philosophy of science.

6.4 Langevin's Traveller in a Rocket

In conclusion, Langevin's personal signature in the history of relativity was to develop a conceptual interpretation of the principle of relativity that translated Einstein's operational approach to the issue of simultaneity into philosophical terms. To be sure Langevin was not the only French physicist with a philosophical mindset. Poincaré and Duhem went further in their philosophical reflections as they invented epistemological theses that deeply marked the philosophy of science. Far from being unique, Langevin's dialogue with philosophers is rather a paradigmatic example of the close ties that existed in early twentieth-century France between the philosophy and science communities. Not only did a number of professional scientists become philosophers but professional philosophers were also very engaged with basic sciences. This was the main feature brought forward to distinguish the French philosophy community from others in international conferences [2, p. 31; 12, p. 242].

In 1911, conditions for a dialogue between physicists and philosophers were optimal. Henri Bergson (Fig. 6.2), star philosopher and professor at the *Collège de France*, described in a very engaging way his conception of the relationship between science and philosophy. While he disapproved of the tendency among some philosophers to seize on ready-made science, attempting the unification of knowledge, he made this remark:

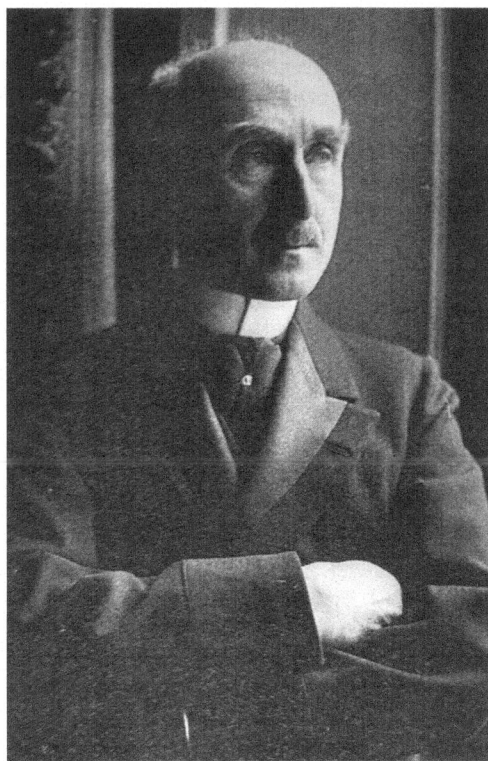

Fig. 6.2 Henri Bergson (1859–1941), professor at the Collège de France, enjoyed great fame at the beginning of the century and his work permeated French philosophy. Langevin made him aware of the theory of relativity in 1911 during the International Congress of Philosophy at Boulogne and in 1922 he discussed theory of relativity with Einstein at the *Société française de philosophie*

Is it not obvious that, if the scientist stops at a certain point on the path of generalization and synthesis, there stops what objective experiment and sure reasoning allow us to advance? And therefore by pretending to go further in the same direction, would we not systematically place ourselves in the arbitrary or at least in the hypothetical? [1, pp. 134–135]

As for the balance of exchanges, this seems extraordinarily fruitful. Langevin has indeed succeeded in inscribing the theory of relativity into the history of philosophy. Directly or indirectly, he is the instigator of a large philosophical activity and numerous debates. It is through Langevin that Bergson became aware of the theory of relativity:

> We take this opportunity to say that it was the communication of Mr. Langevin at the Congress of Bologna that first attracted our attention to Einstein's ideas. We, all those who are interested in the theory of relativity, know what we owe to Mr. Langevin, to his work and his teaching. [3, p. 81]

This encounter led Bergson to publish *Durée et simultanéité* in 1922, a work that fuelled a long controversy until Bergson decided to stop the reprints in 1932. It is also Langevin who led Meyerson to write *La Déduction relativiste*. Meyerson acknowledged his debt in the preface:

> There are many pages in this book for which we cannot claim exclusive ownership. First of all, the initial idea of such work came out of a conversation we had on the eve of Mr. Einstein's arrival in Paris with Mr. Paul Langevin and where we were able to see how much the conception to which the latter had spontaneously arrived on the subject of the realistic essence of relativistic theory agreed with the principles that we believed we could deduce by examining the physical sciences in general and especially their evolution. It is Mr. Langevin also who provided us with part of the documentation we used (…) and who constantly helped me overcome the technical difficulties that arose. [14, p. xv]

Finally, if we recall that Meyerson's *The Relativistic Deduction* triggered Gaston Bachelard to reply, in 1929, with *The Inductive Value of Relativity*, we can measure the importance of the Langevin effect on philosophical productivity. But is this really the result of a dialogue with philosophers, of mutual enrichment?

In striving to bring physics closer to philosophy, Langevin was continuing a French tradition. But, as we will see in Chap. 10, it turned out that the debates about the theory of relativity sounded the death knell for this national tradition.

References

1. Bergson H (1911) La Pensée et le mouvant. Alcan, Paris
2. Bergson H (1915) La philosophie, in La science française a l'exposition de San Francisco. Paris, Ministère de l'instruction publique
3. Bergson H (1922) Durée et simultanéité. Alcan, Paris. Quoted from new edition by Elie During, Paris, PUF, Quadrige, 2009
4. Darrigol O (2004) The mystery of the Einstein-Poincaré connection. Isis 95:614–626
5. Darrigol O (2005) The genesis of the theory of relativity. Séminaire Poincaré:1–22

References

6. Duck F, Thomas A (2022) Paul Langevin (1972–1946): the father of ultrasonics. Medical Physics International Journal 10(1):84–91. In translation: Joliot F (1951) Paul Langevin 1872–1946. Obituary Notices of Fellows of the Royal Society 7:405–419
7. During E (2014) Langevin ou le paradoxe introuvable. Revue de métaphysique et de morale 84:513–527
8. During E (2016) Le paradoxe des jumeaux. Paul Langevin Deux conferences sur la relativité. Presses universitaires de Paris Ouest, Paris
9. Einstein A (1947) Hommage à Paul Langevin. La Pensée 12:13–14
10. Galison P (2003) Einstein's cloks, Poincaré's maps. Empires of time. Cambridge, Harvard University Press
11. Gray J (2013) Henri Poincaré A Scientific Biography. Princeton University Press, pp 367–378
12. Lavelle L (1942) La Philosophie française entre les deux guerres. Aubier, Paris
13. Lévy-Leblond J-M (ed) (2021) "Presentation and annotation of Henri Bergson" *Durée et simultanéité*. Garnier Flammarion, Paris
14. Meyerson E (1925) La Déduction relativiste. Payot, Paris
15. Miller A (1981) Albert Einstein's special theory of relativity. Addison-Wesley, Reading
16. Paty M (1987) The scientific reception of relativity in France. In: Glick TF (ed) The comparative reception of relativity. Reidel, Dordrecht/London, pp 113–167
17. Paty M (1999) Paul Langevin (1872–1946) la relativité et les quanta. Bulletin de la Société française de physique 119:15–20
18. Paty M (2002) Poincaré, Langevin et Einstein. Epistémologiques 2(1):33–74
19. Secord JA (2004) Knowledge in transit. Isis 95:654–672
20. Shapin S (2008) The scientific life: a moral history of a late modern vocation. The University of Chicago Press, Chicago
21. Tonnelat M-A (1971) Histoire du principe de relativité. Flammarion, Paris

Chapter 7
War Service: Underwater Echoes

Abstract The four years of conflict from 1914 to 1918 altered Langevin's scientific focus in two ways. First, he had to set aside the international network of scientists. Second, he applied his talents to support the French war effort. Following encouragement from Jean Perrin and Marie Curie, he developed a proposal from the Russian émigré Constantin Chilowsky for underwater ultrasonic detection and communication. Supported by Victor Colin and Marcel Tournier, by the end of 1915 they had demonstrated that a beam of ultrasound at 100 kHz could be created using a singing condenser. Reception used an underwater microphone. Langevin also developed a new means of measuring ultrasonic power, the torsion balance. The project moved to the Naval Dockyard in Toulon, where Tournier detected the first ultrasonic echoes in June 1916. Chilowsky left, but not before filing a patent in their joint names.

Four years of war will be followed by 20 years fighting for peace. The experience of war was a crucial experience that converted Langevin to pacifism. It was a major turning point, a historical break, forever! The physicist's post-war life will change and never be the same again.

Scientists before 1914 could still think of themselves as participants in the great longstanding endeavour of mankind's adaptation to the outside world. Science embodied progress, civilization and humanization. Scientists ignored borders and linguistic barriers. Langevin himself had been living for 20 years in this transnational community, solidly anchored in international congresses and the international association of academies. Exchanges, research, travel, cooperation were unified. An angelic world, innocent and pure, without friction.

On the surface, at least, because scholars had more than once tasted the fruits of war and nationalist fervours. Nevertheless, Langevin's generation, who grew up in the aftermath of the 1870 Franco-Prussian war, could still believe in the universality of science and its peace-making mission [20]. For this generation, the Great War was the fall from paradise, the brutal collapse of a dream world: because it was hatred and not science that, for 4 years, mobilized everyone and confused everyone. The dream of the civilizing mission of science turned into a nightmare, a satanic parody of universalism.

© The Author(s), under exclusive license to Springer Nature
Switzerland AG 2025
B. Bensaude-Vincent, F. Duck, *Paul Langevin: Physicist and Social Activist*,
Springer Biographies, https://doi.org/10.1007/978-3-031-95260-9_7

7.1 Collapse of a Dream World

The shock was deeper because the scientific community was involved on both sides. Just a few days after the declaration of war, scholars and intellectuals engaged in rhetorical claims and participated in a martial concert. French scientists denounced Teutonic barbarism; they exalted patriotic science, and slandered yesterday's colleagues. Some of them considered they would contribute to national defence by fanning the flames of hatred. They took part in the war of propaganda. The first assault came on 4 October 1914 from the German manifesto, *An die Kulturwelt!* ("To the Civilized World"), translated into ten languages and trumpeted to the four corners of the world.

The text of the manifesto, signed by ninety-three "representatives of German science and German art", including Fritz Haber, Philipp Lenard, Walther Nernst, Wilhelm Ostwald and Max Planck, claimed that it is not true "that Germany was the cause of war"; that German troops "criminally violated the neutrality of Belgium", and "brutally ravaged Louvain"; "that they disregarded international law". It ended up as a defence of German culture:

> *It is not true* that the combat against our so-called militarism is not a combat against our civilization, as our enemies hypocritically pretend it is. Were it not for German militarism, German civilization would long since have been extirpated. For its protection it arose in a land which for centuries had been plagued by bands of robbers as no other land had been. The German Army and the German people are one and today this consciousness fraternizes 70,000,000 Germans, all ranks, positions, and parties being one.
>
> We cannot wrest the poisonous weapon—the lie—out of the hands of our enemies. All we can do is to proclaim to all the world that our enemies are giving false witness against us. You, who know us, who with us have protected the most holy possessions of man, we call to you:
>
> Have faith in us! Believe, that we shall carry on this war to the end as a civilized nation, to whom the legacy of a Goethe, a Beethoven, and a Kant is just as sacred as its own hearths and homes. (https://en.wikipedia.org/wiki/Manifesto_of_the_Ninety-Three)

This protest, according to Planck, was only meant to be a response to the attacks of the international press against the barbarity of the German troops, a gesture of solidarity with the army from intellectuals. But, beyond this intention, it was a symbol of the abdication of science to politics, an act of high treason [20]: a traumatic event that provoked, in France, Britain and elsewhere, a general mobilization of intellectuals to disparage German science. To the naïve claims of the German manifesto, French scholars such as Pierre Duhem [10] and Emile Picard [19] responded with lengthy, erudite arguments, aiming to prove, discipline by discipline, that French science was superior to German science, leading to nationalism and xenophobia. The international scientific community shattered with the first shells. Intellectuals, committed to the war, contributed to the escalation of violence.

And Langevin, in the storm? He who lived with Perrin and the Arcouest group in a friendly, borderless world, he who applauded Jaurès' speeches, what did you expect him to do? Like most intellectuals of France and Germany, he answered the call and devoted himself to his homeland. Certainly, neither Langevin nor his friends ever harboured the slightest thoughts of hatred, nor took part in the nationalist propaganda against the "Teutons". But they were attracted by action and eager to serve their homeland. Langevin commenced a renewed scientific career, just as fruitful and brilliant as the first. The war forced him to engage with applied science. He who had fought, and will go on fighting, for the survival of pure and disinterested research, threw himself with enthusiasm and success into the career of military engineer.

7.2 The Creation of Ultrasonics

At the outbreak of the war, Langevin was living apart from his family, at 11 rue de la Pitié, a small side street in the Latin Quarter of Paris (Fig. 7.1). He was only allowed to meet his children at the weekends. Unlike Perrin, who was serving in the army, Langevin joined the territorial reserve as a sergeant, where he was carrying out noncombat duties in Versailles, while simultaneously also managing courses at EPCI, as students and staff haemorrhaged to the front line.

On 1 January 1915, Marie Curie wrote to Langevin to tell him that she was anxious to set off from Paris with a replacement X-ray van to the front line in the north

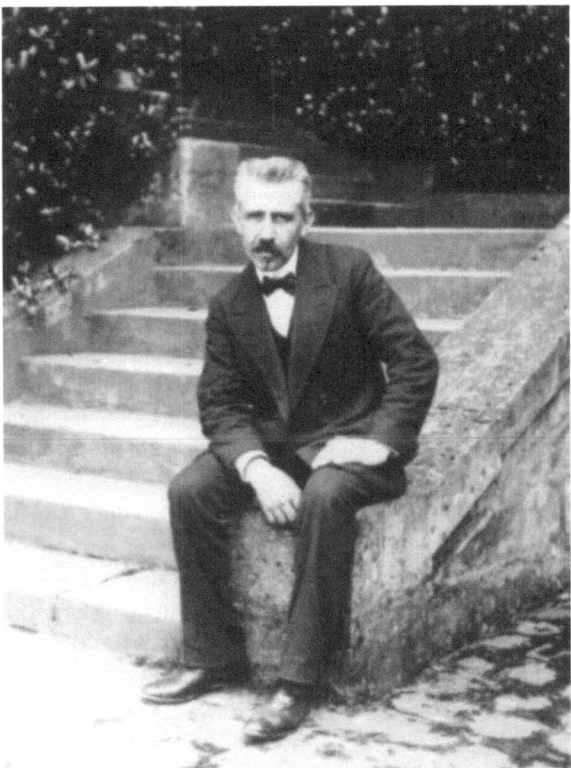

Fig. 7.1 Langevin in 1916 at the *École normale de Sèvres*. (ESPCI)

of France, but that her departure from Paris had been delayed [8, p. 298]. She and Perrin finally got away with two X-ray vans in mid-January. Postcards on 20 January to her daughters Irène and Ève and to Langevin gave news of a delay in Abbeville, about 180 km from Paris, because Perrin's car had hit a tree. The pair reached Dunkirk on 22 January, staying in a "semi-luxurious" hotel, travelling on to Poperinge the next day. During this breathing space, they jointly wrote to Langevin, specifically encouraging him to commit to a new acoustics project [17, pp. 68–69].

Perrin's approach was to appeal to Langevin directly, saying "we think that you should definitely quickly put your idea of the acoustic method into practice". This was the first indication of his future work in ultrasonics, a proposal that was under consideration before they left Paris. Perrin went on to tell his friend that "all other duties go to the second or to the twenty-fifth place! Go for it and neglect everything else". Perrin knew that not only was Langevin covering his duties at EPCI and in the Territorial Reserve, he was a man who often worked on several scientific projects at the same time. In 1913 alone, Langevin had published on the valency of gaseous ions, gas molecular collisions, the inertia of energy and relativity and the physics of electrons. Stop all that, his friend advised, and concentrate on this one project.

Finally, Perrin tried a combination of pressure and flattery:

> We are going through such hard times that a man like you must be keen to render the services that are only possible for him. You can do a great deal and must do so. … By using your intelligence as a PHYSICIST (and your energy can be used to make some first investigations), you can do more service than a thousand sergeants … Sorry to "advise" you, but it is precisely because I admire your intelligence, and all the more as I admire it more.

The accompanying single page letter from Marie Curie is a simple personal appeal. "Cher ami" she wrote to her one-time lover "I have read Perrin's very convincing letter and I think that it is indeed a very nice piece of work that you have before you. I for one would be very happy if this project came to fruition …"

This was not the only time when Marie Curie would be able to persuade Langevin to take on a new role during the war. Ève Curie tells in her biography of her mother how "all the X-ray material that could be used was collected together and then distributed to the hospitals in the region of Paris. Volunteer operators were recruited from amongst the professors, engineers and scientists" [8]. X-ray technology had changed little in the decade since Langevin used x-radiation to investigate gas ionization, so he had no difficulty in the practical art of medical radiology. Thirty years later, when Langevin died of late-diagnosed leukaemia [18], his son André was of the opinion that the radiation dose received at this time caused his terminal illness [17, p. 100].

What were the particular influences that drew Langevin away from his life as an educator and theoretical physicist and into the world of applied physics and subsequent industrial exploitation? The first and perhaps the strongest was that of his closest friends. By now, both Jean Perrin and Marie Curie were fully committed to applying their scientific knowledge to the war effort. Apart from their activities in medical X-rays, Perrin was already developing an acoustic method of locating an

7.2 The Creation of Ultrasonics

enemy gun, and soon he would go further, developing the "myriaphone" for sensitive directional communication.

A second motivation for Langevin was that any project must have a strong scientific challenge, to give the opportunity for the exploration of a new sphere of physics. A project of this calibre, one with a spectrum of potential challenges that quickly engaged his attention, had reached him from his friend, Paul Painlevé, who had by then vacated his academic posts and was fully engaged in wartime politics. Langevin's warmth towards him is clear from his eulogy, describing Painlevé as "a great scholar, ... a profound mathematical genius ... and a man of action of great clarity of mind and unfailing courage". He had a "love of justice ... and a warmth of heart which made him the most charming and the best of friends" (Langevin 1933c).

Jacques Hadamard, mathematician, professor at the *Collège de France* and member of a committee of the Academy of Science in the service of war, approached Langevin and Perrin as being the most appropriate scientists in Paris to voice an opinion about the worth of two proposals that he had recently received [5]. These proposals had arrived on his desk from the economist Edgard Milhaud, a French citizen teaching at Geneva University. Towards the end of 1914, Milhaud himself had been approached by a young Russian engineer Constantin Vasilyevich Chilowsky (1880–1958),[1] whose credentials had been checked by Charles-Eugène Guye, a professor of physics in Geneva [14].

Chilowsky's background was unusual. His father was a senior lawyer in Ryazan, 200 km south east from Moscow. Chilowsky had enrolled to study law at Moscow University in 1900, where he soon became politically active. In March 1903 he was expelled for not paying tuition fees. He was then arrested in June 1903 when he tried unsuccessfully to smuggle Marxist documents into Archangel in barrels of herring on behalf of the Russian Social Democratic Party. Sentenced to 3 years in exile, he was eventually allowed to leave Russia in 1906, with his wife Olga, for medical treatment abroad following a diagnosis of tubercular lungs. In October 1907, still supported by his father, he entered the Physics and Mathematics Department of the University of Strasburg (then in Germany), where he studied for the next five and a half years, taking time off for treatment for his tuberculosis in Switzerland [16]

The first of Chilowsky's two proposals was for submarine detection and communication using ultrasonics. It was titled *On the Possibility of Vision Under Water*. The second was for a method to increase the range of artillery shells, known as the "flame-tipped shell" [6]. The idea was to reduce the air resistance of a shell by causing high temperature gas to be emitted during the first stages of its trajectory, lowering the air density and hence the aerodynamic drag. He, Langevin, considered and recommended both Chilowsky's projects. The first, with its associated challenges of an unexplored part of physics to do with high-frequency acoustics, was of real

---

[1] Константин Васильевич ШКЛОВСКИЙ. Chilowsky, the common Anglicized version of his name, has been used here, The intial sound is soft, as in "chateau". His Russian patronymic, Shklovski, identifies the family as being from Shklov, now in Belarus. Historically, this town was predominantly Jewish.

interest to Langevin. As the war progressed, it will be the second project that would be given the higher priority of the two by Painlevé [11].

7.3 Forming an Expert Team

The 35-year-old Chilowsky, with an expired Russian visa, who has never before experienced permanent employment, was invited to Paris, settling in to 15 rue du Lunain with his wife Olga. He was placed in the physics laboratory at EPCI to work under Langevin's care, "full of charm and enthusiasm … bubbling with ideas and feeding management with countless projects" (Roussel, quoted in Fontanon [11]). Experimental programmes were launched in late March 1915. No time for Langevin to be indignant, or to protest against the war.

Langevin took the lead on the ultrasonics project. Within a couple of months, he had taken three key actions which, together, created the technical and scientific foundation on which the ultrasonics project would be based, and demonstrated his grasp of how to evolve this completely new science and technology, initiating a series of events that led him to be "the originator of the modern science and art of ultrasonics" ([4], p. 5).

Langevin's first action had to do with the generation of a beam of ultrasound. The principle that a torch-like beam of ultrasound is formed if the vibrating source is big enough had been pointed out by Chilowsky and also by the British physicist Lewis Fry Richardson in a 1912 patent. Chilowsky imagined a source up to 1.5 m across, operating over a frequency range from 10 to 100 kHz, using a magnetically driven diaphragm. Langevin predicted that eddy currents would limit the output, and also rejected Richardson's underwater whistle (Langevin 1924e). Instead, Langevin imagined something new, an electrical capacitor, operating in contact with seawater that "sings" when placed in an electrically resonant circuit. For much of the project, until replaced during 1917 by the quartz piezoelectric transducer for which Langevin is famous, this singing capacitor became the bedrock for the early development of ultrasonics. The first design was simple, with one fixed electrode and a second one that was free to vibrate, separated by a small air gap. In due course the design was changed to include a thin mica diaphragm that vibrated when a varying electric potential was applied. A vacuum held the plates in close contact. By operating at 100 kHz, a frequency five times above the limit of human hearing, the design made possible a directional source of ultrasound which was of sufficient intensity and also of manageable dimensions. Langevin understood that he could repurpose wireless technology to drive his "acoustic aerials". It is impossible to overstate the dependence of early ultrasonics on the concurrent developments in radio communications. Langevin estimated that high-frequency voltages of the order of 1 kV would be required and, in order to generate them, he turned to radio technology.

Langevin's second priority was to assemble an expert and competent team. He recruited the French radio pioneer Victor Colin (1868–1941) a naval officer who had been trained in wireless techniques at the *École supérieure d'électricité (Supelec)* in Paris. In 1909, working with Maurice Jeance, Colin had demonstrated a new design of arc transmitter, based on Poulson's design [7], sending a speech-modulated wireless signal from the Eiffel Tower to Villejuiffe in the southern suburbs of Paris [3]. Their design was eventually manufactured for the navy by the *Compagnie générale radiotélégraphique*. Langevin was able to negotiate to have one of the first Colin/Jeance arc systems, which was not being used by the Navy for the moment. He was also able to recruit Colin, now a naval captain in the reserve, to join his laboratory and to look after the arc transmitter.

Colin's was not a trivial apparatus. It required a 650 V dc supply from a petrol-driven dynamo. The arcs were surrounded by hydrogen (made from calcium hydride and water) mixed with acetylene (from calcium carbide and water), and required pumped water to cool the copper electrodes [12, pp. 39–43]. Given the complexity of this apparatus, Langevin's recruitment of Colin to operate and maintain it was essential.

Langevin's third and personal contribution in early 1915 arose from his deep understanding of physics, the direct application of pure science to a technological problem. He might have created a new high-frequency sound beam, but he must also be able to make measurements on it. All obvious measurement methods would be susceptible radio interference. So he adapted a known but little-used phenomenon, acoustic radiation force. His understanding of the associated physics derived from his knowledge of a similar phenomenon, the radiation pressure exerted by a beam of light, which was itself part of his work on the inertia of energy (Langevin 1913c, p. 16). He showed theoretically that the acoustic radiation pressure exerted by a plane wave on a reflecting target is proportional to the energy density and hence to the acoustic power. To measure the small forces he predicted, he adapted the torsion balance that was an established part of experimental electrostatics. He replaced the suspended charged plates of an electrometer with a counterbalanced reflecting disc, 25 mm diameter, placed vertically in the ultrasonic beam: the rotation, measured optically, measured the force and hence the acoustic power. "It is not without emotion", Langevin liked to tell his visitors, "that in this sink of my laboratory I saw, for the first time, deflection of the pendulum … which confirmed the accuracy of my calculations" (Fig. 7.2) [2]. The initial intensities reached a "few tenths of a watt per square centimetre". The first observation of ultrasonic emission was made on 12 July 1915.

They still needed an electronic detector of ultrasound. Failing to make the condenser work as a receiver, the decision was made to use a sealed carbon granular microphone. Electronic amplification would be added as the project progressed, using new military radio amplifiers.

By the end of the summer of 1915, Langevin realized that, while Chilowsky might be an imaginative inventor and "starter" of projects, he was not a good "finisher". Langevin could not afford to place the project at risk. He recruited Marcel Tournier (1888–1964), an ex-student whom he had appointed before the war (1 October 1911) as "Chef de Travaux" in the physics laboratory at EPCI.

As Joliot-Curie later recalled, Tournier brought "youthful enthusiasm, intelligence and experimental ability" [15], and he would play a central role in the ultrasonics project until well after the war is over. With Tournier now taking the lead in the practical implementation of the ultrasonics project, the first successful underwater transmission outside the laboratory was achieved across the River Seine just below the *Pont national,* by the end of the year. All the equipment for Colin's arc

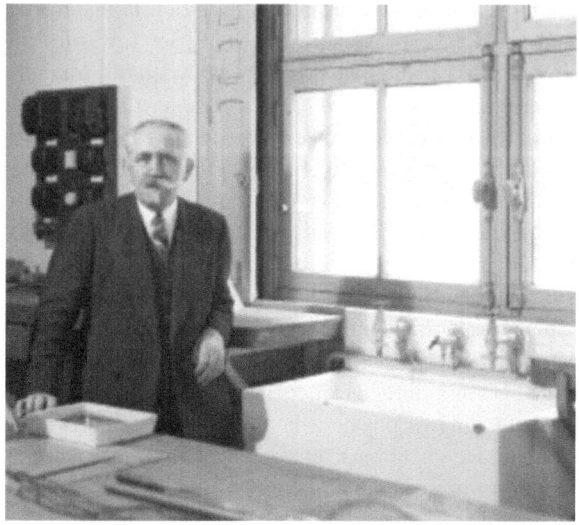

Fig. 7.2 The laboratory sink in EPCI where the first underwater experiments on ultrasonics were carried out. (Paul-Éric Langevin)

transmitter, together with the vacuum pump, were set up in the pinnace *Caducée*, moored on the left bank. The transmitter was placed under water, and the ultrasonic beam was detected by a submerged microphone on the opposite bank. The width of the beam was measured using a microphone mounted on a boat that was borrowed from the *Yacht-Club de France*, sailed back and forth to demonstrate its boundaries. Langevin later observed that it was "this electrostatic solution which permitted the first emissions to be obtained and gave proof of the possibility of emitting ultrasonic waves" (Langevin 1924e, p. 75).

During the first months of the war, both Langevin and Perrin had been rather indignant about the slowness and blunders of an administration incapable of efficiently exploiting the resources of French scientists. The specific arrangements for the ultrasonics project and for its funding remained loose, informal and flexible. Finally, in October 1915, the government fell, and Paul Painlevé became Minister of Public Education and Inventions in the new administration. He organized scientific mobilization and asked for Langevin's advice on scientific organization. On 27 November, Langevin visited London to study scientific mobilization in Britain and to find out about the operation of the British Board of Inventions and Research (BIR), set up in Britain during the previous summer. Langevin's report was sufficiently encouraging for Painlevé to write to the British Naval Attaché in Paris on 31 December suggesting a formal exchange of scientific information [13, p. 39]. The British were unenthusiastic, viewing such liaison as a security risk, and the scheme would only be formally approved on 6 October the following year, when Maurice de Broglie was appointed as the French liaison officer with the BIR.[2]

---

[2] Maurice, duc de Broglie (1875–1916) was an accomplished physicist who had studied under Langevin at the *Collège de France*, and was the elder brother of the physicist Louis de Broglie. He spent 9 years in the French Navy before pursuing a career as an independent researcher, pioneering x-ray diffraction and spectroscopy.

Initially, Painlevé's focus was firmly on supporting the army, overseeing a budget that, for 1916, reached 250,000 Francs. Langevin was placed at the Centre of Artillery Studies, assigned to the Artillery Commission to study ballistics (Langevin 1923a). He also continued to act as consultant on Chilowsky's flame-tipped shell project. With this focus on ballistics, the continuing viability of the ultrasonics project might have been at risk. However, it was protected by the appointments of his friends Jean Perrin and Émile Borel as joint directors of Painlevé's technical committee.

Langevin was now instructed to take his equipment and his team to the Naval Dockyard at Toulon, in order to test its capability over longer ranges, and at sea. The "Langevin-Chilowsky Mission" left Paris on 12 March 1916 (Archives L194/067). Langevin was accompanied by Chilowsky and Tournier, and also by Louis Bournazaud, Langevin's laboratory assistant at the *Collège de France*, and by Giovanni Malfitano, an Italian microbiologist and long-time friend, whose role in this visit is obscure. Colin and his two quartermasters completed the team. The Commandant at Toulon was under instructions to provide assistance, including a laboratory, electrical power and gas lighting and the support of the radio section.

A new Langevin emerges in these circumstances: a team leader, the boss. This is no longer the brilliant theoretician of physics, nor the consummate teacher, who inspires his pupils with his logical presentations. This is not even "the master" of future students who, like Frederic Joliot-Curie, Pierre Biquard and Léon Brillouin, later move on to individual outstanding careers in science. Here is an entrepreneur selecting men of disparate talents, allowing them freedom to test new ideas, giving advice when challenges emerge, creating conditions for mutual support, and whose vision gives confidence in a successful outcome.

The new laboratory was set up in a former floating prison. Transmitting and receiving equipment was installed on two separate *bugalets* (small two-masted ships), which could be moved to test the maximum range for communication. Langevin took a large parabolic mirror—120 cm diameter, focus 70 cm—borrowed from the *Collège de France*, mounting the microphone at its focus. Colin and Tournier increased the acoustic power to 150 W. The initial tests were very encouraging, demonstrating transmission up to 5 km.

7.4 The Chilowsky/Langevin Patent

Chilowsky's relationship with Langevin was always going to be uneasy, bringing a self-view of natural superiority from his background in the Russian nobility. Chilowsky saw himself as a professional inventor, someone who had the ideas, protected them by patents and then licensed the intellectual property to others. He was already armed with three patents, two Russian and one German, when he arrived in Paris in early 1915. He had no interest in being locked into the time-consuming and sometimes tedious business of putting ideas into practice. The move to Toulon in March 1916 did not suit his plans. It took him away from the centre of influence, away from his freedom to exploit his new contacts with senior politicians and scientists. Looking ahead, he pressed Langevin into making an agreement, which they signed on 6 April 1916, that they were joint leaders of the ultrasonics project, that patents would be taken out in their joint names, and that any profits would be shared equally between them [16, p. 54].

On 29 May 1916, a joint patent was filed both in France (using the law firm Armengaud) and in the UK (Langevin 1916b). A year later, on 19 May 1917, the same patent, with minor modifications and a reduced number of claims, was successfully filed in the USA.

In the UK version, Chilowsky describes himself as a chemist. More surprisingly, Langevin is described as a "manufacturer". This clarifies Chilowsky's self-appointed role, a self-view that coloured all his negotiations with Langevin, apparently assigning to his senior colleague the practical engineering jobs of design, testing, construction and marketing, even though it had been Langevin who had initiated the idea of a capacitive transducer, and who had carefully guided the scientific and engineering development during the previous year (Fig. 7.3).

Much of the wording in the patent draws on Chilowsky's original note "on the possibility of vision under water", reinforcing the view that it was he, not Langevin, who was its primary author. Appropriate frequencies, matching layers, the use of continuous and pulsed operation and of Doppler shift are all included, together with the limitation on range resulting from frequency-dependent absorption in seawater. Alternative designs for both magnetic and capacitive ultrasonic transducers are described. The four possible applications for underwater ultrasonics are drawn directly from his original proposal. The first is for "the exchange of directed submarine signals between ships" or from ship to shore. This implies that the use for submarine detection may not have been his primary motivation at this stage. The second use is "for setting up ultra-audible stations with transmitting surfaces of a very large diameter". Application 3 covers "searching for submarine obstacles". Finally the possibility of location from detecting an acoustic shadow is mentioned.

By the time the patent had been filed, Chilowsky had abandoned the work in Toulon and returned to Paris, having achieved all he wanted. Some narratives state that Langevin told him to leave. But, however it came about, the departure suited

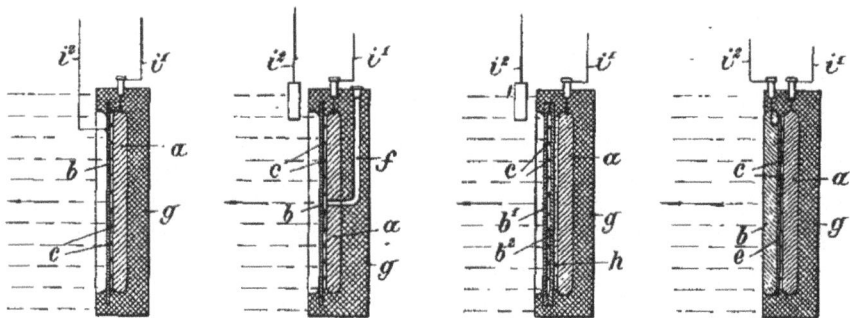

Fig. 7.3 Alternative designs for the singing condenser ultrasonic transducer. (Langevin 1916b) (ESPCI Archives L134/007-03)

both men. Chilowsky now devoted all his efforts on his flame-tipped shell. By this time, Chilowsky was being referred to in Paris as "management's favourite inventor". During 1916, nearly half of the budget was assigned to Chilowsky's ballistics project, which had become the "flagship project of the Directorate of Inventions". He was given laboratory space in the chemistry departments of the EPCI and at the Sorbonne and was assigned two new members of staff to investigate the chemistry of the explosive mixtures to be fired in the nose of the shell.[3] As Langevin had discovered, the Artillery Commission, not the Navy in Toulon, was where the action was, and Chilowsky was motivated to be part of it.

The flame-tipped shell project turned out badly. Chilowsky's team failed to keep proper records. Artillery engineers could not match the performance he claimed and increasingly doubted his scientific integrity. Langevin understood the need for an independent means to measure the aerodynamic forces. He designed and had built a high velocity wind source that used the rapid expansion of heated compressed air, and used it to test the forces on different shell shapes [11].

7.5 The First Echoes

Following Chilowsky's departure, the ultrasonics project was renamed the *Mission Langevin-Colin*. Langevin ensured that arrangements were in place for Tournier to continue the work in Toulon, and returned to his many other responsibilities in Paris, keeping in touch with the 28-year-old Tournier by letters and occasional visits.

On 12 May 1916, Tournier reported his first major break-through: he has detected ultrasonic echoes for the first time. The echoes are from a steel plate, and Tournier "can determine the direction of the obstacle with great precision": a seminal moment in ultrasonic detection, that Langevin, predicting success, leaves to his young colleague. Tournier writes, "Be assured, sir, of my commitment, and let me tell you how happy I am to do such active work, which is as good as it gets" (Archives L194/048).

Tournier's letters to Langevin and to his mother reveal the engineering challenges that he is facing [9]. Are we using the best frequency? Tests will be carried out at 15, 74 and 174 kHz. Can we obtain an echo from the curved surface of a mine? Tournier achieved this in September after adding a three-stage audio amplifier. How can the bulky parabolic mirror be mounted to prevent it coming adrift in bad weather? Is the vacuum necessary behind the mica sheet? Transducers kept failing and electrical interference plagued the experiments. Cross-talk between the transmission pulse and the microphone kept reappearing "like Lady Macbeth's bloodstain" (Archives L194/045).

In spite of the technical difficulties, by December 1916, with the equipment installed on the *Vigoureux* for sea trials, they had achieved a transmission range of

---

[3]A video of this device can be found online: Obus à flamme d'ogive Chilowski. CNRS Images. https://images.cnrs.fr/video/4277

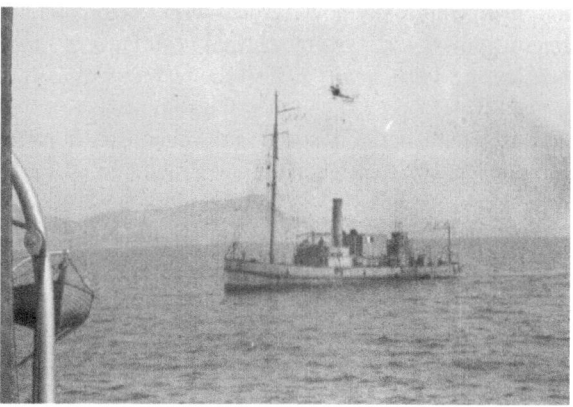

Fig. 7.4 The Vigoureux, on which the first sea trials with ultrasonics were carried out. (ESPCI Archives L166/002)

6000 m. Through each experiment, new knowledge was generated, new challenges appeared (Fig. 7.4).

On 12 February 1917, Maurice de Broglie, now liaison officer to the British Board of Inventions and Research, presented a note on behalf of Langevin at the BIR office in Cockspur Street, London. It was titled *Note on Apparatus for the Detection of Submerged Objects by Waves of High Frequency* (Langevin 1917). He reported:

> (These outcomes) represent the result of two years' continuous work, during which other methods have been tried over and over again without success. Though it is probable that they may be eventually improved, it appears certain that time will be saved by not departing (for the present) from the constructional details hereafter described.

Langevin's capacitive transmitter used a mica sheet 140 mm diameter and 0.1 mm thick, held on to the surface of a metal electrode by a vacuum-filled space and was maintained using a Gaede rotary mercury vacuum pump. Sea-water formed the second electrode. Each new transmitter was tested to ensure uniformity of oscillation across the whole surface but, even so, each had "but an extremely short life".

The mica capacitive ultrasonic transducer continued to be used for about another year as a source of ultrasound in the Toulon anti-submarine programme. But it was about to be superseded. Once Langevin discovered the piezoelectric alternative, he was doubtful that capacitive transducers could ever compete in terms of sensitivity [1]. Even so, modern capacitive micromachined ultrasonic transducers (CMUTs), using silicon rather than mica, share an identical basic structure with Langevin's original design.

References

1. Biquard P (1933) Les ondes ultra-sonores III. Revue Acoustique 2:288–299
2. Biquard P (1972) Generation and detection of ultrasound up to the highest frequencies. The first steps in ultrasound research. Journal de Physique Colloques C6:C6-1–C6-3

References

3. Boyer J (1914) The Colin-Jeance system of wireless telephony. Scientific American 111:352–353
4. Cady WG (1946) Piezoelectricity. McGraw-Hill, New York.
5. Chabert J-L, Gilain C (2024) "Sans amour et sans haine": la Grande Guerre de Jacques Hadamard. Cahiers Franois Viète 3(16). https://journals.openedition.org/cahierscfv/4645
6. Chilowsky C (1918) Improvements in or relating to projectiles. UK Patent 132068. Application 19 Sept 1918. Accepted 11 Sept 1919
7. Colin V (1909) La téléphonie sans fil. Bulletin of the International Society of Electricians Ser 2(9):428–452
8. Curie E (1938) Madame Curie (trans: Sheeham V). Doubleday, New York
9. Dorsay K (2022) Il donnait deux fois parce qu'il donnait vite. David di Napoli 1940–1890 Marcel Tournier 1888–1964. Jean-Jacques Wuillaume
10. Duhem P (1915) La science allemande. Hermann, Paris
11. Fontanon C (2005) L'obus Chilowski et la soufflerie balistique de Paul Langevin: une recherche militaire oubliée de la mobilisation scientifique (1915–1919). In: Pestre D (ed) Deux siècles d'histoire de l'armement en France. CNRS OpenEdition, Paris, pp 81–109
12. Goldsmith AN (1918) Radio telephony. Wireless Press, New York
13. Hackmann W (1984) Seek and strike. Sonar, antisubmarine warfare and the Royal Navy 1914–54. Her Majesty's Stationary Office, London
14. Hunt FV (1982) Electroacoustics the analysis of transduction, and its historical background. American Institute of Physics: Acoustical Society of America, New York
15. Joliot-Curie F (1944) Le professeur Langevin et l'effort scientifique de guerre. La Pensée New series 1:32–37
16. Klyukin II, Shishkov EN (1984) Konstantin Vasilievich Shilovski 1880–1958. Nauka, Leningrad
17. Langevin A (2022) Paul Langevin my father. EDP Sciences, Paris. English edition: Duck F
18. Montel E (1973) Langevin et le rationalisme: le savant hors de la tour d'ivoire. Scientia 2:1–30
19. Picard E (1916) L'histoire des sciences et les pretentions de la science allemande. Hachette Bnf, Reprint Paris (2016)
20. Schroeder-Gudehus B (1978) *Les Scientifiques et la paix*. Presses de l'Université de Montréal. https://books.openedition.org

Chapter 8
The Genesis of Piezoelectric Technology

Abstract In February 1917, Langevin started to investigate the piezoelectricity of x-cut quartz as a receiver of ultrasound, initially using a crystal recovered from the Curies' apparatus. A proposal by Ernest Rutherford to use the *quartz piézoélectrique*, cut along a different plane, led to later claims of priority. By the summer of 1917, the production of a beam of ultrasound using quartz was demonstrated, exploiting piezoelectric resonance. Robert Boyle visited from England, returning there under Langevin's guidance to set up the development of asdic using simple quartz transducers. Langevin designed his resonant quartz sandwich transducer, resulting in successful sea trials in the summer of 1918. He shared his knowledge at the Interallied Conference on Supersonics in Paris in October 1918.

8.1 A Legacy of Pierre Curie

At some time before the end of February 1917, Langevin and Tournier carried out a simple experiment in their Paris laboratory that would eventually lead to the technology of ultrasonics as we now know it.

Eighteen months later, Langevin described how this came about (Langevin 1918c).

> In order to avoid these difficulties I thought (February 1917) of utilizing the piezoelectric properties of quartz, first of all for receiving. Instead of the disposition of it by Pierre Curie in his apparatus for electrostatic measurements using the same property, I thought preferable to make use of the compression of the quartz in the same direction as its electric axis, instead of by traction in a direction perpendicular to the electrical and optical axes.

Langevin's words are precise, clear and deliberate. He recognizes that there are difficulties with the current receiver design. He distinguishes two ways in which the piezoelectricity of quartz could be used for the purpose of receiving ultrasonic waves. He knew from the work of Jacques and Pierre Curie, over 30 years before, about the three electrical axes in a crystal of quartz, spaced by 120° rotation in a single plane. He knew that any steady compression of the crystal generates opposing (polar) charges on the crystal surfaces cut across the ends of these axes. And he knew that Jacques Curie determined a specific crystal orientation for the *quartz piézoélectrique* that Pierre and Marie Curie used to measure the ionization caused by the radiation emitted by radium: the electrical axis was arranged to be perpendicular to the direction of stress, so the charge could be "weighed" [8].

It will be 1944 before anything further is known in public about the experiment that was the genesis of ultrasonics. Details will be included in *Le professeur Langevin et l'effort scientifique de guerre* by Fréderic Joliot-Curie in *La Pensée* [6]:

> Marcel Tournier ... had custody of the precious items from Pierre Curie's experimental work, including a quartz slice used by the great scientist. Paul Langevin asked him to remove this slice to make a microphone. The electrical equipment was assembled quickly in the laboratory. Great was the joy of the experimentalists when, placing a watch on the quartz slice, they heard the ticking of the clock, faithfully reproduced and amplified in the telephone earphones. The next day Tournier brought in an eighteenth century repeater watch, whose delightful, silvery chime was faithfully reproduced by the quartz slice and the amplifier.

The Curies' equipment that Tournier dismantled included two quartz triplets, mounted within a clamp, with which Jacques and Pierre Curie had demonstrated reverse piezoelectricity. One triplet had been connected to a Holtz electrical machine: when a high voltage was applied, the triplet expanded. The other triplet had been attached to an electrometer to measure the generated charge [3]. Unlike the orientation of the *quartz piézoélectrique*, these quartz plates were all cut so that the electric axis was aligned with the axis of compression: this is known as x-cut quartz.

What was the stimulus that caused Langevin to carry out this simple experiment, exactly in February 1917?

The clues to Langevin's thinking are obscure and have led to several interpretations. Perhaps the process of writing the report for the British Board of Inventions and Research (BIR) reminded him of the practical difficulties that would remain by "not departing from the constructional details hereafter described". From a transcribed account of a talk that Langevin gave later (Langevin 1924e), he "thought of returning to a possibility which he had considered in the beginning, but which he had discarded rather hastily", giving as a reason that Rutherford "had likewise dropped it for he believed that it could not solve the problem".[1] But the words "in the beginning" are too vague. Langevin had considered several approaches in 1915 before deciding on the singing capacitor: perhaps quartz was one of them. Perhaps it was in May 1916, part of the reason why Chilowsky left [11]. Joliot-Curie incorrectly places the event with the watch and the Curies' x-cut quartz "towards the autumn of 1916, during a trip to Paris". Langevin's student and biographer Pierre Biquard writes "At the end of the summer of 1916, Langevin had the inspiration of genius which was to overturn the whole problem". In both cases, these accounts may perhaps be seen as understandably partisan attempts to counteract a developing British narrative in favour of a claim of prior discovery by Rutherford.

A plausible explanation of Langevin's renewed interest in quartz is associated with Maurice de Broglie, returning with news from London, where he had just

---

[1] The text mistakenly ascribes this remark to "Sir E Richardson".

presented Langevin's report to the BIR. In order to appreciate the background, it is necessary to return to a meeting between de Broglie and William Bragg[2] in Scotland in May 1916.

8.2　A *Quartz Piézoélectrique* Is Sent to London

De Broglie was the Anglo-French intermediary. In May 1916, he had visited the British Admiralty Experimental Station, then at Hawkcraig, Scotland, meeting William Bragg, who was then the Director of Research there. De Broglie and Bragg had much in common. They were among the elite of European physics, both delegates at the second Solvay Conference in 1913 at which Bragg had presented his breakthrough results on X-ray crystallography, a topic of research interest to de Broglie. In addition, Bragg now had a personal attachment to France: his son William Lawrence has been assigned to work with the French on Nordmann's sound ranging equipment to determine the distance of enemy artillery. Both Bragg and de Broglie were experiencing similar organizational problems at the difficult interface between civilian and military science. This visit initiated a series of events that led to Chilowsky's visit to London in July and the appointment of Boyle to lead British work in ultrasonics.

One of the alternative approaches to either the generation or the reception of ultrasound was to consider piezoelectricity. On 28 September, Ernest Rutherford submitted a brief note to the BIR in which he suggested re-purposing the *quartz piézo-électrique* [12]. Rutherford was well aware of this device from his own work with radioactivity. Having remarked that the Curies used it under static conditions, he stated that, because the changed length "is a molecular effect, there appears to be little doubt that the relation given will hold for alternating potentials of high frequency". In other words, it has the capability of piezoelectric vibration. This is a conclusion that Langevin, also, must reach, although he exploited it in a different way.

At the end of October, de Broglie received a letter from Rutherford, asking "Would it be possible to buy or to borrow such a quartz plate and bring it over to London for me …?". De Broglie immediately sent one crystal and ordered a second, delivered later. Rutherford was not seeking a new receiver of ultrasound: he wanted a new ultrasonic vibrator. In his BIR note, Rutherford suggested two possible new uses of the *quartz piézo-électrique*. The first was to calibrate microphones, to replace, or be used together with, a vibrating metal plate. Boyle found that it worked at audible frequencies but could find no response at ultrasonic frequencies.

---

[2] Sir William Henry Bragg (1862–1942) was a British physicist who shared the 1915 Nobel Prize for Physics with his son Lawrence "for their services in the analysis of crystal structure by means of x-rays". A graduate of Cambridge, he was a life-long friend of Ernest Rutherford, whom he first met in the University of Adelaide in 1895. He held the Cavendish Chair of Physics at Leeds from 1909 to 1915, returning to academic life at University College London after the war was over.

Rutherford retained the second crystal for use in his Manchester laboratory. His second idea was added in a brief paragraph headed "Supersonic Vibrations". Here he states "It seems probable that the Piezo-electrique can be used as a simple generator of super-sonic vibration". One end would be clamped, and a "small stiff plate" attached to the free, vibrating end of the quartz rod. Several such devices might be used in parallel to increase the output. There is no record that this device was ever constructed.

It is plausible, indeed probable, that when de Broglie presented Langevin's report in London in February 1917 he also met Rutherford, and was updated on the use of the quartz that he had supplied for his investigations. He then would have reported back to Langevin on his return to Paris. The timing suggests that it was only then that Langevin realized how to use quartz correctly as a sensitive receiver of ultrasonic waves. He learned that Rutherford was trying to use quartz as a source of vibration. But he realized that he was using quartz in the wrong way. He understood that, while Jacques and Pierre Curie had designed the *quartz piézoélectrique* to maximize strain by applying stress over a small area, he needed to maximize charge generated by a force exerted over a large area. This required x-cut quartz.

In due course, Rutherford's note gained historical traction and will become an important document. It will be cited as evidence that Rutherford thought of using piezoelectricity first. It will be translated into French and used to support the British position in later questions of patent rights. Of course, it was never a question of who thought of it first. Science rarely works in this simple fashion. Ultrasonics was in its infancy, and piezoelectricity was being considered as one of at least six different processes for electromechanical transduction at the time. A legitimate question, which Rutherford addressed, is whether the mechanism causing known piezoelectric behaviour under static conditions would be retained under dynamic conditions. Rutherford's understanding that this would be so, based on Lord Kelvin's interpretation, was correct. The separate question, how to use piezoelectricity to create and detect ultrasonic waves, was one that Rutherford never claimed to answer correctly [7].

Unlike Rutherford, who was seeking to replace Boyle's unsuccessful electromagnetic source of ultrasound, Langevin wanted to replace the unsatisfactory carbon receiver of ultrasound. In writing his BIR report, Langevin noted two requirements: that any new receiver must extend over an area large enough to be directional and the receiver must be polar, responding to both positive and negative oscillations. X-cut quartz promised to solve both requirements.

8.3 From Discovery to Prototype

But Langevin did not know whether the Curies' quartz slice would work not only as microphone at audible frequencies but also as an underwater receiver at a much higher frequency, 100 kHz. Since piezoelectric phenomena were understood to have a molecular origin, the properties might be expected to be retained under oscillatory

8.3 From Discovery to Prototype

conditions. However, Boyle had been unable to observe a response at ultrasonic frequencies. Did this suggest some unknown loss mechanism in the crystal lattice, damping any higher-frequency vibration?

There was no such loss at high frequencies. Shortly after the experiment with the ticking watch, in 2 days according to Joliot-Curie, "the quartz slice microphone was installed in Toulon", and signals were detected from the condenser transmitter at a range of 4 km.

The quartz plate that Tournier removed from the Curies' apparatus was only about 2.5 cm square, much too small to act as a directional receiver at 100 kHz. The first practical challenge was to find a quartz crystal of sufficient purity and volume from which to cut large slices perpendicular to an electrical axis. Langevin obtained this from an established Paris supplier of optical instruments, Ivan Werlein. Originally from Russia, Werlein had settled in Paris by the time the Curie brothers had obtained their quartz slices from him in 1880. Langevin ordered a slice 16 mm thick, 10 cm × 10 cm, to be cut from a large quartz crystal showpiece in Werlein's premises. This slice had a sufficient area to ensure directionality as a receiver at 100 kHz.

At this critical time, Langevin visited London to give the prestigious third Guthrie Lecture at the Physical Society, in the evening of 23 March 1917 (Fig. 8.1). Back in Toulon, Tournier was frustrated about Langevin's absence because he needed help to carry the critical experiment. But Langevin was more focused on his presentation in London, knowing Tournier would be able to cope. He wrote to his son Jean "I was a bit worried about having to speak English in public for the first time, but I heard that I was very well understood" [9, p. 71]. Langevin returned to Toulon briefly at the beginning of April, seemingly more concerned about Tournier's forthcoming marriage than his feelings about the ultrasonic project. He left de Broglie, with his knowledge of crystals, to help work on the quartz receiver, much to Tournier's relief. Meanwhile, Langevin himself spent a few days in the Mediterranean resort of Menton "pour finir un travail de physique" and, no doubt, to relax a little [4, p. 101].

One of those who had attended Langevin's Guthrie lecture was William Bragg. He had a heightened interest in Langevin's work, particularly because Boyle and his colleagues had made no progress in duplicating any of Langevin's results. Bragg's Admiralty Experimental Station was by then installed at Parkeston Quay in Harwich, less than 100 miles north east of London. Bragg invited Langevin to visit this facility, perhaps with a view to hearing how Toulon was organized. They agreed that Boyle should spend time with Langevin, a critical step towards Anglo-French liaison in ultrasonics. Boyle went to France on 20 May, initially for a month, but staying for two, accompanied by a naval officer, Lt. R Saville. Boyle's final report gives a great deal of detail about French progress during these summer months [1].

The comparison between the outcome of Langevin's successful leadership and the inadequate progress in Britain is instructive. It had taken only 3 months in 1915 for Langevin to create and measure a beam of ultrasound, based only on an idea from Chilowsky. Simple small steps had led eventually to the piezoelectric breakthrough. British scientists failed to capitalize on the same advice from Chilowsky.

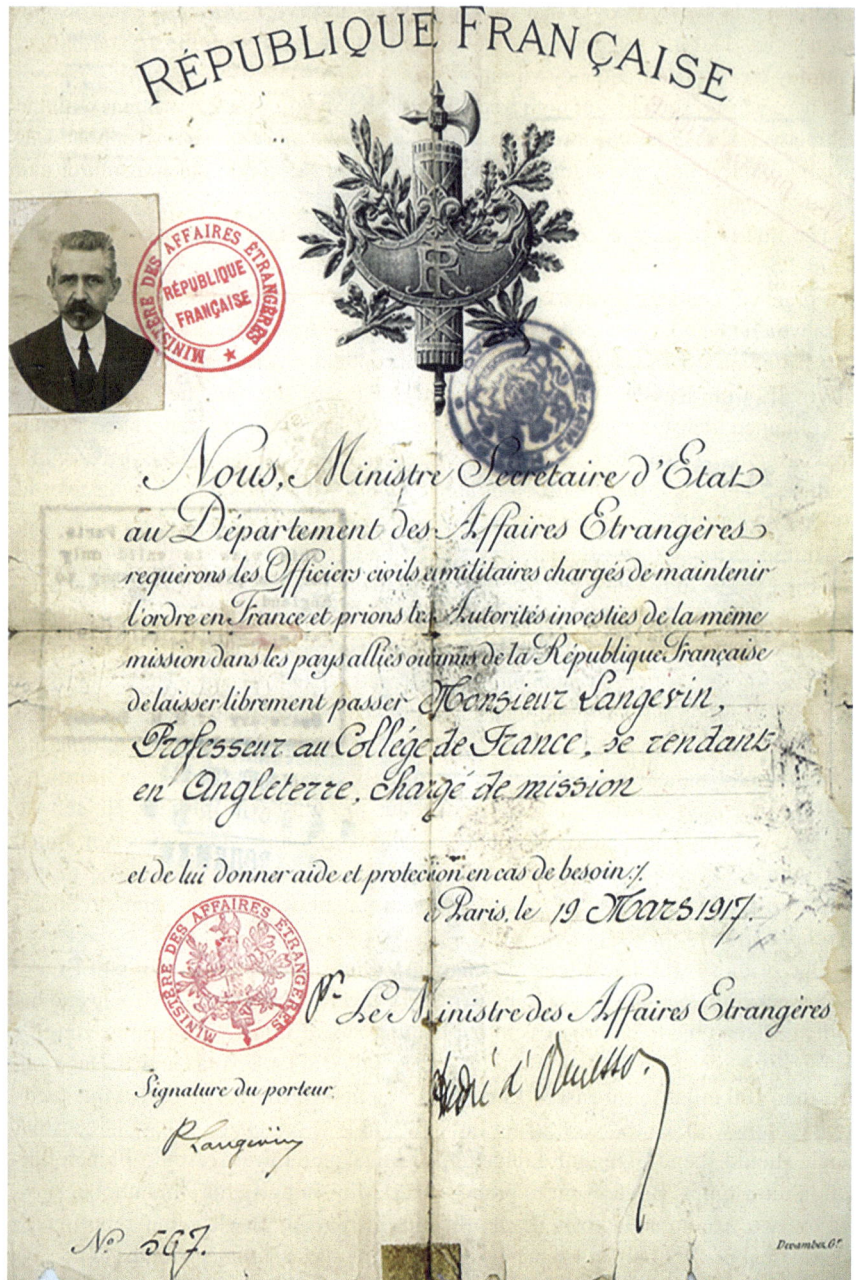

Fig. 8.1 Langevin's pass, in March 1917, for a visit to London to give the Hughes Lecture at the Institute of Physics. During this visit, he discussed further collaboration on the ultrasonic detection of submarines. (ESPCI)

Eventually it took Bragg's personal relationship with Langevin to gain the same leadership in Britain. Later, William Eccles, witness for the British Admiralty against Langevin, is forced under cross-examination to compare the unsuccessful British approach of empirical experimentation with that of Langevin: "Professor Langevin did it the other way, a more creditable way, he envisioned it, looked for it, calculated for it and built his apparatus to perform it" [14].

8.4 The Marvel of Quartz Resonance

The new piezoelectric receiver consists of "a piece of stone, two plates of tinfoil" (Langevin 1924e): a description of such elegant simplicity that Langevin seems to be saying "if you had thought about it a bit more, you too could have come up with the same idea". Of course, it was not just any piece of any stone. More precisely, the new receiver is:

> composed of a thin sheet (of) quartz [or several plates in juxtaposition], placed perpendicularly to an electrical axis, and in contact with the water on one side (either directly, or by the medium of a thin protective sheet attached, mica for example); and on the other side with an insulated metallic plate forming the internal electrode of a condenser in which the quartz formed the dielectric, and the salt-water the external armature, this condenser forming part of a tuned oscillating circuit. (Langevin 1918c)

Within only a few months, Langevin and Tournier would convert this promising idea into a final design for a pulse-echo submarine detector.

The first step was the brilliant, fundamental, insight that opened the door leading to quartz clocks and frequency control: piezoelectric resonance. When Langevin and Tournier tried to tune the new quartz receiver to 100 kHz, the frequency then in use, they found the sensitivity to be greatest when operating at an even higher frequency. Langevin realized that when the thickness of the crystal was exactly one half-wavelength, efficient energy exchange occurred between the electric charge and the strain. The frequency of this electromechanical resonance depended only on this thickness and the speed of sound in quartz.

Langevin's description also included the next stage on the road to success: "several plates in juxtaposition". Seeking a lower resonant frequency and an even greater sensitivity, Langevin's second receiver was a "Curie" triplet of quartz plates in which the polarity of the middle one was reversed with respect to the two outer ones. At the same time, Langevin added another innovation: he used the reciprocal piezoelectric property of quartz to create an efficient emitter of ultrasound.

On 23 June 1917, Tournier sent a three-word telegram to Langevin to inform him that he has succeeded in emitting ultrasound from the new triplet transducer. The next day he wrote:

> To Professor Langevin. Dear Sir, Here are a few words to complete my telegram: I have found a fairly close resonance of the quartz for a frequency of 60,000. Radiation pressure corresponding to an angle of 45° for a pendulum identical with the one used this winter. I will give you a detailed verbal account of my tests.

Langevin has linked the mechanical with the electrical at both microscopic and macroscopic scales. Internal energy exchange was mediated by an external dimension. He created a new fundamental idea that will underpin the future technologies of time measurement and frequency control. He explored one area of science and revealed another.

> If a sheet of quartz of a certain thickness be taken, it will vibrate somewhat like a rod with a frequency in inverse proportion to its thickness; again if, when this quartz plate is excited by an alternating current of a certain frequency, matters be so arranged that the elastic oscillation of the sheet shall be exactly in resonance with the exciting waves, the amplitude of the mechanical movements which the sheet takes up will be augmented. (Langevin 1924e)

Having pointed out that "the sheet must have a thickness of half a wavelength for the frequency under consideration", he gives the example of the first plates he had cut in March 1917:

> The speed of propagation of sound in quartz is about 4,500 metres per second and a sheet of 15 mm in thickness will correspond to a half wave vibration of 150,000 periods.[3]

Fernand Holweck (1890–1941) marvelled at the new phenomenon of quartz resonance when Langevin recruited him at the end of July 1917 to work with Tournier in Toulon. Holweck had been Marie Curie's assistant at the Sorbonne before the war and he had since gained experience in radio communication in the Second Army under Gustave Ferrié. Holweck wrote to Marie Curie on 9 September: "The latest experiment on the elastic resonance of quartz is lovely and you would have to be a very simple physicist to remain insensitive to this beautiful phenomenon" [10].

However, Langevin was still not content. He was already exploring another transducer design. He took a new direction, at first surprising, but logical. He moved on from his discovery of the inherent piezoelectric resonance of a simple plate of quartz. Instead, a quartz slice is bonded onto a single steel block. Each section is one quarter of a wavelength thick, retaining the half-wave overall thickness, but lowering the resonant frequency without using more quartz. The design operated successfully but asymmetry compromised resonance. Nevertheless, Boyle will copy this design for all asdic transducers in Britain, achieving by the war's end performance that will be least as good as the French [5, pp. 88–89].[4]

Bragg realized how important were the French developments. With Boyle still in Toulon, he wrote to Langevin on 15 June 1917 suggesting that a second experimental programme using quartz should be set up in Britain in parallel with that in Toulon. Langevin agreed. On 31 July, Langevin made a second visit to Parkston Quay to advise Boyle and Bragg on how this might be best achieved.

---

[3] Langevin's error in estimating the sound speed in quartz, taken from his knowledge of the speed of sound in steel, suggests that much of the early work on tuning must have been empirical. A 15-mm slice resonates at closer to 180 kHz, so Tournier's observation that the triplet resonates at 60 kHz makes sense. In his August 1917 report, Boyle calculated that it is 5000 m/s, using an incorrect value of the bulk modulus of elasticity (It is 5720 m/s along an x-axis).

[4] Boyle also reports that, during his stay in Toulon in the summer of 1917, "it is possible to telephone through the water, using supersonic waves as the carrier of speech". In March 1926, page 170, the Scientific American published an article titled *Telephoning Beneath the Sea*, describing Harvey Hayes' use of a Langevin quartz sandwich transducer for underwater communications.

Boyle wrote a second report for the BIR later that autumn in which he documented what he had learned from Langevin about the use of piezoelectricity of quartz for ultrasonics. This report is a remarkably detailed account of the piezoelectricity of quartz, its laws, and precise instructions for cutting quartz to exploit this property. The detail suggests that he had been Langevin's very attentive and willing pupil, and that Langevin had been a highly competent and effective teacher. In the absence of French documents, Boyle's two reports open a window onto the status of progress in Toulon at the end of July 1917 [2].

In Toulon, the experimental work progressed steadily, documented by Tournier's letters to his mother and to Langevin, who was "becoming nicer and nicer". On 16 September, Tournier told his mother:

> We were able to transmit our waves with considerable power, ... by putting our hands in the water, next to the source, we can feel a very strange sharp pain, similar to the pain of rheumatism. This kills fish in seconds. This is obviously a very expensive way of fishing. [4, p. 109]

The first outside visitor to observe progress in Toulon was the American physicist Robert Wood, who arrived in Paris in August 1917. Wood had been appointed as a free-lance liaison officer attached to the French Ministry of Inventions. He had a natural affinity for European physics, having been a researcher in Berlin in 1896 when Rontgen announced his discovery of X-rays, and had been the only physicist from the USA to attend the second Solvay Conference in 1913. In Paris, he met Perrin with his "gigantic loudspeaker" and Chilowsky with his flame-tipped shell. But he thought Langevin's work as being much more promising, asking for specific permission to "spend more time with Langevin than the others". He recognized the symmetry between Langevin's work on ultrasound and his own on ultraviolet radiation: he used mercury and sodium vapour lamps to produce light with wavelengths too short and frequencies too high to be seen: Langevin used singing capacitors and quartz plates to produce sound with wavelengths too short and frequencies too high to be heard. The two men visited Toulon, and Wood told Tournier that this time had been "the happiest day of his life".

Wood returned to New York in January 1918, and reported what he had learned about ultrasonic methods to Michael Pupin's anti-submarine group at Colombia University. His recollection of seeing the powerful effects of ultrasonic exposure on fish stimulated his later investigations into high power ultrasonics, with Alfred Loomis at his Tuxedo Park laboratory in New York [13, pp. 196–198].

8.5 The Quartz Sandwich Transducer

Langevin never shared the view that physics existed in separate compartments, one of pure theoretical physics, one of laboratory experimental physics, and one of applied physics in which the discoveries of science can be used for the benefit of mankind and commerce. His life was a continuum of interconnecting facets, each fertilizing the others. The war reinforced this view by direct experience so that, by the end of his life, it was an integral component of his total philosophy of science. In La pensée et l'action, a talk given in the last year of his life, and published in English translation (with the title *Science and Action*) in the American Marxist publication *Science and Society*, he says:

> Furthermore, as the application of the physical and natural sciences has broadened in scope, it has progressively wiped out the originally very sharp distinction between pure science and applied science, between the scientist and the engineer or technician. Their methods of work and characteristics tend to become closer and closer. (Langevin 1946a)

This view was maturing through his experience in exploiting ultrasonics for echolocation. Langevin had taken on the spirit of the *École de physique et de chimie industrielles*. His next invention embodies the ideal of this school, the union of advanced theoretical research and technical innovation. Langevin truly innovated, in the haste and urgency of the war. And he was experiencing, at a very personal level, the fundamental bond between physics and engineering. This experience will drive his future views on science and education. Langevin was no longer the pure physicist, theorizing on the fundamental causes of magnetism: neither was he the experimental physicist, distinguishing heavy from light ions at the top of the Eiffel Tower. Langevin had become a goal-oriented design engineer with a practical job to do: to reach the best possible practical ultrasonic submarine detector.

Langevin was well aware that absorption in seawater increases with frequency. To increase the range he must decrease the frequency. By stacking layers together, Langevin could create thicker transducers that would resonate at lower frequencies. But his 60 kHz layered quartz transducer was already quite thick and, to maintain directionality, all three dimensions must increase in inverse proportion to the frequency: an increase in mass that depends on the inverse cube of the frequency. Langevin selected a target compromise frequency of 40 kHz "principally for reasons of convenience and weight".

Langevin now knew that he could bond quartz to steel using a hot mixture of resin and beeswax and still maintain resonance. But while large blocks of steel are easy to form, quartz crystals of the required diameter were not available. The solution was straightforward: to use an array of many x-cut crystals, all carefully cut to a uniform thickness. Wood reported seeing a transducer made from square plates. Langevin seems to have later understood that this regular array could introduce unwanted coherence, leading to irregularities in the ultrasound beam. His quartz pieces were subsequently cut into a variety of shapes, fitted together into a mosaic, like broken paving slabs.

Langevin asked Tournier to construct a transducer of a new design. Tournier made some practical suggestions, and sketched his ideas (Fig. 8.2). It is the next step from the two-layer idea that Boyle took back to England in July. In this new design, the oscillating plate is made from three layers, but now a thin quartz mosaic layer, about 4 mm thick, is sandwiched between two thicker metal ones. Mechanical resonance is ensured by setting the total thickness to be one half-wavelength. Having first discovered the phenomenon of piezoelectric resonance, Langevin now brilliantly separates piezoelectric transduction from mechanical resonance.

Langevin tested the principle in his laboratory in Paris. Holweck was tasked with building the first working prototype, 20 cm × 20 cm. The transducer was driven

8.5 The Quartz Sandwich Transducer

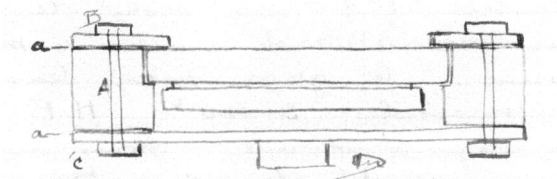

Fig. 8.2 Tournier wrote to Langevin on 2 December 1917, sketching how he proposed to construct a quartz sandwich transducer. (ESPCI, PSL University L194/042)

using a balanced two-valve generator at 3–5 kV. The receiver was a modified 8-valve amplifier from the *Telegraphie militaire*. By 26 February 1918, Tournier was finally able to report to Langevin the successful completion of 2 days' sea trials.

By the middle of May 1918, Colin reported to Langevin that they had achieved transmission to 8 km, and excellent echo detection from a moving and submerged submarine up to a range of 800 m (Archives L194/058). This triggered a decision to set up a formal sea-trial by the French Navy. Starting on 5 June 1918, and lasting over a month, these serious evaluations were the culmination of over 3 years of work by Langevin's dedicated team of scientists and engineers (Archives L194/003).

Success brought other visitors: by the end of August, the ultrasonic detection system had been demonstrated to two more American visitors, and Marie Curie and Henri Abraham both visited. Tournier felt angry that he was generously offering "the fruits of his labours to visitors from America and Italy". He was also irritated that many of the stream of visitors could not speak French.

Boyle's report in October to the Interallied Conference on Supersonics makes abundantly clear his dependence on Langevin's guidance and support. While his was strictly the British ultrasonics project, Langevin was in fact running two European groups, one in Toulon, France and a second in Harwich, England. At each stage, from Boyle's training in the summer of 1917 and Langevin's advice in establishing Boyle's laboratory, from the loan of the first quartz pieces to the provision of French amplifiers, the British success in developing ultrasonics at this time would not have happened without Langevin's input. The two transducer designs differed in one important aspect: Langevin's was resonant, tuned to be efficient at a single frequency: Boyle's was not resonant, designed to operate with lower efficiency but over a wider frequency range. Otherwise, the only contribution that was uniquely British was the term "asdic". This acronym first appeared in the weekly report of experimental work at Parkeston Quay on 6 July 1918. Quartz was known by the secret name "asdivite". Asdic "almost certainly stood for 'pertaining to the Anti-Submarine Division' (or Anti-Submarine Division-ic)" [5, p. xxv]. During WW2 the term will be used to develop a narrative for its origin within the British Navy. It will be retained until the end that war, when the more familiar term SONAR becomes fully adopted.[5]

---

[5] The first newspaper use of the word "asdic" was in a report of the sinking of an enemy submarine on 20 October 1939. On 6 December, in the House of Commons, Churchill reported "The efficacy of the asdic method of detection is increasingly proved". The Admiralty, asked for its meaning, incorrectly stated that it stood for a non-existent "Allied Submarine Detection Investigation Committee". The term "SONAR" was coined by FV Hunt in 1942.

8.6 Interallied Conference on Supersonics (19–22 October 1918)

Langevin was invited to visit the USA during the summer, but he did not accept the invitation. By September, the US Navy was becoming increasingly interested in learning more about this new method of tracking submarines. On 18 September 1918, Edward Raguet, Commander of the US Navy Submarine Chaser Squadron in Gibraltar, made a visit to Toulon. On 26 September, Henry Bumstead, Scientific Attaché to the US Embassy in London, submitted his own report. These high-level contacts resulted in an approach to the French authorities to "supply full specifications and descriptions of the apparatus, together with a certain number of complete sets of the apparatus ready for installation and use on board war ships of the United States Navy". At the time, the French Navy were still in the process of equipping their own ships, clearly not in a position to respond quickly to the American request.

The French reply, no doubt supported by Langevin, was to insist on a small meeting between four representatives each from France, England, the USA and Italy. It was at this meeting in Paris at the end of October that both Langevin and Boyle shared full details of the developments in ultrasonic detection during the past 3 years.

Langevin also shared with the meeting his ideas about future challenges and opportunities: to explore frequencies lower than 40 kHz: to alter the beam-shape to be a fan beam, by changing the shape of the transducer: to improve adhesion by using better glues and by compression: to improve the electronics: to decrease electrical interference: to study underwater wave propagation. With these challenges in mind, and having experienced the British Navy's bid to establish local rights over intellectual property (Chap. 11), Langevin wished to ensure that further developments in ultrasonics would be developed in shared partnership. To this end, the establishment of a Permanent Commission for the Development of Supersonic Methods was proposed. A few days after the armistice, on behalf of the Ministry of the French Navy, Breton suggested that "the fruitful collaboration of scientists, engineers, industrialists, inventors and military personnel of all ranks who have competed in dedication and activity should continue after the cessation of hostilities" (Archives L137/013). But enthusiasm soon waned, and national and commercial interests soon prevailed in the aftermath of the armistice. The proposed Permanent Commission was stillborn.

And yet, no matter how rich they were, these 4 years of war were but an interlude in a life dedicated to peace.

References

1. Boyle R (1917a) Report of mission to France for the Admiralty Board of Invention and Research – May 20th to July 19th, 1917. B.I.R 30061/17. 1 August 1917. UK National Archive, Kew

References

2. Boyle R (1917b) "The piezo-electric phenomenon, with reference to acoustic vibrations" (undated) BIR 38164/17. UK National Archive, Kew
3. Curie J, Curie P (1889) Dilatation électrique du quartz. J Phys 2nd ser. 8:149–170. In translation: Duck F (2009) "The electrical expansion of quartz" by Jacques and Pierre Curie. Ultrasound 17:197–203
4. Dorsay K (2022) Il donnait deux fois parce qu'il donnait vite. David di Napoli 1940–1890 Marcel Tournier 1888–1964. Jean-Jacques Wuillaume
5. Hackmann W (1984) Seek and strike. Sonar, antisubmarine warfare and the Royal Navy 1914–54. Her Majesty's Stationary Office, London
6. Joliot-Curie F (1944) Le professeur Langevin et l'effort scientifique de guerre. La Pensée Oct–Dec 1:32–37
7. Katzir S (2012) Who knew piezoelectricity? Rutherford and Langevin on submarine detection and the invention of sonar. Notes and Records of the Royal Society of London 66:141–157
8. Kelvin L (1893) "Quartz Piezoelectrique de MM. J. et P. Curie". Appendix to: "On the piezo-electric property of quartz". Philosophical Magazine Ser 5 36:331–343
9. Langevin A (2022) Paul Langevin my father. EDP Sciences, Paris. English edition: Duck F
10. Legrand AP (2022) Un réseau social pendant la guerre de 1914. Histoire et patrimoine. Bulletin d'ESPCI Alumni 65:10–13
11. Lewiner J (1991) Langevin and the birth of ultrasonics. Japanese Journal of Applied Physics 30:5–11
12. Rutherford E (1916) "A preliminary notice of a new method of measurement of amplitude of vibration of diaphragm, and of exciting supersonic wave in water" BIR 11738/16. 28 Sept 1916. UK National Archives ASD 2893
13. Seabrook W (1941) Doctor Wood. Modern wizard of the laboratory. Harcourt Brace, New York
14. Zimmerman D (2018) "A more creditable way": the discovery of active sonar, the Langevin-Chilowsky patent dispute and the Royal Commission on Awards to Inventors. War in History 25(1):48–68

Chapter 9
Restoring Science and Peace

Abstract The four years of war were but an interlude. In the 1920s, Langevin entered the public arena to restore international scientific relations and to build a peaceful world by using his scientific reputation. He opposed the boycott of German science that followed the Treaty of Versailles. In October 1919, he signed a petition against the blockade of the USSR. In 1921, he joined the opposition to the court-martial of the mutinous Black Sea sailors. He was curious about what was happening in the USSR, joining the *Amitiés franco-russes* association. Such commitments clearly marked him as "left-wing intellectual". He joined the international movement called *Clarté*, founded in May 1919, comprising European intellectuals opposed to war and seeking social renewal. He was a member of the *Comité international de coopération intellectuelle* to promote international exchanges between academics in the sciences and humanities. In 1931, he was a member of a League of Nations mission to China to advise on the reorganization of the Chinese public education system. For him, science was a collective effort of adaptation of the human species to the outside world. It could not be nationalized.

Work in ultrasonics has many paradoxical effects in Langevin's life. Here is a champion of pure and disinterested science who will find himself embroiled in patent battles with multiple twists and turns (Chap. 11). Here is a staunch enemy of war, who collaborates for years with the French Navy. The height of irony! This powerful theorist, militant pacifist, will receive the highest honours for technical and warlike work: he is awarded the Order of the British Empire, in the third class (CBE); in 1923, Langevin is made a knight of the *Légion d'honneur*, then officer in 1932. Finally, the services rendered by asdic, later called Sonar, will make Langevin a key figure of the Second World War and will contribute greatly to his being considered as a national hero worthy of resting in the Pantheon. And, beyond the solemn tribute of his grateful homeland, it is mainly the applications of the work carried out during the war that made Langevin newsworthy. The quartz watch, and medical ultrasound, ultrasonic cleaning and proximity sensors, fish detectors and food processing have had more impact on day-day living than the reflections of the theorist or the project of school reform. Hence this ultimate paradox, which sums up all the others:

© The Author(s), under exclusive license to Springer Nature Switzerland AG 2025
B. Bensaude-Vincent, F. Duck, *Paul Langevin: Physicist and Social Activist*,
Springer Biographies, https://doi.org/10.1007/978-3-031-95260-9_9

Langevin is better known today for the result of his war work than for his work for peace.

No matter how creative they were, these four years of war were but an interlude in a life dedicated to peace. And Langevin himself will have other concerns: evangelism for relativity (Chap. 10); Council membership of the Solvay Conference (Chap. 14); editor of the *Journal de physique* and managing EPCI (Chap. 13); maintaining his family (Chap. 3).

The war may have been over in 1919, but the armistice signed on 11 November 1918 did not bring back the pre-war life remembered by the scientists who had been involved in wartime activities. Returning to work proved difficult. First, this resulted from the human losses of life, very high in the French population in general and in the student population in particular.[1] The Spanish flu pandemic in 1918–1919 increased the death toll. In common with all countries, France was in mourning and, to maintain the memory of the fallen, monuments were built celebrating the sacrifices made during the war for the country's defence.

Resuming the international contacts between academics throughout Europe was out of question. The Versailles Treaty implied that professional contacts with German and Austrian colleagues were banned. Not only were German scientists no longer invited to international conferences but the measures of boycott also applied to the use of the German language in scientific meetings and journals [8]. The Versailles treaty also imposed reparations on Germany to pay for the financial costs of the war. Because public money was badly needed, not only to reconstruct the devastated zones but also to attract young people into scientific research, the spirit of retaliation against Germany persisted. Return to normal life would imply "demobilizing the mind", especially the mind of those scientists who had taken part in mass destruction to overcome an enemy [9].

L'union sacrée, the political rapprochement that united French people of all political and religious convictions at the outbreak of the war, broke down in the aftermath of the war. The process of demobilization raised political tensions and social unrest. There were strikes in the spring and summer of 1919 and widespread industrial unrest in 1920. The government of the *Bloc national* strongly suppressed these social movements and suspected that they were stirred up from outside by Bolshevists. In 1919, France and its wartime allies launched a military intervention in Russia, which Georges Clemenceau justified as the defence of European civilization against Communist barbarism. The Allied Supreme Council set up an economic blockade of Soviet Russia. So troubled were the years 1919 and 1920 that it is difficult to draw a clear-cut distinction between wartime and peacetime.

---

[1] The French losses amounted to 1.4 million dead (approximately 3.5% of the pre-war population) and 4 million disabled; 450,000 people died in France during the Spanish flu pandemic. Four out of ten ENS students died in war service.

9.1 A Scholar in the Public Arena

In this troubled context, Langevin did not remain inactive. He redirected the zeal he had deployed to defend his homeland during wartime to fight against nationalism and for the restoration of normal scientific relationships. The war had driven him outside the academic community. He would stay in the public arena to build a peaceful world. This now extended to using his scientific reputation and the credibility conferred by his war service to confront governmental initiatives.

In October 1919, he signed a petition "against the blockade" of the USSR. This was published in the left-wing newspaper *L'Humanité*,[2] where he publicly joined the condemnation of the government's attitude (*L'Humanité*, 26 October 1919). Faced with strikes, the government had decided to employ students to replace the striking railwaymen or drivers. In his function of director of studies at EPCI, Langevin refused to suspend classes to break the strike and justified his resistance in a public letter published in *L'Humanité* (Langevin 1920e). The crux of the argument was that students must study. But these professional considerations deceived no one. His refusal was seen as a gesture of solidarity with the working class.

In late 1919, mutinies broke out among the French sailors who were involved in the military intervention against the Soviets. The crew of the French submarine Proteus refused to obey the order to bombard Odessa. French troops were repatriated at the end of 1919 and the Allied Supreme Council decided to lift the economic blockade of Soviet Russia in January 1920. But the mutinous soldiers were tried by a court-martial in 1921. Their fate seemed settled, but public opinion moved in favour of an amnesty. Langevin chaired a meeting in the *Salle Wagram*,[3] alongside Ferdinand Buisson, president of the League of Human Rights and Daniel Renoult, representative of the French Communist Party newly created at the Congress of Tours. Thus, after having supported the Navy during the war, Langevin stood up to it by defending André Marty, organizer of the revolt. In his plea for amnesty, he first invokes the harsh physical and psychological conditions of the sailors, worn out by 4 years of war. Then he describes the October 1917 revolution as "the first realization of hopes of universal liberation" and the dawn of a new era that has been so long awaited (Langevin 1921b).

In these actions, Langevin did not conceal his political sympathies. Like many of those who had experienced the war, and saw in it a collapse of European values, he found a glimmer of hope in what was going on to the east of old Europe. He was curious about what was happening in the USSR (founded in 1922) and keen to counter anti-Bolshevik propaganda. In 1924, Langevin joined the *Amitiés franco-russes* association, later renamed Cercle de la Russie neuve. He chaired the French Committee for scientific relations with the USSR and developed ties with Soviet physicists such as Lev Landau and with Piotr Kapitza whom he met in Cambridge

---

[2] *L'humanité* was a daily newspaper, taken over by the French Communist party on its formation in 1920.
[3] The *Salle Wagram* is a historic auditorium in the 17th arrondissement of Paris.

[4, pp. 86–90]. Like many French intellectuals he made two trips to the Soviet Union in 1928 and 1929, and marvelled at "the excellent work being done here in all fields", as well as at the working conditions of Soviet researchers.

Such commitments clearly marked him as "left-wing intellectual", close to the Communist Party. However he remains on the sidelines of political networks. During the 20 inter-war years he was active in the political sphere without ever being a member of any party or any government. A combative activist but never subservient, such could be the formula that characterizes Langevin as well as a number of leading figures such as Albert Einstein and later Bernard Russell or Jean-Paul Sartre. In short, his was a fairly typical profile of these "intellectuals" as a social group.

9.2 "The Internationale of the Mind"

Langevin joined the international movement called *Clarté*, founded in May 1919 by Henri Barbusse,[4] Raymond Lefebvre and Paul Vaillant Couturier.[5] Their project, which had emerged and matured during the war, gathered European intellectuals who had expressed their hatred for war and their desire for social renewal [7]. Its mission was to:

> Organize the fight against ignorance and those who direct it as an industry ... This movement was born from no political or national influence, it is independent and international; it is sincerely and highly human [1].

The first steering committee brought together international figures from the worlds of literature and sciences: French novelists of the old generation and the young "slaughtered generation": Henri Barbusse, Franci Carco, Roland Dorgelès, Georges Duhamel, Anatole France, Charles Gide, Thomas Hardy, Jules Romains; Claude Autant-Lara, a film maker; the French journalist Séverine; the Belgian J.-H. Rosny elder; the American writer Upton Sinclair, the British writers H.G. Wells and Israel Zangwill and the famous Austrian writer Stefan Zweig. The success of a movement such as this depended on the fame of its members. The committee of *Clarté* did not hide that it needed the "authority of scientists" like Einstein and Langevin. Further, these brilliant scientists were keen on assuming such responsibility.

The *Clarté* movement relied heavily on the conviction that the intellectual elite should work towards the construction of a social order. It had been clearly expressed

---

[4] Henri Barbusse (1873–1935) a French novelist and poet wrote extensively about his war experience and mingled war memories with political reflections. His fame was built on his novel *Le feu* ("Under Fire") (1916) describing the horrors the life in the trenches. After the war, he became anti-war and then an anti-fascism activist and later became a founding member of the French Communist Party.

[5] Raymond Lefebvre (1891–1920) was a student who died young at sea. Paul-Vaillant Couturier (1892–1937) was a writer, journalist and politician, and a member of the French Communist Party.

in a novel by Romain Rolland, *Au-dessus de la mêlée* (1914), which protested against the engagement of the intellectual elite in wartime propaganda. Although he shared Barbusse's anti-war convictions, Rolland refused to join *Clarté* because he disagreed with Barbusse's communism. On 15 March 1918, he published a manifesto "For an Internationale of the Mind" followed in December 1919 by a "Declaration of Intellectual Independence" signed by Benedetto Croce, Einstein, Gorki, Upton Sinclair, Bertrand Russell, Heinrich Mann and others. The same concern about the independence of the mind would re-emerge throughout the interwar period. In 1927, Julien Benda, in *La Trahison des Clercs*, blame intellectuals for having sacrificed the independence of spiritual life by succumbing to the seductions of power or money [3].

At the root of the concern with intellectual independence was the entrance of academics into the public sphere. It was a massive phenomenon, especially in Langevin's scientific environment. However, the paths into the political world were far from uniform, even in the small group formed around the ENS and L'Arcouest. Some academics embarked on a political career: for instance Paul Painlevé the mathematician who became minister during the war, then president of the Council in 1925, or Émile Borel also a mathematician, who became deputy of Aveyron, his native region, and Minister of the Navy in 1925. Other scientists entered politics to promote scientific research. Jean Perrin launched a wide-ranging campaign in the 1920 and 1930s. He was driven by the conviction that it is not only through laboratory work that science advances, but also by walking through the ministries, so as to raise funds and to create research institutes. The socialist *Front Populaire* government created the first secretary of state for scientific research in 1936 and Jean Perrin took the post after Irène Joliot-Curie resigned. In 1939, Perrin's years of effort would finally lead to the creation of the *Centre national de la recherche scientifique*, employing full-time researchers. While he supported Perrin's action for the promotion of science policy, Langevin nevertheless never left the academic world. He was present in the public sphere *in the name of* science rather than doing politics *for* science. Like Einstein and Russell he acted as a missionary whose vision was reconciliation, peace and justice.

9.3 Promoting Cultural Internationalism

How could Langevin combine missionary activism with his professional duties as a scientist? Did he conduct them as two separated, parallel activities in a kind of double life?

In the immediate aftermath of the war, combining these two activities was relatively easy, because the reconciliation between nations was a necessary condition to return to normal scientific life. Scientific research requires international cooperation. It was urgent to put an end to the nationalistic spirit that reigned in scientific communities on opposing sides of the conflict during the 4 years of war.

But the rift in the "Internationale of the Mind", created during the war, was perpetuated by the foundation of the International Research Council (IRC) in 1919. Officially the IRC aimed to replace the international scientific associations that had been closed since the outbreak of the war and to encourage international unions in various branches of science that required multi-national cooperation such as astronomy, geodesy and pure and applied chemistry. In practice, however, the cooperation promoted by the 15 countries that set up the IRC was guided by a principle of exclusion of the defeated countries, Germany, Austria, Hungary and Bulgaria [4]. Scientists from those countries were excluded from scientific meetings and the use of German language was forbidden in scientific journals. In addition, the IRC demanded material reparations in the form of equipment for laboratories. In short, it was like a cold war in science. The universalist ideal that had characterized pre-war international scientific associations gave way to a quarantine for scientists who were held responsible for the war crimes of their home countries [10]. And it lasted even after the official reconciliation at the Locarno agreement in 1925. The ostracism was not lifted until 1926, when the general assembly invited scientists from the defeated countries to join the IRC. Even then, only Hungary accepted the invitation to join the general assembly; Bulgaria could not join for economic reasons; Austria and Germany did not respond. Eventually, in 1931, the IRC was dissolved.

In 1922, as a counterpoint to the ostracism of the IRC, the *Comité international de cooperation intellectuelle* (CICI) was created under the auspices of the League of Nations, to revive the universalist ideal through pragmatic projects of international cooperation. It aimed to promote international exchanges between academics in the sciences or humanities, scholars, teachers and artists. The first chairman was the French philosopher Henri Bergson (1922–1925) followed by the Dutch physicist Henrik Lorentz (1925–1928) and then the British classical scholar Gilbert Murray (1928–1939). With an executive branch (the International Institute of Intellectual Cooperation) set up in Paris in 1926, and most of the financial resources coming from the French government, the CICI was initially dominated by France. It nevertheless reached out to non-western cultures—especially from China and Japan—with an intention to develop a dialogue between civilizations. In 1946, its activities were transferred to UNESCO.

The members were appointed in consideration of their intellectual prestige and high reputation in learned societies, without any discrimination as to their nationality. In addition to Bergson, they included Paul Valéry, Marie Curie, Langevin and Albert Einstein, at that time professor in Berlin. However, Einstein resigned in 1924 in protest against the inefficiency of the CICI. In reality, the participation of Germany posed a real challenge, because Bergson's attitude on this issue was ambiguous [6, p. 235]. Marie Curie and Langevin struggled to convince Einstein to stay in the committee (Archives, L072/007). But Langevin's appeals to other German scientists failed. Fritz Haber, the German industrial chemist who most actively contributed to the German war effort rejected the invitation. He was ready to renew personal ties with foreign scientists, but he considered that, given the political situation in Germany, a collective movement would be more harmful than useful [5, p. 107]. Ostwald refused, arguing that it would be a waste of energy, contrary

9.3 Promoting Cultural Internationalism

to his "energetic imperative" (ibid., pp. 106–107). He considered that one of the missions of the CICI, to develop international biographical tools, was to a certain extent a continuation of the association *Die Brücke* created by him in 1913.

Such responses did not discourage Langevin, who remained a member of the CICI until 1932. For him and for Marie Curie, the CICI was a tool to create a peaceful order through practical initiatives. Curie was proactive in the development of bibliographical instruments, international standards and fellowships in the 1920s. Langevin was active in the sub-committee of intellectual property and took part in the debates on the rights of scientists over the commercial exploitation of their discoveries, an issue that had become familiar to him with his own ultrasonic patents.

He was also active in educational initiatives. In 1931, he was a member of a League of Nations expert mission to China to advise on the reorganization of the Chinese public education system [2]. In this 3-month visit, he was accompanied by the British economist Robert Tawney, the Polish philosopher Marian Falski and the German orientalist Carl Becker (Figs. 9.1, 9.2 and 9.3). Their collective report (Langevin 1932d) warns against the dangers of cultural colonization: this was at the same time as the Colonial Exhibition in Paris celebrated the achievements and benefits of colonialism. The report insists that the Chinese education system should aim to generate a new, appropriate Chinese civilization, independent from European or American influences. The chapter on science, presumably written by Langevin, attempts to resolve the difficulty of the clash between traditional Chinese civilization and modern Western science. It suggests delaying the scientific initiation of students so they have time to assimilate their own culture and to return to its sources of knowledge instead of simply teaching applied sciences. In this way a new China can learn to handle "the powerful instrument of material and spiritual liberation represented by the scientific method". This report reveals the ambiguities of the work of CICI experts, because China was above all seeking assistance from the CICI to attract Europeans and to send students abroad. As Daniel Laqua pointed out:

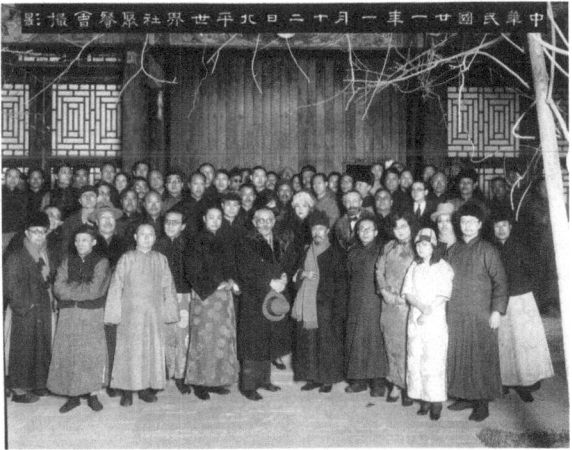

Fig. 9.1 Langevin with a Chinese delegation during the League of Nations visit to China, 1931–1932. (ESPCI)

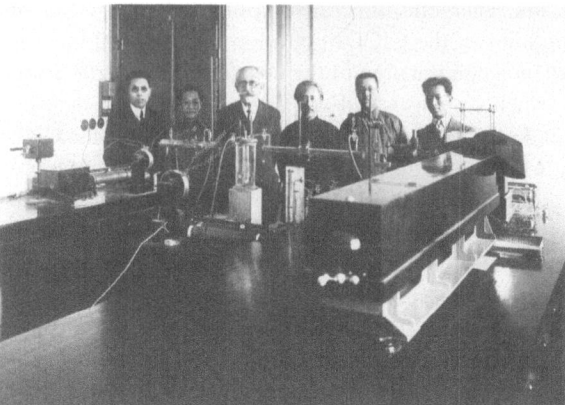

Fig. 9.2 At the National Academy of Science, Peking, 1932. Left to right: Yan Jici, director of the Physics Institute of the National Academy; Ouang Te-Tchao; Paul Langevin; Li Yu Ying, president of the National Academy; Li Lin Yu, president of the Sino-French University in Peking; Zhu GuangCai, physicist. (ESPCI)

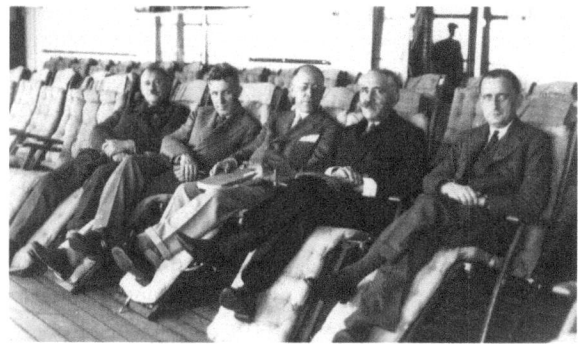

Fig. 9.3 Departure of the mission for China on the Bremen in 1931: Langevin with Tawny, Palsky, Becker and Taylor. (ESPCI)

> The League bodies for intellectual cooperation had to strike a balance between two rather different impulses: the seemingly pragmatic work for the exchange of knowledge, as often desired by governments, and the engagement with more ambitious schemes, as promoted by some intellectuals and associations. [6, p. 239]

Langevin himself struggled to strike the balance between idealism and pragmatism through his various commitments in the education system (Chap. 20).

9.4 Challenging the Boycott of German Science

In his activities as a physicist, he implemented practical measures to promote the reconciliation of nations although he faced a strong resistance from scientific institutions. In 1920, he became editor-in-chief of the Journal de physique which then merged with *Le Radium*. He challenged the IRC measures of boycott since he opened the journal to scientists "from all countries" and reserved about half of each issue for reviews of French and foreign books. However, he insisted that everything be published in the French language and stated in the editorial that the mission of the journal was "to represent, in its various events, the activity of French-speaking physicists" [5, p. 82].

9.4 Challenging the Boycott of German Science

When he became a member of the scientific committee of the Solvay Councils of Physics, the measures aimed at excluding Germany were relaxed. The decision made in 1920 to publish all reports in a single language, French, did not a priori exclude references to research carried out by German scientists. In April 1923, Lorentz, chair of the scientific committee that authorized notes written by German scientists in the reports, declared that he was ready to invite Einstein "if he has dealt with the subject that we want to choose". But the committee still refused, although more softly than in 1920, to choose relativity as the theme of the next conference.

Inviting Einstein to present the theory of relativity in 1922 was a more spectacular gesture of defiance of the IRC boycott measures. On 18 February 1922, Langevin wrote to Einstein:

> Scientific interest requires that relations be restored between German-speaking scholars and us. You can help better than anyone, you will render a very great service to your colleagues in Germany and France and above all, to our common ideal by accepting (…) We would be very happy if you could come before June and that your first visit to Paris is made for an exclusively scientific purpose. This will be the best way to work towards the appeasement that we all desire. [5, p. 76]

This letter clearly suggests that political and scientific motivations merged in the invitation to give a lecture at the *Collège de France*. Einstein initially refused because it was difficult, given his situation in Germany, to subordinate politics to science:

> You know that I am of the opinion that relations between scholars should not suffer for political reasons and that the consideration of the scientific working community should come before all others. You also know that I am unreservedly animated by internationalist sentiments (…) But after scrupulous reflection I have come to the conviction that in this period of political tension, my visit to Paris would have more harmful consequences than favourable ones. (27 February 1922 Archives 072/024)

Einstein did not want to appear disloyal in the eyes of his German colleagues who suffered from isolation due to the boycott imposed by IRC, and he also feared protests in Paris. He could no longer believe that science could supersede the feelings of hatred and resentment generated by nationalism:

> The general public and politics have long since seized my theory and my person and have endeavoured to adapt both to their goals in one way or another. There would be a considerable number of people who would watch every free word from me to throw it to newspaper readers with a sauce of their own making; my experiences in this regard in recent times make me judge this danger as very serious. The final effect is always hatred and hostility instead of reason and benevolence. (Ibid.)

Einstein was very pessimistic; he seemed to be overwhelmed by the interference of politics in science. From then on, only political pressure could make him reconsider his refusal. On the advice of the German Minister Walter Rathenau, he finally agreed to travel to Paris. In the name of "the superior interest of the mind", Langevin thanked him (8 March 1922). Langevin's plan was risky and adventurous. Einstein was not wrong. Langevin managed to circumvent the measures of the boycott because the invitation came from the *Collège de France* whereas the *Société française de physique* strictly applied the rules imposed by IRC.

Perhaps Einstein and Langevin have never been closer to each other than in 1922, during the rich hours of Einstein's visit, when they shared scientific ideas and political ideals. And yet never has the contrast of their characters been more pronounced: Einstein behaved as a prudent loyal citizen matured by adversities, while Langevin's optimism could testify to his idealism and naivety. But, for once, naivety was going to pay off and triumph over lucidity.

In conclusion, Langevin worked hard to restore the pre-war universalist ideals through a wide spectrum of fields of action. For him, science would always remain a collective effort of adaptation of the human species to the outside world. It could not be nationalized. The 4-year state of exception due to the war had to be closed and give way to a global peaceful order constructed through science and education.

References

1. Barbusse H (1920) La Lueur dans l'ablîme. Clarté, Paris
2. Becker CH, Falski M, Langevin P, Tawney RH (1932) The reorganisation of education in China. League of Nations' Institute of Intellectual Cooperation, Paris
3. Benda J (1927) La trahison des clercs. Grasset, Paris
4. Fox R (2019) The International Research Council and its unions: 1919–1931. Chemistry International 41:7–8. https://doi.org/10.1515/ci-2019-0303
5. Langevin A (2022) Paul Langevin my father. EDP Sciences, Paris. English edition: Duck F
6. Laqua D (2011) Transnational intellectual cooperation, the League of Nations and the problem of order. J Glob Hist 6:223–247
7. Racine N (1967) The *Clarté* movement in France 1919-21. J Contemp Hist 2(2):195–208
8. Reinbothe R (2010) L'exclusion des scientifiques allemands et de la langue allemande des congrès internationaux après la Première Guerre Mondiale. Rev Ger Int 12:193–208
9. Schroeder-Gudehus B (1978) Les scientifiques et la paix. Presses de l'Université de Montréal. https://books.openedition.org
10. Schroeder-Gudehus B (1990) Nationalism and internationalism. In: Olby RC et al (eds) Companion to the history of modern science. Routledge, London, pp 909–919

Chapter 10
Einstein in Paris

Abstract In inviting Einstein to lecture on relativity theory in Paris, Langevin challenged the post-war boycott of German science. His visit in April 1922 was a Parisian social event and a political gesture that gained media attention. From a scientific perspective, it was the crowning achievement of Langevin's long battle for disseminating the theory of relativity in the physics community and for discussing the notion of time with French philosophers. The tense debate with Henri Bergson at the Societé française de philosophie had a tremendous cultural impact in France. It was the acme of the French tradition of dialogue between scientists and philosophers although it ended in a series of monologues.

10.1 A Major Media Event

Einstein arrived in Paris on 28 March 1922 at midnight, to avoid the crowd of reporters who expected him at the Gare du Nord at noon. Langevin and Charles Nordmann, a French astronomer and populariser of Einstein's theory, had travelled to the Belgian border to escort Einstein because they feared public protests upon his arrival (Fig. 10.1) [12]. His visit had been announced in the daily Parisian press and raised a turmoil in public opinion [6]. A professor from Berlin, a member of the Academy of Prussia and a Jew to boot, arriving in Paris: what a scandal! L'Action française jumped on it to rekindle anti-Semitism with some high-class sneering pamphlets. Léon Daudet, referred to Langevin as "*Langepasvin*", presented Einstein as an "ambassador of German-Swiss-circumcised thought", and Jean Druault insinuated that the Collège de France was not "de France", but "de Judée". Left-wing newspapers announced the visit of a Jewish-German professor in Paris as a good sign of revival of scientific internationalism after 4 years of war.

Media attention was heightened because Einstein was no longer an obscure scientist. His theory no longer was a principle of relativity pointing to the horizon of physics. By 1922, the "general theory of relativity", developed by Einstein between 1907 and 1915, incorporates gravity within the relativistic framework. The field equations presented by Einstein before the Prussian Academy of Science in

© The Author(s), under exclusive license to Springer Nature
Switzerland AG 2025
B. Bensaude-Vincent, F. Duck, *Paul Langevin: Physicist and Social Activist*,
Springer Biographies, https://doi.org/10.1007/978-3-031-95260-9_10

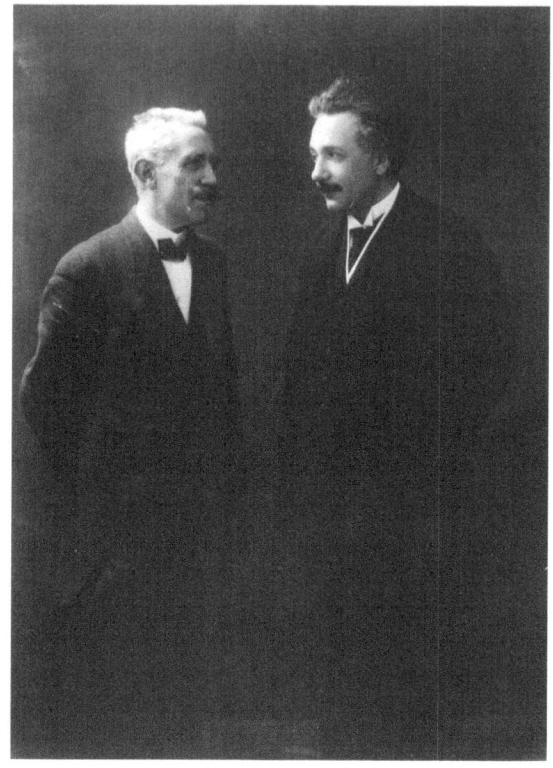

Fig. 10.1 Einstein and Langevin in 1922. Close friends, Einstein and Langevin shared and promoted the same views about the theory of relativity. (Hebrew University of Jerusalem)

November 1915 include Newtonian attraction between masses as an effect of a geometrical deformation of space and time by these masses. In 1917, Einstein extends his theory to the whole universe, thus initiating a relativistic cosmology.

Moreover, the theory, involving geometry, astronomy and cosmology, was by this time firmly established on experimental grounds. Two British scientific expeditions had been conducted on the occasion of the solar eclipse in May 1919 to test one of the consequences of Einstein's general relativity: the deflection of light rays by the gravitational field of the sun. Arthur Eddington, British astrophysicist, travelled to the equatorial island of Principe off the west coast of Africa, part of the Portuguese colonial empire, while Frank Dyson, the Royal Astronomer, went to Sobral in the northeast of Brazil [10], These expeditions anticipated the "big science" that would become a feature of twentieth-century scientific research. They required precision instruments and involved, in addition to the British academics, many technicians, and local workers, as well as the use of colonial plantations, and the active participation of Brazilian and Portuguese scientific institutions. The results were widely reported in the local and international press as a specifically scientific achievement, although their success relied on a complex web connecting science, religion, politics, society and colonialism [19].

10.2 A Busy Week of Lectures

The experimental confirmation of one of Einstein's predictions had a tremendous effect on the physics community. Langevin resumed and intensified his campaign. From 1919 to 1922, his course at the *Collège de France* was about "Relativity and gravitation". He gave a lecture at the French Society of Electricians (Langevin 1919b), another one at the French Society of Physics (Langevin 1920a, 1921c) and one at the French Society of Philosophy (Langevin 1922c). Langevin was no longer alone. In 1922, the theory of relativity was taught at the National Museum of Natural History and at the Polytechnic School [3]. Charles Nordmann, astronomer at the Observatory, also embarked on a dissemination campaign [16, 17]. No less than 21 books on the theory of relativity were published in French language in the 1920s [13, pp. 28–30]. How could a highly mathematical theory of physics draw such public media attention?

10.2 A Busy Week of Lectures

Einstein and Langevin had a busy week of lectures and discussions (Fig. 10.2). On 30 March, Einstein attended a lecture on the general theory of relativity, delivered by Langevin at the General Association of Paris students. This lecture had been planned for several months, in view of a publication in the April–May issue of the monthly *Bulletin* of this dynamic association (Langevin 1922b). The auditorium was already overcrowded.

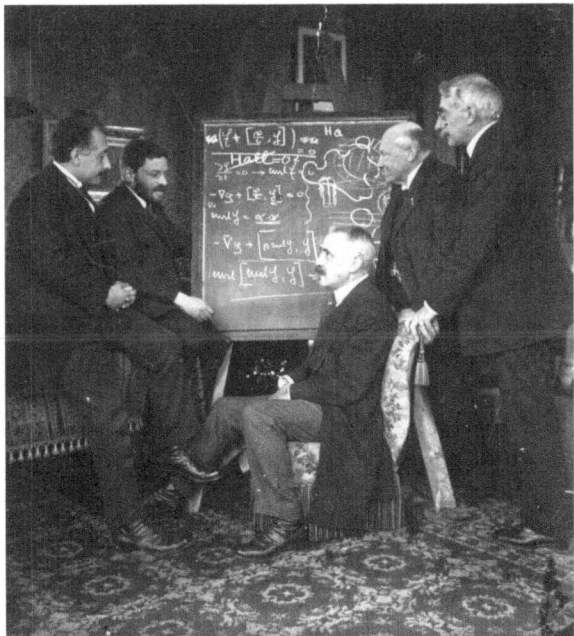

Fig. 10.2 Einstein and Langevin in debate. (Hebrew University of Jerusalem)

On 31 March at 5.30 p.m., Einstein delivered the Michonis lecture at the *Collège de France* to an audience of more than 350 people. Einstein first clearly distinguished special from general relativity, while insisting on the central role played by mathematics. He then clearly developed five points: the invariance of the velocity of light, the relation between mass and energy, the concept of space and time, the impossible simultaneity of two distant events, and finally the equality of inertial and gravitational masses. The following morning's newspapers marvelled at the clarity of Einstein's presentation. The public lecture was followed by three expert sessions, on 3, 5 and 7 April at the *Collège de France*. Despite the technical nature of the discussions, the press duly reported the objections raised by Georges Sagnac, Paul Painlevé and Edouard Guillaume and the responses made by Einstein, with the support of Langevin, Nordmann and Borel. Finally, the programme included a session of discussion with philosophers at the *Société française de philosophie*, on 6 April (Figs. 10.3 and 10.4).

To discuss Einstein's lecture on 31 March at the *Collège de France*, Langevin had carefully selected a number of critics and opponents of the theory of relativity. They developed their objections during the sessions between experts [6, pp. 20–25]. Einstein first confronted the physicist Georges Sagnac who, in 1913, had set up an experiment to prove the existence of the luminiferous ether, which had been made superfluous by special relativity [18].[1] Although Langevin had explained the Sagnac effect in the terms of general relativity in the *Comptes rendus de l'Académie des sciences* (Langevin 1921b), Sagnac reiterated his argument without convincing anyone. Then, the mathematician Paul Painlevé objected that the "Langevin's traveller" paradox was in contradiction with the reciprocity implied by the principle of relativity. This classical objection rests on a confusion between Einstein's principle of relativity and the Galilean principle which effectively implies the equivalence of

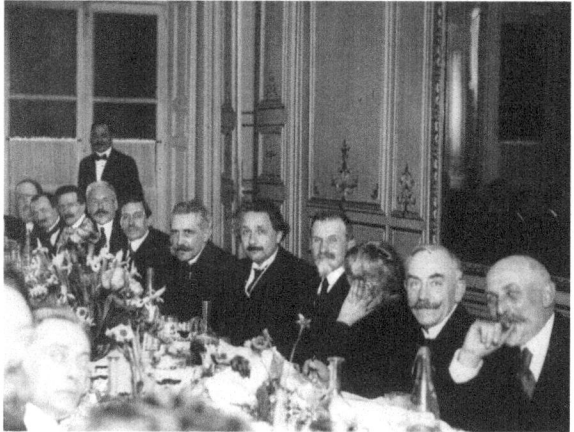

Fig. 10.3 Einstein's visit to Paris in April 1922. Einstein is sitting here between Langevin and Bergson. (Hebrew University of Jerusalem)

---

[1] The Sagnac effect, implemented in the ring interferometer, has applications today in the Global Positioning System [18].

10.2 A Busy Week of Lectures

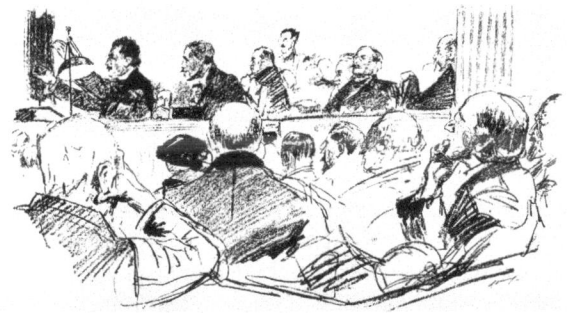

Fig. 10.4 Einstein and Langevin at the *Collège de France* (*Science et Vigilance*)

frames of reference in uniform movement. The next session, on 5 April, opened with a retraction by Painlevé, who said that the previous day's discussion had cleared up any misunderstandings. Then Edouard Guillaume, a Swiss physicist from Geneva challenged the principle of the constancy of the velocity of light in vacuum. His objections were quickly dismantled for using non-consistent premises. This was followed by a discussion about the new dynamics, led by Langevin and involving Charles Nordmann and Jacques Hadamard.

Let us explore how Langevin presented the new theory (that Einstein named "general relativity") during his lecture at the General Association of Paris students (Langevin 1922b).[2] Langevin could no longer present the theory of relativity as an electrodynamic synthesis of physics. By integrating gravitation, which had not been included in the earlier theory of relativity (that Einstein renamed "special relativity" in 1916), general relativity opened up a radically new dynamics and a new cosmology.

From the beginning, Langevin insists on the discontinuity between special and general relativity, even suggesting that it is a kind of Copernican revolution:

> We have more than a discovery here, it is a change of viewpoint comparable only to that introduced by Copernicus when he put the Earth in its place in the system of the world. (Ibid., p. 135)

The analogy is based on the common idea of a reversal of perspective. First, it is an inversion of our representation of celestial movements. Instead of explaining, as in a Euclidean universe, the trajectory of the Moon by the attraction exerted by the Earth on it, in general relativity the Earth produces a modification of the properties of space around the Moon, which affects its spontaneous movement. It is a revolution, Langevin went on, because general relativity implies a reversal of the positivist hierarchy. Auguste Comte's famous classification, which proceeds from mathematics to astronomy and physics, could seem definitively established like mechanics itself. However, the theory of general relativity shakes the edifice by removing the priority of geometry over physics (ibid., pp. 145–146). The properties of space, the laws of geometry, depend on the bodies that are there, that is to say, of physics.

---

[2] This lecture should have been delivered in Einstein's presence, but apparently he was not able to attend, according to Xavier Léon's remark in his introduction to the next session at the *Société française de philosophie* (Langevin 1922c).

It is the very conclusion of the theory of General Relativity that the very properties of the universe are determined by the matter and energy present, are relative to what is there or what is happening there. (Ibid., p. 136)

Inversion, reversal: at first glance, Langevin's discourse sounds more revolutionary than in 1911. Yet the allusion to the Copernican revolution does not suggest in any way the idea of an epochal break. The theoretical shift consists primarily of a reversal of the relationship between disciplines and a plurality of geometries. In Langevin's view, the advancement of physics is even more continuous than ever, because the theory of general relativity is a unifying synthesis that crowns the historical quest for the unity of science. This is the key message of Langevin's presentation. The theory of general relativity is both elegant and powerful. It allows empirical predictions and unites the three principles of conservation, mass, energy and momentum, into one single concept of space-time. Langevin insists that it unifies and simplifies at the same time, abandoning the a priori and absolute postulates that underlie classical mechanics (ibid., p. 144).

By getting rid of old notions, the general theory offers a simple explanation of the world. The new dynamics is simpler than the old one (ibid., p. 162). Langevin notes that electromagnetic phenomena, usually considered as more obscure and mysterious than mechanical ones because they are perceived only through instruments, nevertheless have a strong explanatory power. The simple, adds Langevin, never comes first; it results from a long process of scientific development. "We see that it is not at all the most anciently known and most familiar phenomena that are the simplest from the point of view of an explanatory theoretical construction" (ibid., pp. 150–151). Simple is not synonymous with familiar or intuitive. This epistemological remark suggests that the progress of knowledge is not linear although it is oriented towards the search for identity, for an invariant in all frames of reference.[3] Curiously, however, Langevin did not develop this epistemological consideration when he addressed philosophers in the session at the French Society of Philosophy (Langevin 1922c).

10.3 A Memorable Session at the *Société française de philosophie*

Xavier Léon, president of the French Society of Philosophy, opened the meeting with these words: "The date of April 6, 1922, will go down in the annals of our Society as an epoch-making event, and the presence of the brilliant author of the theory of special and general relativity is an honour of which it is fully aware"

---

[3] This epistemological remark could proceed from Langevin's conversations with Emile Meyerson, a philosopher who frequently visited at EPCI in the early 1920s to discuss issues of relativity. Meyerson assumed that, in science as in common knowledge, the human mind is driven by a quest for identity involving a reduction of diversity [4, 14]. Simplicity is the result of this rational impulse.

(ibid., p. 349). Einstein's French was not very good, so the session was introduced by Langevin.

He begins with an insistent emphasis on the physical dimension of the theory of relativity: "The theory of relativity is first and foremost a physical theory; it starts from known facts and leads to the prediction of new facts; it is essentially experimental" (ibid., p. 351). At first glance, the positivistic tone of this opening remark seems almost rhetorical because he moves on to present the difference between the axioms underlying the special relativity and those of general relativity. Axioms and experiments, Langevin strikes a balance between the empirical and the mathematical interpretations of the general relativity. He plays on two fronts: on the one hand, he insists on the consistency and beauty of a theory capable of embracing a multitude of phenomena on the basis of a few axioms. On the other hand, he insists on its experimental foundations to respond to those, Duhem and Mach among others,[4] who considered Einstein's theory as a mathematical game that defies common sense and cultivates paradox.

Above all, Langevin wants to convince the philosophical audience of the realism of the new notion of time emerging from the theory of relativity.

> For special relativity, each system of inertia had its own particular time. In generalised relativity, on the other hand, the systems of inertia disappear, and this disappearance makes it impossible for there to be a common time for all reference systems. All that remains is the notion of proper time measured by the arc of the trajectory of the universe described by a given material point; but it is not possible to establish unequivocal relationships between the proper times of different material points. (Ibid., p. 352)

In thus insisting on the physicality or reality of Einstein's notion of time, Langevin sought to rekindle the debate with philosophers that he had initiated in 1911. How did the audience react?

10.4 Dialogue and Misunderstandings

The debate was opened after Langevin's talk. It followed a protocol based on a tacit hierarchy of disciplines. The mathematicians first took the floor, Jacques Hadamard, Elie Cartan, Paul Painlevé, followed by the physicists, Paul Lévy, Perrin and Langevin.

Finally, the floor was open for the guest philosophers. Léon Brunschvicg seeks to clarify the relationship between relativity theory and Kantianism. Instead of talking about the Kantian conception of space and time (outdated by relativistic physics), he argues that in the Einsteinian world it is impossible to distinguish between the container (the forms of space and time) and the contents (events and substances).

---

[4] During World War One, Duhem dismissed the relativity theory as an exemplar of the algebraic and deductive excesses of the "Germanic spirit" [8, pp. 134–139]. Mach, shortly before his death, was indignant at being sometimes considered as a precursor of this new dogmatism far removed from experience.

Like a magician Einstein gets rid of Kant's antinomies of pure reason (ibid., pp. 357–358). He thus causes great joy among philosophers. Brunschvicg claims that Einstein's theory is revolutionary in the sense that it fully accomplishes the connection that Kant outlined between mathematics and physics. Einstein replies with a touch of irony: "I think every philosopher has his own Kant" (ibid., p. 359). For him, Kant is more about a priori categories and in this respect the relativity theory is incompatible with Kantianism.

Then, Edouard Leroy makes a short comment arguing that the time of philosophers and the time of the physicists are two different things and he quickly leaves the floor to Bergson (ibid., p. 359).

Bergson raises no objections to the relativistic concept of time, but he endorses the common sense hypothesis of a universal time, common to consciousness and things. He claims that the multiple times of relativity exclude neither the intuition of duration nor the philosopher's time on the simultaneity of events. Bergson agrees with Einstein's operational definition of simultaneity by the synchronization of clocks:

> If we take the simultaneity from this standpoint—and this is what the theory of relativity does—it is clear that simultaneity has nothing absolute about it, and that the same events will be simulated or successive depending on the point of view from which they are considered. (Ibid., p. 362)

Bergson suggests that the simultaneity proceeding from the indications of two clocks is a purely contingent or conventional procedure of measurement. He is more concerned with the perception of simultaneity between an event E and a clock H, a problem that is not addressed by the physicist's definition of simultaneity. Bergson concludes: "Once the theory of relativity as a physical theory has been accepted, everything is not finished. [...] What remains to be done is to determine what is real and what is conventional in the results it produces, or rather in the intermediaries it establishes between the position and the solution of the problem" (ibid., p. 364). And he ends on a tentative conciliation: "I believe that the theory of relativity is not incompatible with the ideas of common sense".

Einstein replies that the time common to consciousness and to things and the simultaneity of events, are nothing but local, mental constructions. So for him there is nothing like a philosopher's time; there is only a psychological time, different from the physicist's time. It's a brutal response, particularly indelicate when you're the guest of a society of philosophers! Undoubtedly, Einstein disagreed with the conventionalist overtones of Bergson's interpretation of the physicist's time. He presumably tries to prevent purely formalist interpretations of the theory of relativity. And he obviously lacked nuance in his handling of the French language.[5] Even so, his response denied philosophers the right to talk about time.

After this exchange, which must have made the audience cringe, Meyerson pacifies the debate. He modestly asks Einstein for clarification but nevertheless raises

---

[5] According to Jean Langevin, Einstein whispered in Paul Langevin's ear that he didn't understand a word in Bergson's talk [12].

two serious criticisms. He disapproves of the concept of time as a "fourth dimension" of space, because it is incompatible with the second principle of thermodynamics that implies the irreversibility of time. He finds the term "relativity" equally inappropriate, because in his view the theory of relativity is fundamentally realist, aiming for the absolute and should be disconnected from Mach's positivism. Einstein agrees on both points adding that "Mach was good at mechanics", but that he was "a miserable philosopher" (ibid., pp. 368–369).

10.5 Impacts of Einstein's Visit

To conclude this chapter, let us try to assess the impact of these few days of intense debates in Paris. Einstein's visit was, first and foremost, a Parisian social event and a political event for the public at large, who saw in this visit the symbol of the "Internationale of the Mind". In this respect, it was a success. For an entire week science triumphed over nationalist passions. It was also a great moment in Langevin's individual life, one of those rare moments when he managed to pursue several of his dearest struggles in a single week: building peace, advancing physics theory and sharing knowledge across boundaries. Langevin will never again have the opportunity to pursue all his ambitions in one week.

The combination of scientific and political struggles was no longer possible when Langevin visited Berlin the next year as a member of the League of Human Rights. He arrived in Berlin, accompanied by Jean, his eldest son. They were certainly well received, both at Einstein's home and by the crowd of activists of the *Nie wieder krieg* movement. But so intense was the popular resentment that Langevin could not give a public talk in person (although he was fluent in German). His message was read by the leader of the German movement. The French press reported that "The police prefect forbade Mr. Langevin from speaking, because as a Frenchman he could cause trouble" (Fig. 10.5).

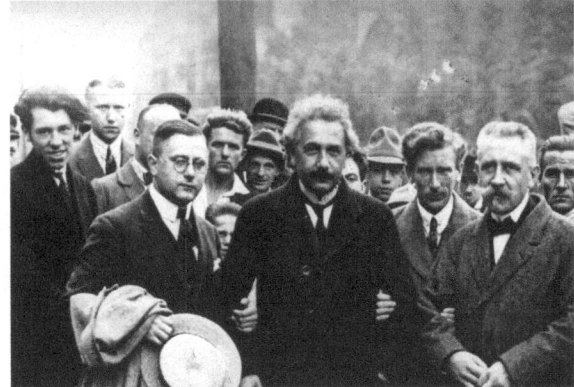

Fig. 10.5 Einstein and Langevin in Berlin 1923. (Hebrew University of Jerusalem)

On his return, he wrote a rather pessimistic report describing the miserable condition of the Germans, the queues in the shops, the empty trams, the soaring prices. To conclude, he firmly condemned the attitude of the French occupying troops and closed with a pathetic warning: "The higher intellectual functions are compromised, the brain substance in the country threatens not to renew itself" (Archives L028/048). So, in retrospect, 1922 appears as a unique moment, a fragile and quasi miracle conjunction of the two planets science and politics.

From a scientific perspective, Einstein's visit was the crowning event of Langevin's long battle for the new physics that had commenced before the war. During the debates at the *Collège de France*, which were lively and sometimes tumultuous, Einstein, supported by Langevin and Charles Nordmann, certainly did not manage to convince the entire physics community. But the conversion of Painlevé to relativity after the first discussion was a decisive conquest because he had a high scientific authority and a high political position.

However, was it really a triumph of the theory of relativity or the success of a certain image of science, symbolized by Einstein's smile? The lay public could hardly follow the discussions between experts and, for most people, the theory of relativity remained incomprehensible. Still, these scholarly meetings were enjoyable. They demonstrated that there are still minds that live on the heights, above the fray. The spirit is still alive. It did not die in the trenches.[6] It survived the atrocities of war. Perhaps the debates over the theory of relativity were reassuring precisely because they were understandable. It is comforting, when one feels blind and helpless, to know that there are people who see clearly, "visionaries" experienced in dealing with the greatest intellectual challenges, capable of leading the crowd and guiding humanity: in short, an enlightened elite. It is even better to discover that such "visionaries", or magi, are also human. The press often concentrated on Einstein's smile, his humour and fantasy [6, p. 43], a figure of hope that announced salvation. It is almost as though it was the Messiah that was given a Paris welcome in Spring 1922.

Finally, the debate at the French Society of Philosophy had a tremendous cultural impact in France. It was the acme of the French tradition of dialogue between scientists and philosophers although it ended in a series of monologues. The difficulties of communication proceeded from overlapping interests between scientists and philosophers. Ironically, the two communities were suddenly too close for them to understand each other and cooperate. Einstein's humiliating reply to Bergson marked the beginning of a divorce between French philosophers and scientists [7]. The controversy sparked during Einstein's visit turned into a campaign of attacks when Bergson developed his views in *Durée et simultanéité*, after the debate [5]. Jean Becquerel and André Metz, a young career officer, waged a bitter campaign to demonstrate that Bergson misunderstood the paradox of Langevin's traveller. "In the name of truth", Metz joined forces with Einstein to ridicule Bergson who

---

[6] Leopold Infeld, one of Einstein's close collaborators, explained the public enthusiasm for his theory by the social aspiration to forget about the horrors of the war and to focus on ideas and people that transcend the patriotic interests (Infeld quoted in Lévy-Leblond [13, p. 26]).

responded head on in the appendices of the reprints of the book. He decided to interrupt the reprints of *Durée et simultanéité* in 1932. This measure stopped the fierce attacks but did not put an end to the controversy. Remarkably, one century later, the debate is still going and has aroused enough interest among physicists and philosophers to justify two recent critical reprints of *Durée et simultanéité* in 2009 and 2021 [9, 13]. Both editors defend Bergson's arguments, while acknowledging a few errors in his interpretation of Langevin's paradox.

Meyerson, who was better able to enter into conversations with Langevin and Einstein, also sparked a fierce controversy. In 1925, he published *La déduction relativiste*, a book inspired by Langevin's interpretation, as he acknowledged in the preface:

> There are many pages in this book for which we cannot claim exclusive ownership. First of all, the initial idea of such work came out of a conversation we had on the eve of Mr. Einstein's arrival in Paris with Mr. Paul Langevin and where we were able to see how much the conception to which the latter had spontaneously arrived on the subject of the realistic essence of the theory of relativity agreed with the principles that we believed we could deduce by examining the physical sciences in general and especially their evolution. Mr. Langevin also provided us with part of the documentation we have used (…) and constantly helped me overcome the technical difficulties that arose. [15, p. XV]

While Bergson focused on the question of time, Meyerson concentrates on the question of space. In his view, relativity is a spatialization of phenomena. The identification of inertia and gravitation requires the identification of physics and geometry. For Meyerson the theory of relativity is not driven by experimental results. It is above all a deductive science based on a minimum of axioms, a form of pan-mathematism. Meyerson presents the theory of relativity as an exemplar of the aspirations of the human intellect to deduce reality from reason. Einstein read Meyerson's book and seemed to recognize himself in this portrait of a realistic metaphysician although he raised a few objections [2]. He nevertheless wrote a positive review of the book [11].[7]

Meyerson's *The Relativistic Deduction* triggered an alternative interpretation of the theory of relativity by Gaston Bachelard, who opposed Meyerson in *The Inductive Value of Relativity* [1]. We can thus appreciate the extent of Langevin's influence in the history of French philosophy.

References

1. Bachelard G (1929) La Valeur inductive de la relativité. Vrin, Paris. (reprint 2014)
2. Balibar F (2010) Meyerson et Einstein, éloges et malentendus. Corpus Revue de Philosophie 58:63–79
3. Becquerel J (1922) Principe de relativité et théorie de la gravitation. Gauthier-Villars, Paris

---

[7] In fact, Meyerson took advantage of Metz's revision of the translation to propose changes that mitigated Einstein's objections (see Bensaude-Vincent and Telkès-Klein [4], p. 187).

4. Bensaude-Vincent B, Telkes-Klein E (2017) Les identités multiples d'Emile Meyerson. Champion, Paris
5. Bergson H (1922) Durée et simultanéité. Payot, Paris. English trans: Duration and simultaneity. Clinamen Press (1999)
6. Biezunski M (1981) Einstein à Paris. Presses de l'Université de Vincennes, Paris
7. Canales J (2016) The physicist and the philosopher: Einstein, Bergson, and the debate that changed our understanding of time. Princeton, Princeton University Press
8. Duhem P (1915) La Science allemande. Hermann, Paris.
9. During E (2009) Presentation and annotation of Henri Bergson *Durée et simultanéité*. PUF Quadrige, Paris
10. Eddington A (1923) Mathematical theory of relativity. Cambridge University Press, Cambridge
11. Einstein A (1928) A propos de la *Déduction relativiste*. Revue philosophique de la France et de l'étranger 105(3/4):161–166
12. Langevin J (1979) Le séjour d'Einstein à Paris. Cahiers Fundamenta Scientiae 93(1979):91–113
13. Lévy-Leblond J-M (ed) (2021) Presentation and annotation of Henri Bergson *Durée et simultanéité*. Garnier Flammarion, Paris
14. Meyerson E (1908) Identité et réalité. Alcan, Paris. English trans: Identity and reality. Allen and Unwin/Macmillan, London/New York (1930)
15. Meyerson E (1925) La Déduction relativiste. Payot, Paris. English trans: The relativistic deduction. Reidel Publishing, Dordrecht (1985)
16. Nordmann C (1921) Einstein et l'univers. Une lueur dans le mystère des choses. Hachette, Paris
17. Nordmann C (1923) Notre maître le temps. Hachette, Paris
18. Pascoli G (2017) "The Sagnac effect and its interpretation by Paul Langevin". *Comptes-rendus de l'Académie des sciences*. C R Phys 18:563–569. https://comptes-rendus.academie-sciences. fr/physique/articles/10.1016/j.crhy.2017.10.010/
19. Simões A, Sousa AM (2019) The global adventure of science: Einstein, Eddington and the eclipse. Chili com Carne, Lisbon

Chapter 11
Ultrasonics in Peacetime

Abstract Langevin continued his activities in ultrasonics well into the 1920s. He successfully patented his quartz sandwich transducer in Europe, although failed in the USA as a result of prior patents by Nicolson and Pupin, based on the trans-Atlantic wartime transfer of knowledge. Langevin remained an external advisor to the Naval laboratory in Toulon, which focused attention on ultrasonic transducer design and measurement. He advised on hydrophone design, and a novel power meter with Ishimoto, visiting from Japan. He patented the "Langevin stack" transducer. He gave a course on ultrasonics at the *Collège de France* in 1924. Driven in part by Chilowsky, echo sounding was developed commercially by SCAM, their two patents assigned under license. Langevin failed to gain significant remuneration on behalf of Chilowsky from the British Admiralty. The ultrasonic investigations of Wood, Boyle, Brillouin and Biquard were all inspired by Langevin.

Ultrasonic detection of enemy submarines was never used in action by either the French or the British navy during the First World War. In some ways, the wartime work of Langevin was an operational failure. At that time, the modest financial investment in the development of this entirely novel technology saved no lives and prevented no sinkings.

Nevertheless, there were two, linked peacetime outcomes from Langevin's wartime foray into applied physics and engineering. The first, negative, taking much of his time and resources, was his involvement with claims and counterclaims concerning patents. The second and positive outcome was the successful development of ultrasonic echo-sounding, the first commercial outcome of ultrasonic technology. Langevin took part in both these activities during much of the 1920s. But, to set the context, it is necessary to return to the wartime developments in ultrasonics.

11.1 International Patent Competition

Most historical narratives have suggested that Langevin was not only the "originator of the science and art of modern ultrasonics" but that he also pursued patents for personal gain [7, 12]. Certainly, there were some at the time who were seeking financial gain, either personal or corporate. Langevin himself ensured that others, such as Chilowsky and Jacques Curie, benefitted from these developments. But, although in due course he would receive considerable income from the commercial exploitation of his discoveries and inventions, the evidence suggests that he did not initiate negotiations, and largely accepted the outcome when others set a monetary value on his input. In this chapter, we explore how these events played out.

On 7 July 1917, towards the end of Boyle's stay in Toulon, Tournier had shared with Langevin his concerns on the ownership of the intellectual property of piezoelectric transduction in ultrasonics.

> If you do not forthwith obtain a patent ensuring your ownership of all the details, there will perhaps shortly appear, and perchance in England … another Marconi who will procure for himself all possible advantages hereafter. [16]

As Tournier was aware, Chilowsky and Langevin had already filed for patents in France, Britain and the USA that covered the basic principles of directional ultrasonic detection and communication, and descriptions of capacitor transducers. His new concern is to protect the use of quartz for ultrasonic transduction. But Langevin had a reputation for delaying publication until he had explored a topic to his full satisfaction. The 60 kHz laminated resonant quartz transducer that Tournier identified as in need of patent protection was only one stage in Langevin's careful progression towards a device that would be as complete as he could imagine. For the present, Langevin did nothing.

Tournier was correct, of course. It was not, however, in England that "another Marconi" appeared, but in the USA. By the time Tournier wrote to Langevin in July 1917, it was already too late to prevent others claiming "title of ownership".

The USA had declared war on Germany on 6 April 1917. This action opened official channels of communication between the USA and the other Allies, France, Britain and Italy, on all matters to do with the war, specifically sharing details of military scientific and technical activities. A joint Anglo-French delegation was arranged, to inform the new American colleagues of the current status of Allied military research and to seek assistance from American finance, organization and expertise. In this way, the news of Langevin's breakthrough using quartz transduction crossed the Atlantic.

The Anglo-French mission set off to the USA in the middle of May 1917. The British mission was led by Ernest Rutherford and the French contingent by Charles Fabry, professor at the Sorbonne. Langevin did not go. Rutherford visited him in Paris on 18 May, to ensure that he was fully informed on the status of the French progress. It was Tournier's opinion that, when Fabry and Rutherford spoke in Washington on 15 June, Rutherford undoubtedly communicated what he had

11.1 International Patent Competition

learned from Langevin during his Paris visit (Archives L142/008). Those attending these presentations included representatives from American military, academia and industry [7, p. 51].

It is unsurprising, therefore, that one outcome was exactly what Tournier had feared. More than one anticipated "Marconi" emerged. The first was a Serbian-born physicist and engineer, Michael Pupin, from Columbia University, who was leading a group on submarine detection. He was also a prolific patentee. Robert Wood, on his return from France in January 1918, updated Pupin on all he had learned from his visits to Langevin's laboratories. On 4 February 1918, Pupin filed for a patent that included a thin x-cut quartz crystal as a receiver of sound waves up to 100 kHz [15]. In doing so, he claimed for himself the discovery that Langevin had made a year earlier. Adding insult to injury, he also successfully filed for a French patent.

The other patentee was an Argentinian-born Englishman, working for the Western Electric Company in New York, Alexander McLean Nicolson, a talented engineer who had already taken out patents on the design and use of thermionic valves. Just before Rutherford returned to England at the end of his visit to North America he was invited to return to the Western Electric Company, and it is fair to assume that it was during these visits that Nicolson's interest was aroused in the scientific and commercial possibilities presented by the piezoelectric properties of some crystals, as revealed by Langevin's preliminary results.

Less than a year later, on 2 and 10 April 1918, Nicolson applied for two patents on the production and use of piezoelectric transducers made from Rochelle salt, sodium potassium tartrate, a crystal with very strong piezoelectric properties. The first explained how to grow such crystals. The second, titled *Piezophony*, proposed their use for "telephone transmitters and receivers, repeaters, loud speakers, generators and modulators of alternating currents and the like" [13]. It alluded to the "purely experimental work" of Pierre Curie but added not a word about Langevin. The patent states "It has been discovered that piezo-electrical crystals may be used to particular advantage in submarine signaling and for the detection of hostile submarines" a direct reference to work that was, at this date, secret and still incomplete. Together with Pupin's patent, Nicolson's patent, with its 36 claims, will be used to successfully block Langevin's 1920 patent application in the USA.

Tournier also wanted to protect his own the intellectual property arising from the work being carried out in Toulon. In July 1918, following the successful completion of sea trials, a French patent application was submitted in the joint names of Langevin, Colin, Tournier and Holweck, to protect their electronic design for heterodyne transmission. The *Télégraphie militaire* challenged this application, stating that the work was done for national defense, drawing on confidential information while working for the Navy. Langevin withdrew the application, saying that it was submitted in good faith, and apologized for his clumsiness. The application was most likely intended to give credit to his co-workers, who had designed and tested the circuit (Archives L137).

11.2 Langevin's 1918 Patent

Finally, on 18 September 1918, Langevin filed his own patent for his quartz sandwich transducer. The motivation for this patent was very different from that of the Chilowsky and Langevin patent 2 years earlier.

The background lies in the personal trust and friendship between Langevin and William Bragg. With Langevin's guidance, Bragg had successfully re-launched the British ultrasonics project. But, in January 1918, Bragg had been appointed as Scientific Advisor to the Admiralty and was replaced by the physicist Arthur S Eve. Then, in a letter of 24 June 1918, Eve raised the question of patent rights, from an understandable concern over the protection of the intellectual property being now freely exchanged between the Allies. But, unlike his own predecessor Bragg and the ultrasonics lead Boyle, Eve had no close association with the ultrasonic project and so he was in no position to separate the possible claims of those who had been involved. He did admit, though, that "the advance has been a general one in which M. Langevin has played an outstanding part".

On 28 August, writing from Toulon, de Broglie warned Langevin that Bragg had told him the British Admiralty were thinking of taking out patents in the names of Rutherford and Boyle, although insisting that "your name appear on them and that they would contact you" (Archives L194/051).

Langevin recognized the difference between his own resonant quartz transducer and the non-resonant design that Boyle had used. So he decided to file a patent that covered only that part of the work that was uniquely his, carried out in Paris and Toulon and was not duplicated in any way by Boyle and the British team.

Eve knew Rutherford well, having worked with him in the physics department at McGill in Montreal, Canada, when they were both there in the early 1900s. The reintroduction of Rutherford's name, someone who had had no direct involvement with the ultrasonics project, is entirely due to Eve. As he noted in his later biography of Rutherford:

> Some of us advocated the view that Rutherford had originated the scheme of the piezoelectric-submarine detector, whereas Langevin had claimed priority. Rutherford's reply to me was short and final "If Langevin says the idea was his, then the idea was Langevin's". [4, p. 307]

Only 3 weeks after he heard from Bragg, Langevin applied for a French patent in which he set out a detailed specification of his resonant quartz sandwich transducer (Langevin 1918a). In a letter to the Admiral Lacaze, Naval Prefect of Toulon, on 2 October, he acknowledged the British plan, and included a copy of his own patent application on "the invention as I communicated it through Dr Boyle" to be forwarded to the English Admiralty. He left open the possibility of additions arising from Boyle's and Rutherford's "improvements based on what I regard to be my personal contribution", in which case he offered to consider modifying "my original intention in the manner desired by the English Admiralty" (Archives L138/176). Unsurprisingly, this never happened.

11.2 Langevin's 1918 Patent

Nevertheless, Eve's claim on Rutherford's behalf persisted and grew. As late as 1983, in a lengthy biography of Rutherford, it was still claimed that "the official record bears out Rutherford's unmade claim to be at least the co-inventor of sonar" [17, p. 375]. Nothing could be further from the truth. There was no correspondence on ultrasonics between Rutherford and Langevin. With one notable exception, there is no mention of Rutherford's ideas about ultrasonics in the official papers. Numerous letters were written to Langevin and to the French Navy from senior British scientists, including Eve, Eccles, Paget and Bragg, but not one from Rutherford. Apart from their briefing meeting in May 1917, prior to the mission to the USA, Rutherford never met Langevin for the purpose of discussing the ultrasonics project. The sole contribution, noted in Chap. 8, was Rutherford's proposal to the BIR in September 1916 to repurpose a Curie *piézoeléctrique* as a possible source of ultrasound.

Langevin's concise three-page patent describes all the essential components of his resonant quartz piezoelectric sandwich transducer. The physics of ultrasound propagation, described in the previous patent, is assumed. The preliminary claims include ultrasonic waves generated by x-cut quartz and by using the natural resonance of a quartz slice. The specific claims are supported by three figures, each showing one of the key functional elements (Fig. 11.1).

Thus, concisely, Langevin described his quartz sandwich transducer (Fig. 11.2). He made no attempt to cover Boyle's non-resonant layered design, with its rugged

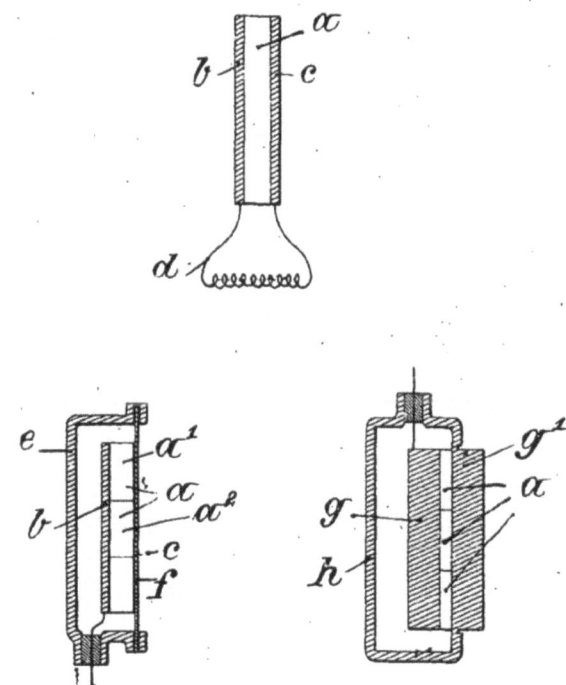

Fig. 11.1 Langevin filed for a patent in 1918 for his quartz piezoelectric ultrasound transducer. (1) A single x-cut quartz plate in electrical resonance with an appropriate coil, operating either as an emitter or a receiver of elastic waves. (2) A quartz mosaic, half-wave resonant: one electrode is sea-water separated from the quartz by a thin mica sheet, the other is backed by air. (3) Air-backed resonant sandwich transducer, quartz mosaic between steel plates. (ESPCI, PSL University L167/035)

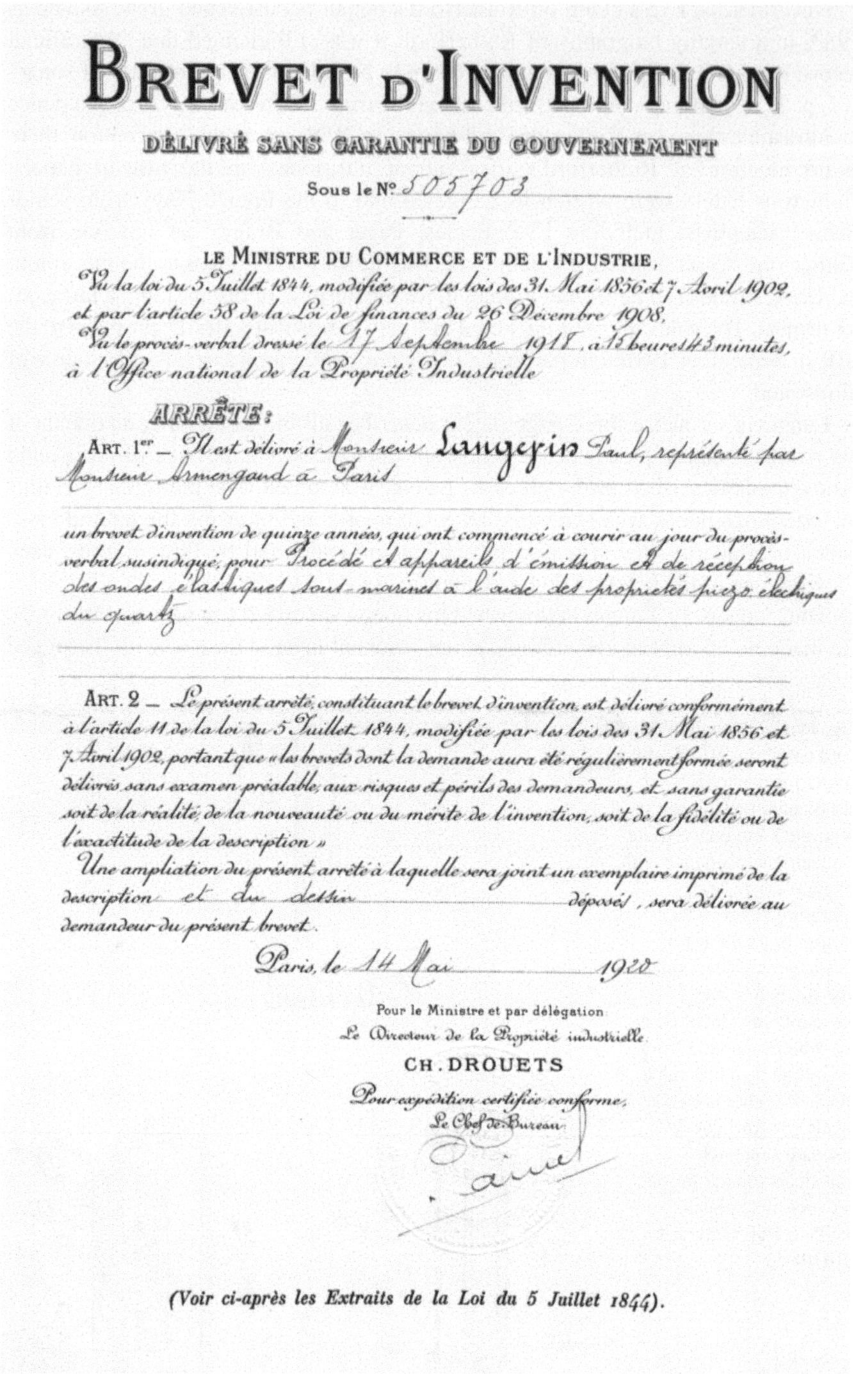

BREVET D'INVENTION

DÉLIVRÉ SANS GARANTIE DU GOUVERNEMENT

Sous le N° 505703

LE MINISTRE DU COMMERCE ET DE L'INDUSTRIE,

Vu la loi du 5 Juillet 1844, modifiée par les lois des 31 Mai 1856 et 7 Avril 1902, et par l'article 38 de la Loi de finances du 26 Décembre 1908,

Vu le procès-verbal dressé le 17 Septembre 1918, à 15 heures 43 minutes, à l'Office national de la Propriété Industrielle

ARRÊTE :

ART. 1er — Il est délivré à Monsieur **Langevin** Paul, représenté par Monsieur Armengaud à Paris

un brevet d'invention de quinze années, qui ont commencé à courir au jour du procès-verbal susindiqué, pour Procédé et appareils d'émission et de réception des ondes élastiques sous-marines à l'aide des propriétés piézo-électriques du quartz.

ART. 2 — Le présent arrêté, constituant le brevet d'invention, est délivré conformément à l'article 11 de la loi du 5 Juillet 1844, modifiée par les lois des 31 Mai 1856 et 7 Avril 1902, portant que « les brevets dont la demande aura été régulièrement formée seront délivrés sans examen préalable, aux risques et périls des demandeurs, et sans garantie soit de la réalité, de la nouveauté ou du mérite de l'invention, soit de la fidélité ou de l'exactitude de la description »

Une ampliation du présent arrêté à laquelle sera joint un exemplaire imprimé de la description et du dessin déposés, sera délivrée au demandeur du présent brevet.

Paris, le 14 Mai 1920

Pour le Ministre et par délégation
Le Directeur de la Propriété industrielle

CH. DROUETS

Pour expédition certifiée conforme,
Le Chef de Bureau

(Voir ci-après les Extraits de la Loi du 5 Juillet 1844).

Fig. 11.2 The French patent for the piezoelectric quartz ultrasonic transducer was awarded on 14 May 1920. (ESPCI, PSL University L167/035)

resin encapsulation. He left a loophole open for the British Admiralty to file its own complementary patent, if it so wished. But, soon, Boyle returned to Canada and Rutherford, even if he had wished to pursue the matter, had taken up the prestigious position as Cavendish Chair of Experimental Physics at Cambridge, replacing J.J. Thomson.

After considerable discussion, documented elsewhere [12], an equivalent UK patent application was filed on 30 June 1920 (Langevin 1920). With interest growing in commercial exploitation, patent applications in other countries followed, successful in Germany and Italy, unsuccessful in Japan and the USA.

Did Langevin intend any personal gain in filing his patent? This seems unlikely. The Interallied Meeting on Supersonics, noted: "Owing to the financial disinterestedness of the French and English inventors (i.e. Langevin and Boyle) it was desirable to take steps to prevent profiteering or construction or patent royalties by other parties". Langevin's son André went further in his biography of his father.

> No man was more disinterested than he was and he had no love of money. As soon as he had a little, he spent it with pleasure; he loved to give gifts to his family and friends, he was incapable of resisting a sponger, and as the members of this honourable guild of hangers-on communicated to each other, my father assembled a very large number of lawyers. [10, p. 73]

11.3 Ultrasonics Survives

Will ultrasonics research and development survive in France into peacetime? Scarce financial resources will need to be carefully directed and protected. During the first months of peace, Langevin makes regular visits to Toulon, guiding Tournier and Holweck, under Captain Moysan's supervision, ensuring that the ultrasonic laboratory is not disbanded. But quite the opposite happens. The war-time laboratory of submarine warfare is reconfigured and extended to become the *Laboratoire du centre d'études de Toulon* (LCET), adding activities including coastal artillery, optics and telemetry, mines and grenades, radio and submarines. This multi-faceted laboratory becomes the scientific and technical interface between the navy, academia and industry. The staff of about 30 is given contracts, a salary structure and prospects. The centre has facilities for research and prototyping, a library and workshops. Langevin and his academic colleagues, Perrin, Tournier, Holweck, Brillouin and Becquerel, become "external collaborators".

Under continuing guidance from Langevin, LCET concentrates on the measurement of ultrasound output and on new transducer designs. As systems for echosounding and ultrasonic navigation became manufactured for the navy and for commercial use, transducers are sent to LCET for certification. In this way, LCET becomes the first independent testing laboratory for ultrasonics [3]. Even so, Langevin has to be persistent. He proposes a design for a quartz hydrophone, to measure the distribution of local intensity in the ultrasonic beam. There is no interest and this project is cancelled until Langevin intervenes personally.

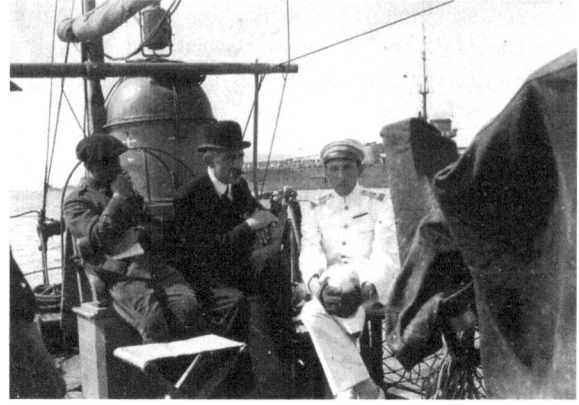

Fig. 11.3 Collaboration between Langevin and the French Navy continued after the war, and he regularly visited Toulon for discussions. Here he is seen on board the ship *l'Orage* in 1919. (ESPCI)

Ultrasonics itself was revitalized by echo-sounding. If the beam from Langevin's 40 kHz quartz sandwich transducer were to be directed downwards, instead of horizontally towards a submarine or mine, naval captains would have a new tool for navigation, especially useful in shallow water. Following the demobilization of Tournier and Holweck in 1919, and their return to Paris, the electrical engineer Charles-Louis Florisson took the lead in re-purposing the ultrasonic submarine hunter (Langevin 1923b). He was tasked by Langevin to redesign the equipment to emit very short pulses, to be capable of high precision time measurement, and to be operated by relatively inexperienced personnel. The first successful sea-trials were carried out off Cicié near Toulon in the early summer of 1920, reaching a depth of 1100 m with a precision of 5 m. This was followed by an official demonstration off Nice in October 1920 (Fig. 11.3).

In December 1920, Langevin met Pierre Marti of the French Hydrographic Service, who had been asked by Moysan to create a continuous-reading depth recorder, plotting the change in echo with time as the boat moved. His first device, a drum recorder using smoked paper, adapted from one manufactured by Georges Boulitte for blood pressure recording, was finished in April 1921 [11]. At the same time, Florisson developed his own optical analyzer, more accurate for spot soundings but without continuous recording. Both recording systems were given extensive sea-trials during the summer of 1922.

The work remained secret, under the control of the Navy. Langevin visits, advises, encourages, guides, negotiates, but cannot freely inform others. Marti also wanted to publish details of his recorder in *Comptes rendus*, but the navy refused, unless details of the apparatus are omitted to prevent foreign competition gaining an advantage.

11.4 Chilowsky Reappears

On 17 September 1919, an agreement had been concluded between Chilowsky, Langevin and the Minister of the Navy for the sale of a licence to use their joint patent. The French Government acquired the license, and the Ministry paid Chilowsky

11.4 Chilowsky Reappears

100,000 francs. Langevin assigned all the rights belonging to him to the State, free of charge, receiving only minor expenses [8, p. 71].

This lump sum allowed Chilowsky to set himself up as a freelance inventor. During the next 3 years, he filed five patents on topics as diverse as sound recording (1919) processing heavy engine fuel (1921) and Doppler measurement for absolute ship speed (1921). Several were also protected in Britain, the USA, Germany and Sweden. This all came with legal costs and, without finding any new backing, Chilowsky was looking to an uncertain financial future.

So he was highly motivated to find a way to commercialize the echo-sounder that had been developed for the navy in Toulon. On 5 August 1922, a project was awarded to the SFR (*Société Française Radio-électrique*) to arrange a 6-year manufacturing contract for the civilian use of ultrasonic technology on behalf of Langevin and Chilowsky. The agreement provided for the use of the device for measuring sea depth, directional telephony, direction finding and searching for navigational obstacles. It took until 3 February 1923 for Langevin to gain an agreement with Chilowsky about how any future income should be shared. And it took an arbitration commission that included Paul Painlevé, Jules Breton and Charles Morin to adjudicate: "That in any application thereof involving piezoelectric transmission devices ... whether problems of navigation, medical problems, or others, the possible income shall be divided as follows: one third to Chilowsky, two thirds to Langevin". This ratio was based on an estimated relative value of the original proposal by Chilowsky compared with the value of the practical solution by Langevin. A final stipulation was that "Negotiations on the use of ultrasound will be carried out through a third party appointed by the arbitrators". The person appointed was the organic chemist Philippe Landrieu[1] from the *Collège de France*. Both patents were transferred to a holding company, for which Chilowsky and Langevin received 100,000 Francs.

Several companies made bids for the work. On 11 July 1923, the contract was awarded to the *Société de Condensation et d'Applications Méchaniques* (SCAM), a company without electronics expertise, but with a high level of specialist skill in cutting quartz and granite. Florisson was appointed as the chief engineer. Thus, without taking the lead, Langevin became central in the negotiations to create a commercial version of the depth-sounder and inevitably was drawn deeper into plans for further patent protection.

The sums received by the inventors as a result of this commercialization were substantial. From the first sales, in the second half of 1924, SCAM paid 15% or 5956.15 Francs. This was divided as follows: Langevin 46.5%, Chilowsky 24%, Florisson 10%, and Tournier 4.5%. Langevin allocated some of his share to others. He was still close to Marie Curie and her family, and ensured that some of this revenue was shared between her daughters, Irene and Ève (2.5% each) and with Pierre's brother Jacques (5%), whose PhD had originally described the *quartz piézo-électrique*. The Office of Inventions took the remainder. Lelong has estimated that,

---

[1] Philippe Landrieu (1873–1926), assistant professor at the *Collège de France*, was a Protestant intellectual socialist. Apart from his work as a scientist, he contributed to, and then managed, the socialist newspaper *l'Humanité*.

during the second half of the 1920s, Langevin received each year a sum of the order of 180,000 Francs, adding, however, that "we cannot deduce from this that Langevin made a fortune from ultrasonic detection: the archives give no evidence on his use of these receipts" [11].

Langevin was retained as a consultant by SCAM. Commercial interests required that any new intellectual property needed to be protected both in France and around the world: patents were filed in Great Britain, Germany, Italy, Holland, Sweden, Denmark, the United States, Japan and the USSR. A further patent by Langevin and Florisson was filed in December 1923 that declared the details of the commercial echo-sounder, including Florisson's depth indicator (Langevin 1923b). An associated patent, filed in January 1924, Langevin's alone, demonstrated his developed skills in electronic circuit design, giving a detailed description of two valve circuits suitable for timing the returning echo (Langevin 1924a).

The sounder entered Naval service in May 1924 (Archives L136/002). By the late 1920s, the *Sondeur Ultra-sonore Langevin-Florisson-Marti* was being widely installed on merchant and passenger ships (Fig. 11.4). "Langevin" had become a maritime brand name.

11.4 Chilowsky Reappears

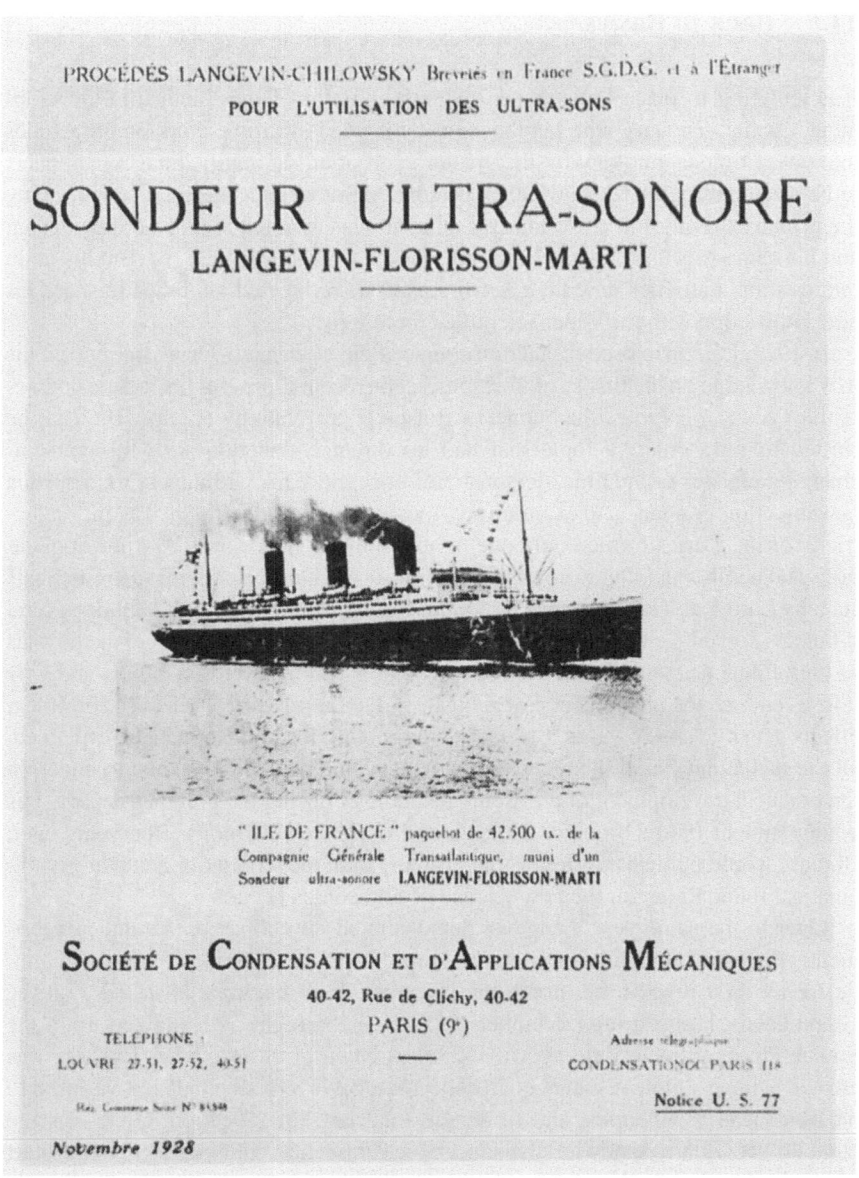

Fig. 11.4 *Le sondeur Langevin-Florisson-Marti* was the first civil application of ultrasonics and was installed by SCAM on many liners, including the *Ile de France (Science et Vigilance)*

11.5 Back to Basics

It is tempting to place Langevin as the sole initiator of these industrial developments, as the visionary who led the conversion of his wartime work on ultrasonics into peace-time technology for the greater good of all. In reality, Langevin appears to be a tolerant partner, Chilowsky's personal drive to gain financial benefit being the primary driving force. Certainly, Langevin was retained as a scientific advisor, and his name was used for publicity, e.g. for the Calais beacon [5, 6]. But his main interests and activities now lay elsewhere and he redirected his focus to share his new knowledge with the wider scientific community.

In 1923, Langevin used his lecture course at the *Collège de France* to present his new knowledge on the theory of ultrasonics. His recent topics for his lecture courses at the *Collège de France* had concerned aspects of relativity (Chap. 10). That he shifted to ultrasonics, a topic that had no direct connection with the concept-changing physics of the time, demonstrates once more his willingness to identify a new direction in science, to examine previously unexplored territory. The piezoelectricity of the Curies formed only one minor theme in his course. Wartime applications and depth-sounding were never mentioned. He built on classical acoustic texts such as Lord Rayleigh's *Theory of Sound*, extending the theory to include several problems solved for the first time. His theme was fundamental science, the physics of high frequency sound: how it propagates, how beams are formed, how and why it loses energy, the phenomenon of acoustic radiation pressure, even how non-linear effects generate shock waves. Langevin brought into the public arena, he explained, all the mathematics, all the theoretical analysis, that he had developed to underpin the practical development of ultrasonic technology during the previous decade. His young student Pierre Biquard attended, and made detailed notes. Ten years later, Biquard would publish a series of four articles, a unique record of Langevin's mathematical foundations for the new science of ultrasonics [1].

Later in the same year, Langevin demonstrated how to set up a simple experiment with an ultrasound beam in the laboratory. The experiment was shown in public for the first time at the month-long *Exposition de physique et de T.S.F* at the Grand Palais, Paris during December 1923, to celebrate the 50th anniversary of the French Physical Society (Langevin 1923c). A beam of ultrasound at 150 kHz was created using a simple resonant quartz slice. Langevin's torsion balance was used to measure beam boundaries, and to demonstrate laws of reflection. Gone was the large 40 kHz quartz sandwich transducer used for echo-sounding. Here is the start of experimental ultrasonics.

At the same meeting, Langevin introduced a visiting scientist from Japan, who had been working with him on a novel piezoelectric device for the measurement of ultrasonic power (Langevin 1923d). The torsion balance was perfect for measurements in the laboratory, but no use for making measurements at sea. A visit by the Japanese physicist Mishio Ishimoto allowed Langevin to take forward an idea for a robust electronic power balance. The detector was a quartz plate mounted so that acoustic force is applied perpendicularly to the electric axis. Ishimoto's visit was

11.5 Back to Basics

part of a general expansion in Franco-Japanese post-war scientific and cultural links and coincides with that of Nobuo Yamada to work at the Radium Institute with Marie Curie. Ishimoto's school friend Lt. Takeshi Nawa of the Japanese Navy was also in Paris and so learned of Langevin's work, a contact that will eventually lead to the Japanese Navy's interest in purchasing ultrasonic equipment from SCAM [14].

The date 27 January 1926 marks the end of Langevin's primary contributions to ultrasonics. He has shared with others all he has discovered about this new sector of theoretical and applied science. It is time to move on. On this day he filed one more patent, in his own name, into which he placed several innovative transducer designs and metrological advances, drawn together into a single document (Fig. 11.5). It was filed in two parts in Britain the following year (Langevin 1926b). More a scientific paper than a patent, it presents a careful theoretical analysis of the

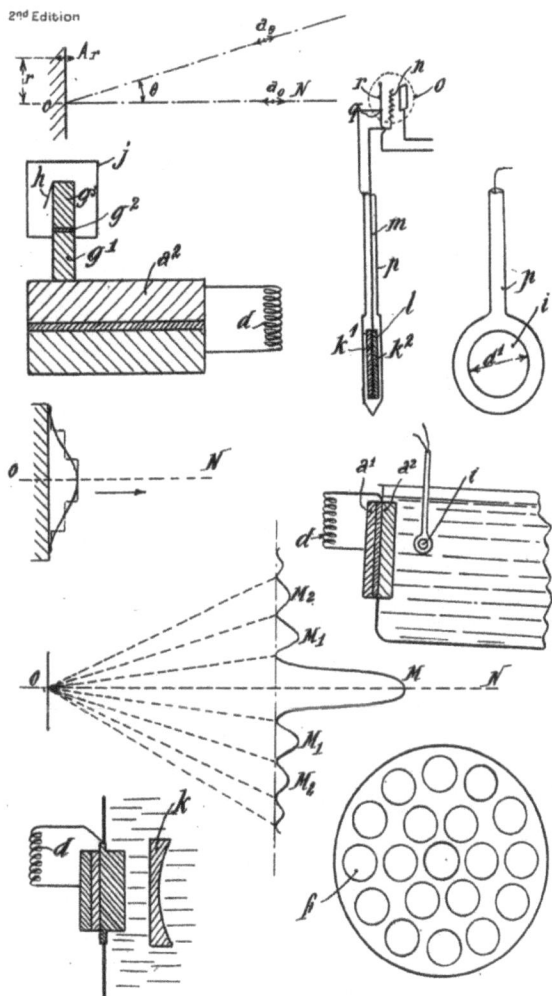

Fig. 11.5 Langevin's 1926 patent included several new innovations. (1) Theoretical definitions. (2) Probe for mapping surface vibration. (3)–(5) Screened broadband hydrophone. (6) Side lobes from circular piston source. (7) and (8) Array and apodization. (9) Acoustic lens. (Langevin 1926b; ESPCI, PSL University L139/044)

electromechanical losses in a quartz/steel sandwich transducer and, as a result, comes up with a many-layered design of improved efficiency, a design still known as the "Langevin stack". Additionally, Langevin describes two ways in which the beam may be modified, either using an acoustic lens, or an apodized array. Finally, two means of measurement are described, the first, resonant, to investigate the vibrating surface of the transducer, and the second, a thin screened quartz hydrophone to measure the acoustic field at any frequency.

Later that year, in May, Langevin visited Rutherford in Cambridge and give "an informal talk for an hour on 'supersonics'". Rutherford explained that the members of the Cambridge Physical Society had "not had papers on that subject" (Archives L076/045). Notes in English, perhaps for a different talk, reveal the level of mathematical detail he would have used (Fig. 11.6).

He retained an active interest in piezoelectricity, filing three more patents on various uses of quartz (Langevin 1927b, c, d). He also retained an interest in the difficult challenges posed by underwater acoustics (Langevin 1929d, 1931g). Eventually, as the time he devoted to political activities took their toll, he inspired both his son-in-law Jacques Solomon and his son André to add their own contributions to this new branch of physics (Langevin 1935b) [9].

11.6 Claims and Counterclaims

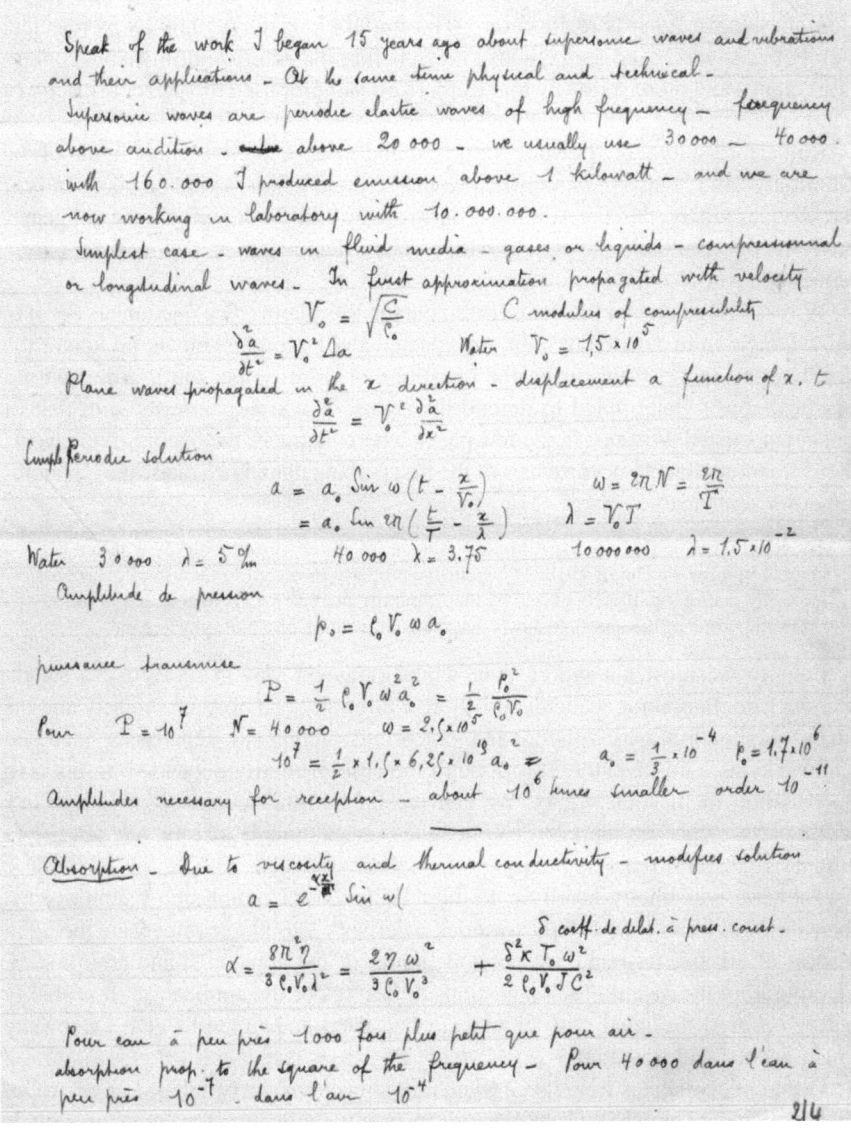

Fig. 11.6 Langevin's notes for a lecture in English on ultrasonics, c. 1930. (ESPCI, PSL University L174/002)

11.6 Claims and Counterclaims

During this same post-war period, Langevin had pursued negotiations with the British Admiralty, on behalf of Chilowsky and himself, for compensation for the benefit to the British Admiralty from ultrasonic developments during and after the war [18]. In October 1923, the Admiralty passed the claim on to the British Royal Commission on Awards to Inventors. The initial claim for £50,000 was rejected, stating that it was based on methods known before the war (a legitimate but contentious claim) and more seriously that Rutherford had proposed the piezoelectricity of quartz prior to the date of Langevin's first use.

Rutherford wrote that he was "surprised and disappointed by the attitude of the Admiralty" and "that a great injustice would be done to Langevin and his country if the services rendered to the Admiralty during a most difficult period were not generously recognized" (Archives L139/126). They decided to resubmit their claim, reducing it to £10,000.

Why is Langevin making the effort to pursue this claim? The documents seem to show Langevin in a different light, unexpected and largely unknown: no longer the disinterested theorist, despising the questions of priority, but the inventor with a practical sense, determined to defend his rights. The style contrasts with that of Langevin's usual writings: in the few pages where he traces the history of the work, there are more than 35 occurrences of the first person, namely "I" and "me", punctuate every sentence:

> The research undertaken at the Admiralty was on my initiative and with my constant collaboration until the end of 1918. My exclusive property in regard to the use of quartz has moreover been formally recognized by the Admiralty in 1920 (...) A historical and technical examination of the question shows that it is an invention of Chilowsky and me.

Equally we must not ignore that, while Langevin was in receipt of a steady income from his senior academic position, Chilowsky had no such security and his financial situation was volatile and precarious. Langevin generously included Chilowsky as a co-inventor, even though the case primarily depended on his own introduction of piezoelectricity. We can see here further evidence of Langevin's willingness to act in support of colleagues, even though history has tended to emphasize the clash of personality between these two men.

The case was finally heard on 19 July 1926.[2] The Commission recommended that Chilowsky and Langevin be awarded a derisory £2000 to compensate them "in respect of all use, past and present and future, of the apparatus, and arts thereof, incorporating the inventions, suggestions or designs of the applicants". It probably barely covered the legal costs. Langevin had tried and failed to give Chilowsky much-needed additional income.

Different challenges were faced when pursuing claims on behalf of Langevin and Florisson in the United States of America. A patent application for Langevin's sandwich transducer was filed in 1920, but then became embroiled in a separate patent battle between Alexander Nicolson and Walter Cady.[3] It was refused in 1924, and

---

[2] Tragically, Chilowsky's wife Olga had died earlier that year from injuries sustained in a subway accident.

[3] Walter Guyton Cady (1874–1974) was an American physicist and electrical engineer who completed his doctorate in Berlin in 1900 before returning to Weslyan University in Connecticut, USA. In 1921, he designed the first circuit to control frequency using a quartz crystal.

11.6 Claims and Counterclaims

Langevin had no great personal motivation to continue this legal battle. From an American historical perspective, Langevin "had not taken adequate steps to protect his American patent interests" [7, p. 56], anathema to the American way of doing business. In fact, Langevin's patent firm Armengaud did its best. They invoked the testimony of Charles Fabry, to produce the exact date of his arrival in the USA, the nature of the information communicated, specify whether it was orally or in writing, and so on. Armengaud managed to have the dispute considered as a "case of interference" and not of priority. Despite this, the procedures dragged on: in 1930, Fabry was again summoned to testify under oath at the US consulate. The US Patent Office rejected the further patent applications filed on behalf of Langevin. Finally, after 8 years of expensive legal wrangling, the joint patent with Florisson describing the SCAM echo-sounder was awarded on 17 May 1932.

But it will be 20 years before the United States patent courts find in Langevin's favour over his original patent. By then he will be under house arrest in German-occupied France. The final financial settlement will be agreed the day before he dies in December 1946 (Archives L144/23). Langevin's compatriots were justifiably aggrieved, but misunderstood what had happened. Pierre Biquard blamed Boyle, who he believed to be American, for leaking technical details across the Atlantic. In reality, once the general possibility of electromechanical transduction using piezo-electricity was known, it was only a matter of time before the wider scientific and technical implications were being investigated. It was too large a discovery to be kept secret, and Langevin had opposed all attempts to do so.

Langevin allowed himself one speculative addition to his original 1918 patent. For the first time, he mentioned that the invention may be used also "for medical and other uses of elastic waves of high frequency". While he may have been funded on a military project, he knew that his scientific and technical achievements had the potential to reach far beyond submarine detection and secret signalling. During the next decade, he took the first steps to make his vision a reality. Slowly, the study of ultrasonics begun to catch the attention of scientists, industry and the military. Still in its infancy, it offered a host of theoretical and experimental challenges, an open field of possible applications to be explored for the benefit of mankind.

Most of the scientists who started to investigate ultrasonics during the 1920s mentioned that their inspiration arose from Langevin: Robert Boyle, now home in the University of Alberta, investigated acoustic cavitation and metrology: the American Robert Wood, working with Alfred Lee Loomis at his private laboratory at Tuxedo Park, studied the chemical and biological effects of ultrasound at very high intensities: in Paris, Léon Brillouin explored optical diffraction using ultrasound and proposed micro-massage: Pierre Biquard investigated ultrasonic loss and non-linearity. All their experimental studies used x-cut quartz transducers to create beams of ultrasound, as Langevin had shown. Langevin had seen clearly when he perceived how widely his wartime work could spread [2].

References

1. Biquard P (1932) Les ondes ultra-sonores. Revue Acoustique 1:93–109. and 315–335; 2:288–299 and (1933) 3:104–132
2. Duck F (2020) Ultrasound – the first fifty years. Medical Physics International Journal Special Issue History of Medical Physics 5:470–498
3. Duck F (2023) Langevin's ultrasonic metrology. IEEE Transactions on Ultrasonics Ferroelectrics and Frequency Control 70(2):173–180
4. Eve AS (1939) Rutherford. University Press, Cambridge
5. Florisson C-L (1925) Improvements in method and apparatus of the combined radio and ultra-audible type, for navigation purposes. UK Patent 258235. (French Convention 8 Sept 1925) UK Application 4 Aug 1926, Accepted 29 Sept 1927
6. Florisson C-L (1927) Les applications des ultrasons à la navigation. Association Technique Maritime et Aéronautique, pp 1–16
7. Hunt FV (1982) Electroacoustics: the analysis of transduction, and its historical background. American Institute of Physics/Acoustical Society of America
8. Klyukin II, Shishkov EN (1984) Konstantin Vasilievich Shilovski 1880–1958. Leningrad, Nauka (in Russian)
9. Langevin A (1935) Utilization du quartz piézoélectrique pour l'étude des pressions variable et des vibrations à fréquences élevées. Revue général de l'electricité 38:3–10
10. Langevin A (2022) Paul Langevin my father. EDP Sciences, Paris. English edition: Duck F
11. Lelong B (2002) Paul Langevin et la détection sous-marin, 1914-1929. Un physicien acteur de l'innovation industrielle et militaire. Épistémologiques 2:205–232
12. Lewiner J (1991) Paul Langevin and the birth of ultrasonics. Japanese Journal of Applied Physics 30(1):5–11
13. Nicolson AM (1918) Piezophony. US Patent 1495429, Filed 10 Apr 1918, Awarded 27 May 1924
14. Nirei K (1991) Introduction to Japan of the technology of the echo sounder and active sonar developed by professor Paul Langevin. Japanese Journal of Applied Physics 30(1):3–4
15. Pupin MI (1918) Wave signalling system. US Patent 1,561,278, Filed 4 Feb 1918, Renewed 26 Jan 1921, Granted 10 Nov 1925. Also UK Patent 130,496, Appl. 25 Feb 1920, Accepted 25 May 1921. French Patent 507,608, Filed 20 Dec 1919, Delivered 29 June 1920
16. Tournier M (1917) to Langevin July 7 1917. UK National Archives T173/16
17. Wilson D (1983) Rutherford. Simple genius. Hodder and Stoughton, London
18. Zimmerman D (2018) "A more creditable way": the discovery of active sonar, the Langevin-Chilowsky patent dispute and the Royal Commission on Awards to Inventors. War in History 25(1):48–68

Chapter 12
Figures of Science and Rationalism

Abstract "Through science, for peace" could be Langevin's motto in the immediate aftermath of the First World War. There was a spontaneous alliance between the interests of the scholar and those of the pacifist. Doing science already soothed the grudges. This chapter explores the convictions and moral values underlying Langevin's peace activism. Like many of his contemporary intellectuals, he reflected on the shock of the world war and on the part that science played in it. He consequently forged a mental world centred on the moral value of science and its social and political function as "mother and daughter of democracy" and "elder sister of social justice".

"Through science, for peace": such could be the Langevin's motto. Provided that we add that the meaning of the formula changes over the years. In the early 1920s, there was a spontaneous alliance between the interests of the scholar and those of the pacifist. Doing science already soothed the grudges. But very quickly this proved insufficient. Because international tension persisted and increased: as early as 1927, fascism emerged in Italy.

Then the commitments of the peace activist became overwhelming. As an active member of several organizations, constantly solicited for a petition, a speech and a campaign, Langevin was caught on a treadmill that he couldn't stop. The more renowned he became, the more responsibilities were entrusted to him: President of the French Society for Education from 1922; vice-president of the League of Human Rights from 1927; president of the French section of the International League for New Education (*Groupe français d'education nouvelle*) in 1928; vice-president of the *Union rationaliste* in 1930; co-president of the World Committee against War and Fascism in 1932… The list grew over the years.

A frenetic, exhausting, daily life. But this activism was driven by thoughts about the roots of war. Like many of his contemporary intellectuals, Langevin reflected on the shock of the world war and on the part that science played in it. Under the pressure of circumstances, he gradually forged a consistent set of philosophical views, which were sufficient to develop and support his efforts.

By retracing the genesis of this mental world, we will focus on his convictions and moral values. This chapter will discuss two questions. On the one hand, to what extent did Langevin's dedication to the service of peace proceed from a feeling of guilt about his actions during the war? On the other hand, to what extent did this faith in science survive the shock of the First World War?

12.1 The Prostitution of Science

Science can spread horror, violence and death. Langevin did not wait for the Hiroshima bomb to make this statement. Twenty years earlier, he raised the alarm, in a motion of the League of Human Rights (Archives L018/003):

> Scientific and technical effort has increased considerably and increases daily the power of men to do good as well as to harm. By an automatic process against which all attempts at partial regulation have remained without outcome, the results of this effort have been used, since the most distant past, to perfect the art of killing.
>
> The recent war saw the birth of new means of destruction and we are promised, in the case of a new catastrophe, incomparable horrors under the name of chemical or microbial warfare.
>
> There is a danger, for the human species and for its civilization, that could make it possible to doubt the moral value of scientific progress and there are those who are beginning to think that just the possibility of another war is insufficient cause to rise in opposition.
>
> The undersigned consider it a primary duty to denounce the terrible danger that the preparation of new scientific wars represents for humanity as a whole, and especially for the most civilized nations, the *prostitution of science to war*.
>
> As it is unthinkable to limit science, we must absolutely fight against war. It is indeed impossible to stop the work of adapting thought to the facts that life imposes on us, and there is a deep *instinct* that drives us to continue to develop with each passing day. Those who have dedicated their lives to it see, with pain, the results of their efforts placed at the service of traditions of violence: they must and want to be the first to fight against the danger they have unwillingly contributed in creating.
>
> Experience has shown that all international conventions that have aimed at limiting the applications of science to war are ineffective. They introduce arbitrary distinctions, because they do not go to the root of the evil. Nothing can prevent a nation that believes that it is in a state of legitimate defence from using all the available resources offered by nature and by human efforts.
>
> The only effective action must aim at eliminating war, denouncing the fallacy of seeking security in armaments, and ardently propagating the conviction that the immediate establishment of international justice is a matter of life or death for the human species.
>
> It is necessary, through multiple associations and tireless propaganda, to educate public opinion, to convince it that peace must be created and that justice must be constructed by the common will of all nations. It is necessary to exert a constant pressure on governments to lead them to conclude agreements and to create the necessary international bodies.
>
> For these reasons and for these purposes, the undersigned declare that the first duty of the present hour is to protest against the very principle of war, against the use it makes of the best results of scientific work and against the influence of prejudices or interests that tend to maintain the barbaric tradition of employing violence to resolve international difficulties. (Professor Paul Langevin, Paris, May 1925)

Let us fully understand the scope of these words. Science is prostituted, and it is not a passing vice since it has always served the art of killing. In truth, it is demonic because the scientific development which is, for Langevin, a process of adaptation driven by an "instinct", serves life and death, progress and barbarism indiscriminately. It's an infernal machine, an uncontrollable automaton.

Is this science fiction? No, it is a call, a cry, that should not sound too desperate. Langevin assumes that we cannot stop science, that it is an autonomous, inevitable process. We cannot even judge it, put it on trial, as it is seen as the product of an instinct beyond good and evil, irresponsible, amoral. We cannot hope for a regulation of its use, a limitation of armaments. The catastrophe seems inevitable.

The proposed solution, to "eliminate war", seems somewhat angelic after the realistic picture of the situation. A pious wish followed by active measures such as "educating public opinion" and "exercising constant pressure on governments". In brief, fighting in education, at the Human Rights League or at the League of Nations are the only remedies. Langevin saw no alternative because of his conviction that the link between science and war is only conjectural. It is a "prostitution", a regrettable deviation of an "instinct" of adaptation.

12.2   "Science, Mother and Daughter of Democracy"

As threats increased, ironically, Langevin saw a way out of this uncomfortable position. Fascism clearly altered values and allowed science to be whitewashed. By discovering a deep link between fascism and war, Langevin could stretch, dissolve almost, the conjectural link between science and war. In 1926, he presented them as two opposing forces, two rival instincts.

This new argument emerged in a brief paper published in the *Frankfurter Zeitung*, titled *Fascismus und Demokratie*. Fascism is described as an instinct of regression to brute force, to bestial violence; and nationalism as the "rebirth in collective form of an ancestral selfishness". Democracy and justice embody, on the contrary, progressive instincts that had gradually emerged in history. Their rise, slow and always precarious, requires material conditions, "a minimum of living conditions and security", and a spiritual effort, namely science: "In this process of actions and reactions an essential role is played by science, in both cause and effect, the mother and daughter of democracy" (Langevin 1926e).

Fascism, with its declared aversion for peace, science and freedom, is an offence to Langevin's dearest values. As scientist and peace activist, he had no choice but to combat fascism: A fight that he would like to be non-violent in response to their glorification of violence. He opted for an opposition that would respect legality and institutions.

> An energetic collaboration, but without nervousness, without the violent agitation that always favours forms of regression (…) Even if we judge our institutions too imbued with the errors of the past we must not only trust them but constantly seek to perfect them. (Ibid.)

Where is he to find a non-violent force capable of opposing the rise of violence and fascism? In science. Langevin firmly believed in the moral value of science. After having briefly doubted this, because of its "prostitution" during the war, he exonerated science, and expected that it would restore peace and freedom. The idea emerged in a talk he gave in Buenos Aires (Langevin 1928a). Science, Langevin argues, can serve good as well as evil, but he does not mean that it is neutral in the sense of dual use because he adds: "From the excess of evil must come the remedy. Science contributes to the elimination of war."

How is it possible that the prostitution of science generates peace, freedom and justice? On his return from Argentina, Langevin developed a whole new perspective. Science, always singular in his words, is no longer just "cause and effect, mother and daughter" of democracy. It is the driving force of all historical evolution, the primary source of all progress.

> In fact, the stages of development of human societies are determined by their understanding of the physical and moral world. Social transformations are necessarily preceded by the diffusion of new intellectual and emotional concepts. (Langevin 1932g)

This is a strong philosophical claim. Ideas and emotions govern the world. Among all human concepts, it is science that has had the greatest influence on political history following the emergence of modern scientific method:

> Greek civilization and legislation were imbued with the same spirit that Greek science had introduced. The liberation of minds at the Renaissance and the Reformation represented a reaction against the abuses of scholasticism and deductive mysticism. It cannot be denied that Newton played a significant role in social evolution during the eighteenth century: the encyclopaedists, precursors of the French Revolution, drew their inspiration from the works of this English scholar. (Langevin 1926c, pp. 193–194)

Langevin implicitly suggests an increasing influence of science on socio-political history: In Greece, society was imbued with the spirit of science; in the Renaissance, science and religion cooperated to the emancipation of mankind; finally, in the eighteenth century, science alone, embodied in Newton, triggered the French Revolution and the Declaration of Human Rights.

Significantly, Langevin does not attribute this crescendo of influence to technological progress. Technology is, for him, only an "additional gain", a secondary benefit rather the natural consequence and, even less, the purpose of modern science. Langevin marks, on several occasions, his distance from "what has been called positivism in the narrow sense of the word", the one that tries to limit the goal of science to prediction and to action. For Langevin, the contribution of science is primarily spiritual: by its spirit and its methods, by the constant contact with reality, it strengthens reason and emancipates the human mind (Langevin 1931c, pp. 8–13).

But is this enough to make science the driving force of Western civilization? How can science manage to shake and move the entire edifice of culture and society? Langevin provides a partial response to this objection. There is an inner "force of expansion" in scientific doctrines. Already, in his 1904 lectures, he had criticized the mechanical theoretical framework for its ambition to conquer and dominate the

12.2 "Science, Mother and Daughter of Democracy"

whole of physics. In 1926, he turns this one-off remark into a general law of history which could be dubbed the "law of exaggeration":

> At each step of human evolution we find the same tendency to exaggerate the value of the results obtained and to believe that we possess the key to the world. (Langevin 1926c, p. 188)

Every novelty tends to overflow the limits of its domain of validity to conquer the entirety of the cultural field. This abusive generalization is inevitable, and immediately science tips into mysticism. To support his claim, Langevin mentions a few examples, taking a quick glimpse at the evolution of human societies. In the works of ethnologists such as James Frazer and Lucien Lévy-Bruhl, he picks up the first manifestation of this force of expansion: the mastery of language generates magic (ibid., p. 189). In Ancient science, he finds two examples: the discovery of number and nascent arithmetic tip into Pythagorean mysticism and Kabbalah. The development of astronomy gives rise to astrology. A fourth example comes from medieval science: the powerful Aristotelian logic becomes scholasticism. Experimental physics itself, after Newton, turns into a kind of mechanistic mysticism. Finally, thermodynamics engendered energetics, another kind of mysticism (ibid., p. 193). Like many mythological heroes, the scientific spirit is prone to excess, to "hubris". The scientific spirit is never well formed; it is always in a process of deformation and denaturation. Its growing influence in human history results less from its wisdom than from its repeated follies.

Here is a decidedly strange vision of the progress of reason! Certainly, Langevin assumed that there is progress, in the sense of a better adaptation of the mind to reality. But it is not a serene ascent. It is a wavering, oscillating, uncertain march. Scientific thinking can never drive out religious thinking, since it repeatedly generates new mysticisms. Therefore, if we understand Langevin correctly, we should revise Auguste Comte's famous law of the three phases, which states that society as a whole, and each particular science, develop through three mentally conceived stages: (1) the theological stage, (2) the metaphysical stage and (3) the positive stage. For Langevin, humans never leave the theological stage; science always brings it back there.

Indeed, Comte himself had a more nuanced vision of the progress of science. Under the overall schema of the law of three phases, he perceived "unequal and variable oscillations" [2, pp. II, 135]; he too thought that excess and exaggeration are integral to science. However, for Comte, the excesses are follies of youth. It is the founders who tend to exaggerate the scope of their theory; the successors then sweep away the metaphysical slag, correct excesses, normalize science. The excess of genius provides the momentum and then everything falls into order. For Langevin, the process is reversed and, as a result, more disturbing. Wisdom belongs only to the founding geniuses; but the horde of successors inevitably damage their doctrine through attempts at expansion and colonization of other territories. The source is pure, and then aging scientific doctrines become crazy, senile.

Through a variety of talks addressed to a variety of audiences, Langevin ended up composing a personal grand narrative in the 1920s and 1930s. It distinctively belongs to the category of idealistic philosophies of history, because the course of history is driven by ideas in the human mind, and especially by scientific doctrines. The driving force of science in history is expressed in uncontrolled excesses of scientific thinking that end up in mysticism. Because of this "law of exaggeration", there is no linear progress. The march of the human mind and human societies towards emancipation is not straightforward, and the future remains uncertain. In this case, is it reasonable to propose science as a remedy for social disorders? Can we cure evil with evil?

12.3 "Science, Elder Sister of Justice"

Science, as it advances, guides society. It shows the way forward. Langevin first justified this idea by invoking the competence acquired through the experience of crises in physics (Fig. 12.1):

> I consider myself somewhat qualified by this necessary experience on the scientific side to come and tell you: our generation must bring to the problem of war and peace a comparable effort to that which physicists have brought to their own problems. We must not shy away from the necessary effort to rework the received wisdom, to revise notions and to adapt them to new conditions. (Langevin 1931e, p. 54)

Langevin ventures a second argument about general culture in 1932 at the inaugural lecture of a Congress of Education. Indeed, science might be the source of evil because it provides the military with means of destruction and machines for warfare. Science is not to blame, however, because the root of the problem is the lack of unity in culture. Due to the imbalance between the rapid pace of technical advances and the slow pace of moral and social progress, there is a dangerous gap between the material and the spiritual. "Science", he explains, "has today taken a considerable and dangerous lead over justice" (Langevin 1932a, p. 235). The root of crisis of social justice lies, according to Langevin, in "the absence of a link between the

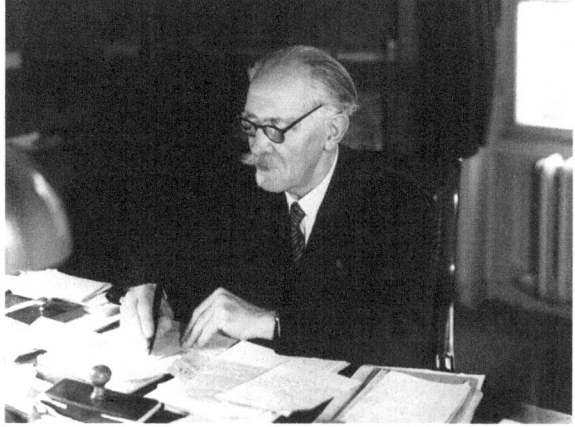

Fig. 12.1 Langevin at his desk. (ESPCI)

12.3 "Science, Elder Sister of Justice"

intellectual and the emotional, between science and justice, between the two too clearly separate aspects of general culture" (ibid., p. 236). Henri Bergson developed a similar perspective at the end of *Les deux sources de la morale et de la religion* [1]. But the remedy proposed by Langevin has nothing to do with the "soul supplement" Bergson was hoping for: far from calling on mysticism to rescue "mechanics", he wants to ground morality and society on the foundations of science.

If the source of the crisis lies in the gap between science and morality, what can be done to bridge this gap? Slow down scientific progress? Langevin cannot envisage this option because he views the advancement of science as a necessary process, driven by an "instinct". Therefore, he claims that morality and justice should be raised to the level of science through education, through "a broader introduction of science, conceived in its spirit more than in its results". It is not just about developing the teaching of the sciences and their history. It is in fact about applying science to the problems of society:

> If … justice, reputed to be lame, is lagging behind science, my deep conviction is that it is up to the latter to extend a fraternal hand to its companion to allow it to regain lost ground. If human institutions are lagging behind technical progress, it is important that we apply to the study of the former the spirit and methods that have allowed the latter, which none of us would want to give up since it represents our only possibility of material liberation of men, a necessary and preliminary condition for their moral liberation. (Langevin 1932a, p. 238)

Far from being the hellish power responsible for violence and social disorders, natural science can guide political emancipation through solidarity and mutual support from Darwin's theory of biological evolution (ibid., p. 239). In fact, Langevin referred to an alternative view of biological evolution. Darwinism was widely discussed and criticized in France in the 1930s when it was not unusual to say that it was bankrupt.[1] In line with French contemporary biologists, he considered Darwinism as a "myth", an outdated theory superseded by more recent doctrines.

> Fortunately, we are no longer there: we know that conflict has never created anything and only knows how to destroy. *What allows the appearance of new and higher forms of life, is on the contrary the process of association and mutual aid.* It is through this that the primitive protozoa came together to become a multicellular being, that the individuals thus constituted have become progressively complicated by the differentiation of primitive elements that were initially identical and then, at the next level, have associated to constitute animal or human societies with differentiation and increasing specialization for enrichment and mutual aid. It is this process that must, in the current circumstances, lead to an even higher level, to the grouping of different and united nations. (Langevin 1934a, pp. 49–50)

---

[1] For instance, Jean Rostand, a French biologist and populariser (1897–1974), assumed that "Lamarck and Darwin have largely failed". Lucien Cuénot advocated a pre-adaptation theory. Pierre-Paul Grassé who worked with Langevin in the collaborative project of the *Encyclopédie française* was Lamarckian (*Encyclopédie française*, 5-24-12). Langevin may have found the idea of evolution by mutual aid in Piotr Kropotkin, an anarchist thinker. In *L'Entraide, un facteur de l'évolution* (French edition, Paris, 1906) Kropotkin assumed that, in extreme environments, like Siberia, mutual aid can be more determinant for the evolution of the species than the struggle for life. Langevin discovered this work through Aline Ménard-Dorian, a member of the *Comité d'honneur Piotr Kropotkin*.

Langevin's view of science as a moral guide allowed him to overcome the moral crisis generated by the First World War. He escaped conflicts and remorse by whitewashing science of all its crimes. He altered the image of prostituted, dangerous and demonic science into one of an innocent, gentle and maternal science. He even evoked the delight of "feeding on the good milk of science, also full of human tenderness" (Langevin 1932a, p. 239).

12.4 Rationalism or Scientism?

As a scientist who dreams of reorganizing society, of extending the empire of science to solve social and political issues, Langevin seems a direct descendant of the French tradition of scientism often dated back to Ernest Renan, who claimed in *L'Avenir de la science*: "To organize humanity scientifically: this is the final word of modern science, this is its audacious but legitimate claim" [7, p. 757].

The term "scientism", introduced in the late nineteenth century, and too often confused with positivism [6], refers to a movement that can be summarily characterized by three distinctive traits: the idea that science is the only legitimate knowledge about the world; the conviction that it is morally good and should guide mankind; and, finally, an immoderate confidence in the powers of science to bring about solutions to all kinds of problems [8]. Langevin fulfilled all criteria except the first one. He set science as a moral guide and claimed to find political resources in it.

The creation of the *Union rationaliste* in 1930 marked the revival of this tradition in France. The association was established on 10 March 1930, with Henri Roger, Dean of the Paris Faculty of Medicine as President, and Langevin vice-president. The initiative was taken during a dinner between Albert Bayet[2] and Langevin. They soon attracted many of their close friends: Emile Borel, Jean Perrin, Louis Lapicque, Henri Laugier, Célestin Bouglé and others. The origins of the *Union rationaliste* suggest a continuity with the French movement of Freethought (*la Libre pensée*), which was very influential in the establishment of secularism by the Third Republic [4]. It seems that the project emerged with David Jahia, a member of *la Libre pensée*, and of similar circles in the early twentieth century (Langevin 1946d, p. 58). Like the scientism of the 1890s, the rationalist movement of the 1930s was strongly tinged with anticlericalism and offensive secularism. The *Union rationaliste* valued science as the only legitimate form of knowledge and fought against what they considered as pseudo-sciences. However, the major threat, in the 1930s, was the rise of fascism. The autos-da-fé in Germany and the exile of thousands of scientists appeared as an obscurantist reaction against the progress of reason. Moreover, the crisis of determinism in quantum physics generated a wave of discourse on the bankruptcy of science in Germany. In less than one year, the Rationalist Union had

---

[2] Albert Bayet (1880–1961), a French sociologist Professor at the Sorbonne and at the *Ecole pratique des hautes études*, was a member of the Human Rights League and later in 1949 President of the *Ligue de l'enseignement*.

12.4 Rationalism or Scientism?

1000 members and the movement reached 3000 members by 1935, most of them recruited among teachers and left-wing intellectuals [5].

Its programme, outlined in the first issue of *Les Cahiers rationalistes*, the monthly published by the Union, was:

> To defend and spread among the general public the spirit and methods of Science in order to combat irrationalism, and even more so, ignorance, by grouping together a number of scientists willing to give up a few hours of their personal research to devote themselves to this work of education.

The rationalist impetus culminated in 1937 with two events during the *Exposition Nationale des Arts et Techniques dans la Vie Moderne*: the foundation of the *Palais de la découverte* by Jean Perrin, an active member of the *Union rationaliste* and author of *La Science et l'espérance*; and the Congress of Philosophy, which celebrated the tricentennial of Descartes *Discourse on the Method*.

Although Langevin was associated with this consecration of science his personal rationalism did not triumph. In Langevin's texts, the words "worry", "security", "comfort" and "trust" keep returning. Everything expresses the feeling of danger and weighty threat. One of Langevin's favourite metaphors in the 1930s, possibly introduced by Lucien Febvre,[3] is that of mankind embarked on the immensity of the ocean (Langevin 1932a, p. 244). This image indicates the limits of trust in science. It is not about blind faith in an all-powerful science. Science cannot calm the waves, does not perform miracles. It does not remove the danger, it just reassures the passengers. That's all. It cannot solve all the problems that threaten humans. It is up to people to unite to solve them:

> This human adventure of a species isolated on the ship of Earth, in the immensity of space and time can, depending on our actions and our will, end tragically or continue in a wonderful way. And more and more we must all feel solidarity, be convinced that we will all be lost or saved at the same time. (Ibid., p. 244)

Langevin took science as a guide, but he had no illusions about its power or effectiveness. It was just a way out of anxiety. While he praised scientific competence, Langevin did not give scientists any prerogatives in political matters. Science does not naturally prepare scientists for public affairs. They are like philosophers reluctant to be distracted from the contemplation of the "World of Ideas" in Plato's *Republic*, who had to be forced to descend back into the cave to guide the prisoners. Langevin exhorted them to act on the world around them, to be responsible. In short, he reminds them of being human.

---

[3] Lucien Febvre (1878–1956), historian, founder of the *Annales of economic history and social* (1929), was with Marc Bloch the craftsman of a renewal of historical studies in France. He interacted with Langevin on several occasions: first he was, like him, a professor at the *Collège de France*; he was also an active member of the *Centre International de Synthèse*; he chaired the Committee of the *Encyclopédie française* of which Langevin took part (see Chap. 15); finally, he participated in the Langevin-Wallon Commission for educational reform (see Chap. 20).

12.5 A Religion of Reason

Was it a credo, a new religion? Langevin spoke of "salvation" and never ceased to proclaim his "faith". He also sometimes used terms such as "devotion" and "holy curiosity". This vocabulary is not accidental because there is clearly an apostle in Langevin: A will for secular apostolate particularly marked in his talk "Science and secularism". Langevin openly criticized the Christian doctrine, which he judged as individualistic, selfish, and he wanted to replace it with a more generous scientific morality, more human and more stimulating (Langevin 1931c, pp. 22–23).

After Langevin death, Einstein wrote: "Reason was his religion, to bring not only light but also redemption" [3]. Yes, Einstein was right: Reason was to take the place of religion. But the meaning of "religion" in Langevin's context must be clarified. It is not the worship or adoration of an idol, but a deliberate act of trust: "We must believe." Langevin endorsed Pasteur's credo: "I believe unshakably that science and human solidarity will overcome ignorance and war" (Langevin 1921b, p. 259). For him, this faith is a duty that becomes imperative to confront the rising tide of fascism in Europe. Langevin seems increasingly convinced that the rational analysis of the causes of war is no longer sufficient, albeit necessary. To counterbalance the mystique of force created by military propaganda, more than reason is needed; it requires faith. Langevin explicitly stated that "justice comes after science and presupposes faith" (Langevin 1932g, p. 651). Émile Zola embodied this effective alliance:

> The example of Zola's life and work teaches us that the knowledge of new facts and the acceptance of new ideas are not enough to achieve this creation. We must add acts of courage and love for the emergence and the propagation of a faith, for an educational work that translates these ideas into a living reality, and which alone would allow the necessary mutation. (Ibid., p. 653)

Ironically, Langevin's faith was based on doubt, on the awareness of the limits of the power of science. Faith must come to the aid of reason. It is a voluntary attitude of "active optimism", a resolution to believe and to act in order to escape the torpor of despair.

Langevin's rationalist credo belongs to a religion that rejects the sanctification of science. Langevin has experienced the sacred terror that science inspires, when it becomes a blind, uncontrollable power, commanding humanity's destiny. Science was for him like an implacable, unpredictable deity, bringing discord or concord: Mars and Venus, at the same time. Therefore, all his efforts aimed to break the isolation of scientists by imposing on them the duty to share their knowledge and securing strong links between science and culture in the field of education. Langevin sought to prevent the gap from widening between an ignorant crowd and an elite of scholars. He judged, indeed, that an elite, even very knowledgeable or enlightened, constitutes a danger as soon as it becomes isolated.

> The government of scholars that Renan thought of would be, indeed, as dangerous as any other dictatorship of a man or an oligarchy. Experience shows us that a man with excessive power, political or financial, becomes unbalanced: scholars would not be an exception and would also become dangerous madmen. (Langevin 1946a, p. 356)

Langevin's rationalist credo is therefore not a resurgence of nineteenth-century scientism. In his effort to restore the value of science he was aware of the risks raised by the power of science. He promoted reason in the face of rising violence with a view to controlling science, putting it back in its place in culture to prevent future disasters.

References

1. Bergson H (1932) Les deux sources de la morale et de la religion. English trans: The two sources of morality and religion. Paris, Notre Dame University Press, Paris (1977)
2. Comte A (1830) Cours de philosophie positive. New edition (1975). Hermann, Paris
3. Einstein A (1947) Hommage à Paul Langevin. La Pensée 12:13–14
4. Lalouette J (1997) La Libre-pensée en France, 1848–1940. Albin Michel, Paris
5. Laurens S (2019) Militer pour la science. Les mouvements rationalistes en France (1930–2005). éditions de l'EHESS, Paris
6. Petit A (2023) Un siècle de positivisme, vol 1. Hermann, Paris
7. Renan E (1849) *L'Avenir de la science*, quoted from *Oeuvres complètes* (ed: Psichari H), vol 3. Calmann Lévy, Paris (1949)
8. Schöttler P (2013) Scientisme, sur l'histoire d'un concept difficile. Rev Synth 134:89–113. https://doi.org/10.1007/s11873-013-0212-4

Chapter 13
Career Profile

Abstract In surveying Langevin's engagement in the World Committee Against War and Fascism and in the *Comité de vigilance des intellectuels antifascistes*, this chapter raises the question whether his scientific activity suffered from his commitments in the political sphere. It argues that despite his frenetic activism, Langevin maintained an intense scientific activity, even though he no longer carried out his own original research. His professional activity was divided between teaching, research training of engineers at EPCI, the management of two research units, and above all scientific consultancy through discussion with young physicists and scholars in the humanities. We argue that his career profile is typical of the French scientific establishment which favours the accumulation of functions and responsibilities among senior scientists.

In 1934, Langevin's name featured in the columns of newspapers under two strangely contrasting faces, activist and scientist.

As a leader of the peace movement, he was harassing the French government by campaigning against its passive defence propaganda. On 5 March, Langevin appeared in the media alongside the ethnologist Paul Rivet and the philosopher Emile Chartier (known by his pen name Alain), as co-founders of the Watchfulness Committee of Antifascist Intellectuals (*Comité de vigilance des intellectuels antifascistes*, CVIA).

On 25 June the same year, Langevin reappeared in the press because of his election to the *Académie des sciences*. This was a late recognition of his contributions to science. Langevin had presented his candidacy to the Academy at least four times, in 1921, 1922, 1923 and 1927 before finally being elected in 1934 with 30 votes, ahead of Henri Abraham (13 votes) and Jean Becquerel (12 votes).

The press presented two sides of Langevin: the famous physicist who was elected to the *Académie des sciences* on 25 June 1934 and active protestor leading a campaign against "the gas war". Jules Moch, a deputy member of SFIO, a leftist party, wrote in *L'Oeuvre* 28 June 1934, under the headline "From Moral Sciences to the Morality of the Sciences":

The French, still attached to cerebral things, have just experienced a pleasant surprise: the *Institut de France* has opened its doors to a man not only worthy of being admitted but who, in hindsight, is astonished that he was not, for a long time, a member. The Académie des sciences has broken a tradition established by other learned societies: that of the cult of incompetence. In the first round of voting, with a strong majority and against two other physicists who are also eminent, it has allowed itself to admit Professor Langevin, whose reputation extends beyond both the geographical borders of our country and the intellectual limits of pure science.

L'Oeuvre did not hesitate, however, to open its columns to a certain R. Maurecourt who accused Langevin of "creating unpatriotic teachers" because a schoolteacher had opposed or sabotaged an official demonstration of passive defence. He wrote:

> Observe a Langevin spreading his sinister defeatist propaganda, and teaching the crowds, from the top of his pulpit, the leader adorned with his diplomas […] See a Langevin transform a *Société française de pédagogie* into a pacifism shop, and expel the founding general secretary, a secular teacher, guilty of patriotic sentiments!
>
> I witnessed the execution of this brave comrade, Alfred Moulin, in the hall of the pedagogical museum. The whole fanfare of pacifism, defeatism and university Masonism, from the Sorbonne or from the primary school, was there, assembled, making a bodyguard to the defeatist pontificator. By a vote of one hundred to one, France in the person of Alfred Moulin had to give way to anti-France.
>
> Disgusting spectacle!
>
> And it was under the orders of the same Bolshevik Langevin that a few days before, with a revolting savagery, the pacifist anti-national union of teachers, represented by its most notorious leaders, and effectively helped by Berlin, punched our comrade Dufrenne and expelled or insulted the patriotic protesters

The conjunction of these two profiles—the activist close to the Communist Party and the respectable scientific authority—raised many comments in the media. It raised a storm of protest among the right wing. Senator Hervey even suggested that Langevin had dishonoured his title of professor (Fig. 13.1, Archives L028/021). The left-wing press seized the opportunity to mock and ridicule the government. Moch added: "Langevin's victory poses an immediate legal problem: either the government recognizes the authority of the scholar and, following his advice, condemns the propaganda for gas masks; or the government admits that Langevin is wrong, that he is guilty of high treason because he tends to discourage the population, and deserves the High Court" (Archives L102/020). As for the supporters of peace movements, they described him as a man of all qualities, a revolutionary because he is reasonable and because he is wise.

Langevin's Janus profile comes from his intimate conviction that:

> All those who have had the good fortune of a scientific training cannot separate themselves from what is happening outside, although it is more comfortable to stay in the peace of the laboratories, although never has the progress of pure science and of its material applications been faster or more captivating. (Langevin 1932a, p. 242)

It is a duty for scientists to get out of their ivory tower, into the public arena and confront the power to defend their intimate political convictions.

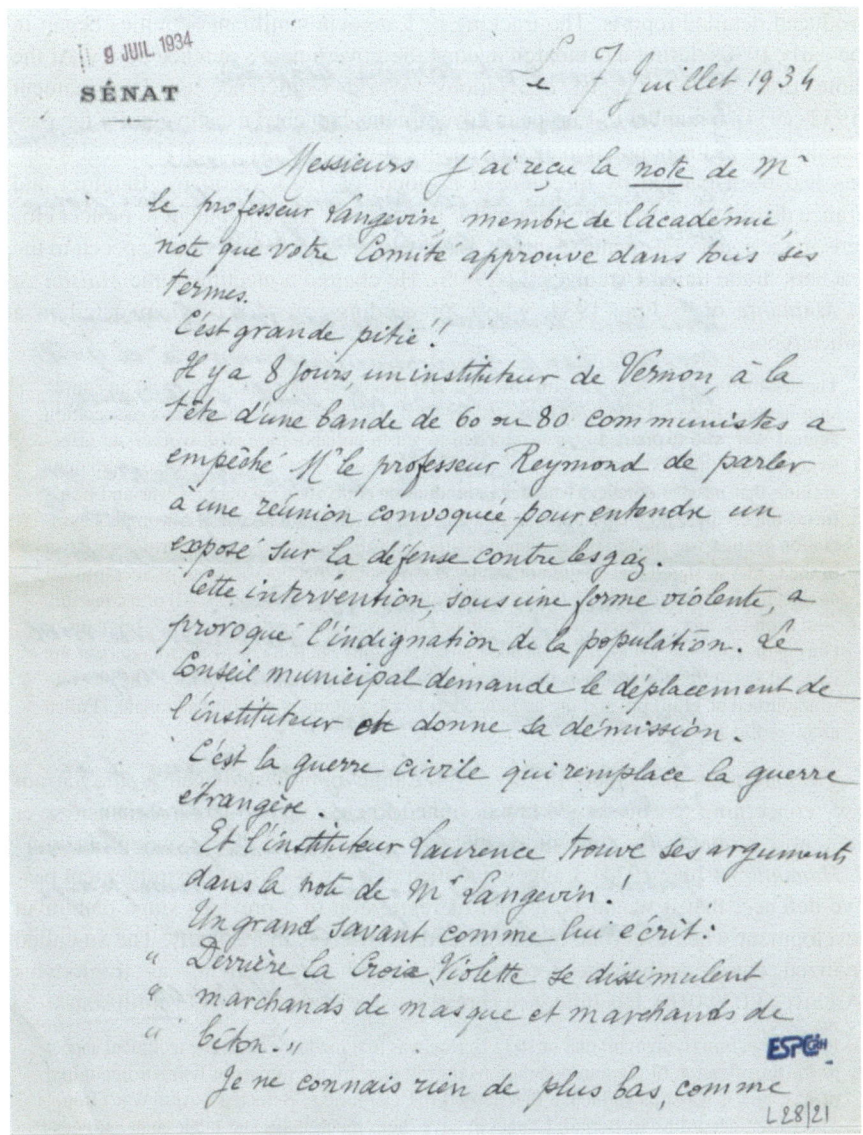

Fig. 13.1 Hervey's letter, 7 July 1934 (*Science et Vigilance*)

13.1 Intensifying Activism for Peace

From 1934 on, Langevin's name appeared not only in newspapers but also in police files. He was closely monitored by the *Renseignements généraux*. They drew up a list of all the associations of which he was a member (many more than appear in Langevin's personal archives). Police officers attended his public meetings and produced detailed reports. The tracking of Langevin's militant activities began in the early 1930s during a campaign against the government's defence policy. At the same time as the League of Nations' World Conference on Disarmament (1932–1934), a number of European governments launched a campaign for the passive defence of the population against chemical weapons. Although chemical weapons had been banned by the Geneva Protocol of 1925, Germany, Belgium and France distributed posters giving precise instructions and equipment to protect citizens in the event of a chemical attack. Langevin protested in 1931 in a speech to the teachers' trade union (Archives, L029/05). He chaired a meeting at the *Maison de la Mutualité* on 6 June 1934, whose proceedings are described in detail in a police report.

> The session opens at 9.30 pm with around 2,700 people in attendance, who paid an admission fee of 3 Francs. Langevin is assisted by Dr d'Alsace from the Physicians Association against War who explained how it intended to act in collaboration with workers to effectively combat the scourge of war. Then a Pr. Chassigneux criticizes the defensive campaigns arguing that passive defence, whether individual or collective, encourages war and transforms the civilian, population into combatants. Leo Wanner, on behalf of a woman's association against war invited the audience to attend a rally on 4 to 6 August. Professor Rivet of the CVIA declared that he did not want gas masks, but that he wanted to protect himself against the lies spread daily by the General Staff in the mainstream press. All of us, he said, "intellectuals and workers, will fight against the war and against fascism" (applause). During the exchanges with the audience Langevin points out that one of the founders of the national gas protection league is the director of a protective equipment factory. The meeting is adjourned at 11.40 pm and the audience left to the singing of the Internationale. (Police archives file 4929)

The campaign intensified. In July 1934, Langevin protested against "the Sarraut law" concerning gas masks, "a law designed to create petty authoritarianism over the entire country through individual or collective local passive protection" (*L'Humanité*, 4 June 1934). Langevin argued that it was difficult to implement passive defence, that it would be a kind of regression to a previous stage of human development when everyone had to defend themselves individually. The so-called civilized countries become fortresses, with inhabitants living as troglodytes (Archives L029/016). His influence spread outside France. As Goldsmith states:

> It was from him (Langevin) that in 1935 Bernal was first made aware of the technical aspect of the terrorization of civilian populations during war, by the threats of bombardment and of gas, and it was that influence that started the Cambridge Scientists' Anti-War Group. Thereafter, according to Bernal, Langevin gave them much help, and made many suggestions for practical work. [2, p. 126]

Beyond this campaign against a government measure, Langevin was deeply involved in a broad international movement that had been started in 1932 by Henri Barbusse. This activist writer had already launched *Clarté* in 1919, *Monde* in 1928, and organized an anti-fascist congress in Berlin in 1929. He wanted a powerful movement coordinating local initiatives and standing "above parties". Accordingly, he composed a politically neutral French steering committee, with Romain Rolland, the novelist Victor Margueritte, the philosopher and journalist Félicien Challaye, and Langevin [7]. The movement quickly attracted the support of numerous parties

13.1 Intensifying Activism for Peace

and associations, with the exception of the SFIO (*Section française de l'Internationale ouvrière*). The international committee included the same well-known names who had started *Clarté* in 1919: Bertrand Russell, Albert Einstein, Henrich Mann, Karl Krauss, Maxim Gorki, John Dos Passos, Upton Sinclair, ... all intellectuals who hoped to convince nations of the absurdity of war, thanks to their prestige and moral authority. Their success was prodigious. Between May and October, the movement gathered nearly 15,000 members, including 10,000 French middle class, civil servants and teachers. The first congress was held in Amsterdam in August 1932 and a second Congress at the Pleyel Hall in Paris on 4–6 June 1933. The success of these meetings further directed the committee towards the fight against fascism.

Soon, however, conflicts emerged within the movement. First, between Barbusse and Rolland, who disagreed on two points of the manifesto (no legitimation of the status of conscientious objector and no mention of Gandhi). Second, as the Amsterdam Manifesto declared that capitalism was responsible for war and denounced "the armed crusade" against the USSR, political divisions broke out. The French Communist Party (PCF) represented a third of the participants at Pleyel, and the participation of socialists dropped between Amsterdam and Pleyel. Was it the communist predominance that encouraged some members of the Committee to create another movement? In any case, in June 1933, a new manifesto appeared in *Le Monde*, proposing to investigate the causes of fascism and to organize a plan of struggle and self-defence groups. The official secretaries of this initiative were Gaston Bergery—former radical deputy—and Langevin.

What prompted Langevin's decision? It could be a discomfort from Barbusse's repeated attacks against the League of Nations, denouncing "the ridiculous parody and odiousness of official pacifism and institutions such as the League of Nations which, under the guise of peace, is in reality the instrument of the great imperialists" (Archives L030). Langevin was still a member of the League of Nations in 1933 and he was not ready to give up the hope of international justice. He nevertheless remained very active in the Amsterdam-Pleyel Committee, soon renamed the Committee Against War and Fascism. He even became co-president, with Rolland and Francis Jourdain, in 1936, after the death of Barbusse. The direct attacks against capitalism were replaced with softer statements saying that world peace requires "a profound transformation of the social state".

His responsibility in the Amsterdam-Pleyel Committee did not prevent Langevin from participating in other movements. In political commitments as in scientific research, he adopted the strategy of maximum dispersion.

On the one hand, Langevin was simultaneously active in many organizations. He remained vice-president of the League of Human Rights and member of the League of Nations, he participated in the National Institute for the Study of Fascism where he learned about methods of political propaganda (Archives L030 and L031); he co-directed the monthly *Clarté* with Rolland and Angell (Archives L030), and he did not hesitate to create new committees of struggle in response to events. Thanks to the police files, we are aware that he was also chair of *L'Entente féminine* in 1934; in 1935, he was the honorary president of *the Comité d'aide aux victimes du fascisme hitlérien*, and vice-president of the *Ligue humanitaire* and member of the

Association concorde et progrès. Langevin was a frequent speaker at meetings held by these latter groups and often chaired meetings and conferences organized against war and fascism.

On the other hand, Langevin also diversified the targets of his campaigns: against Japan, against colonial wars in 1933; for aid to Jewish refugees from Germany and in support of Dimitrov and Thaelmann;[1] against the Italian aggression in Ethiopia in 1935; for a reform of colonial administration and for the Spanish Republicans in 1936; for the independence of Austria, against the coup in Brazil and for China in 1937; for Romania in 1938 (Archives L032).

His correspondence with foreigners was strictly scrutinized by police. For instance, in 1936, a national security officer forwarded to the Prefect of Police a telegram sent by Langevin to Norman Angell in London inviting him to attend a meeting. The Prefect replied in July 1936 that the telegram concerned the meeting "For Peace and for the League of Nations" held on 12 June at 8 p.m. in the Buffalo Stadium and attended by an English delegation led by Lord Robert Cecil. This confidential correspondence testifies to a strict official observation of Langevin's activities.

Langevin worked hand in hand with British activists. In June 1937, the British press published a letter from Langevin to publicize a meeting in the Albert Hall in London to raise support for Basque refugee children (Archives L032/065). The dozen or so eminent men and women who added their names to this letter described themselves as "a few of the thousands of members of the academic and artistic professions who have been watching with profound alarm the recent events in Spain". His name was followed by Henri Matisse, then Pablo Picasso, whose stark painting Guernica had just appeared in the International Exhibition in Paris. Several of the Bloomsbury Group also signed, including Virginia Woolf and Vanessa Bell, as did the pacifist actress Sybil Thorndike. His presence in this group, as a scientist, sets him apart from many colleagues who may have shared his views but kept silent.

Langevin's major initiative in France was the Comité de vigilance des intellectuelles antifascistes (CVIA), created on 4 March 1934 in the wake of the bloody riots of 6 February.[2] To face the sudden resurgence of the fascist threat, many intellectuals of the Dreyfusard tradition gathered around three leaders: Paul Rivet, ethnologist, founder of the *Musée de l'Homme* in 1937; Alain (pen name of the philosopher Emile Chartier) who seems to have suggested the term "vigilance"; and Langevin, who would have preferred to remove "intellectuals" from the title of the Committee to open it to all social categories.

On 5 March 1934, the CVIA launched a "Manifesto to the Workers", *Aux travailleurs*, recommending solidarity between intellectuals and workers. This founding

---

[1] A campaign launched by the *Secours rouge international* to fight the Nazi campaign against the German Communist Party. Dimitrov proposed that Thaelemann, whom the Nazis had arrested and imprisoned, along with other communist functionaries, be summoned, so that he turned the court into a public debate.

[2] On 6 February 1934, an anti-parliamentarist street demonstration organized by far-right leagues in Paris ended up in riots on the *Place de la Concorde*. It led to the fall of the second *Cartel des gauches* and a political crisis that threatened the Republican regime.

13.1 Intensifying Activism for Peace

text of the CVIA had an immediate success among left-wing intellectuals [8, 9]. In a few weeks, the CVIA boasted 2300 members (mainly teachers, writers, journalists, etc.), and at the end of 1934, had reached more than 6000 members, including workers and the youth. These mass memberships might have been due to the political eclecticism visible in the choice of the triple patronage: Rivet was close to the Socialist Party, Alain close to the Radical Party, and Langevin was viewed as close to the Communist Party for having participated often in demonstrations that were organized by the communists. The composition of the permanent officers, established on 8 May 1934, reflects the support of a wide spectrum of left-wing parties.[3] Barbusse himself recommended joining the Vigilance committees en masse and, on 27 July 1934, a Pact of Unity of Action was signed with the Amsterdam-Pleyel Committee.

Ignoring parties and factions, the CVIA fought against war and fascism that appeared as one and the same target. In 1934, war and fascism were a single phenomenon, an unleashing of passions that must be opposed by wise reason.

> Our vigilance is exercised on armaments, on propaganda and on fascist pressures. Our intellectual struggle is waged against the errors that are spread in the nation by avowed or hidden fascists and those who serve the cause, consciously or not. Fascism appeals to the passions of men to nullify their critical intelligence: it disguises facts; it blurs ideas. Our goal is to restore the truthfulness of facts and the clarity of ideas. (*Vigilance*, 1, 28 April 1934, 1)

The fight in the name of truth and in defense of "facts" proved particularly effective. On 8 June 1935, Langevin chaired a meeting of all left-wing organizations, who formed a coalition, the *Comité national de rassemblement populaire*. A large parade was organized on 14 July, the French national day, at the Buffalo Stadium (Fig. 13.2, Archives L030). This parade, where Langevin marched side by side with Maurice Thorez, Léon Blum, Daladier, Barbusse, still remains today a symbol of the power of large, convergent political action. Thus Langevin played a key role in the victory of the *Front Populaire* which came into power in the Parliamentary elections of June 1936. And his influence was not restricted to his homeland. As he had many English friends and contacts, he was the obvious choice to disseminate this French left-wing success, speaking about the *Front Populaire* at the Liberal Summer School in Cambridge in July 1937.

Between 1932 and 1939, Langevin was speaking everywhere, fighting on many front at the same time. Although he had a remarkable gift of ubiquity [3], his strategy of dispersion was not always fruitful. Langevin's health also suffered from overwork. A police file of 31 March 1936 reported that: "Professor Langevin coordinator of the CVIA is currently unwell. He has had to suspend his lectures at the *Collège de France* and will be living in the Fontainebleau region for 2 months". In

---

[3] It included P. Langevin, P. Abraham, J. Alexandre, J. Baby, V. Basch, A. Bayet, F. Dominois, R. Fernandez, Alain, P. Gérôme, G. Fournier, G. Lapierre, G.-H. Luquet, M. Prenant, E. Renard, H. Wallon and A. Wurmser. The eclecticism of the movement was even more evident in the fate of its members during the Second World War: some like F. Delaisi and L. Emery supported the Vichy government, while others like Rivet and Gérôme supported the Resistance.

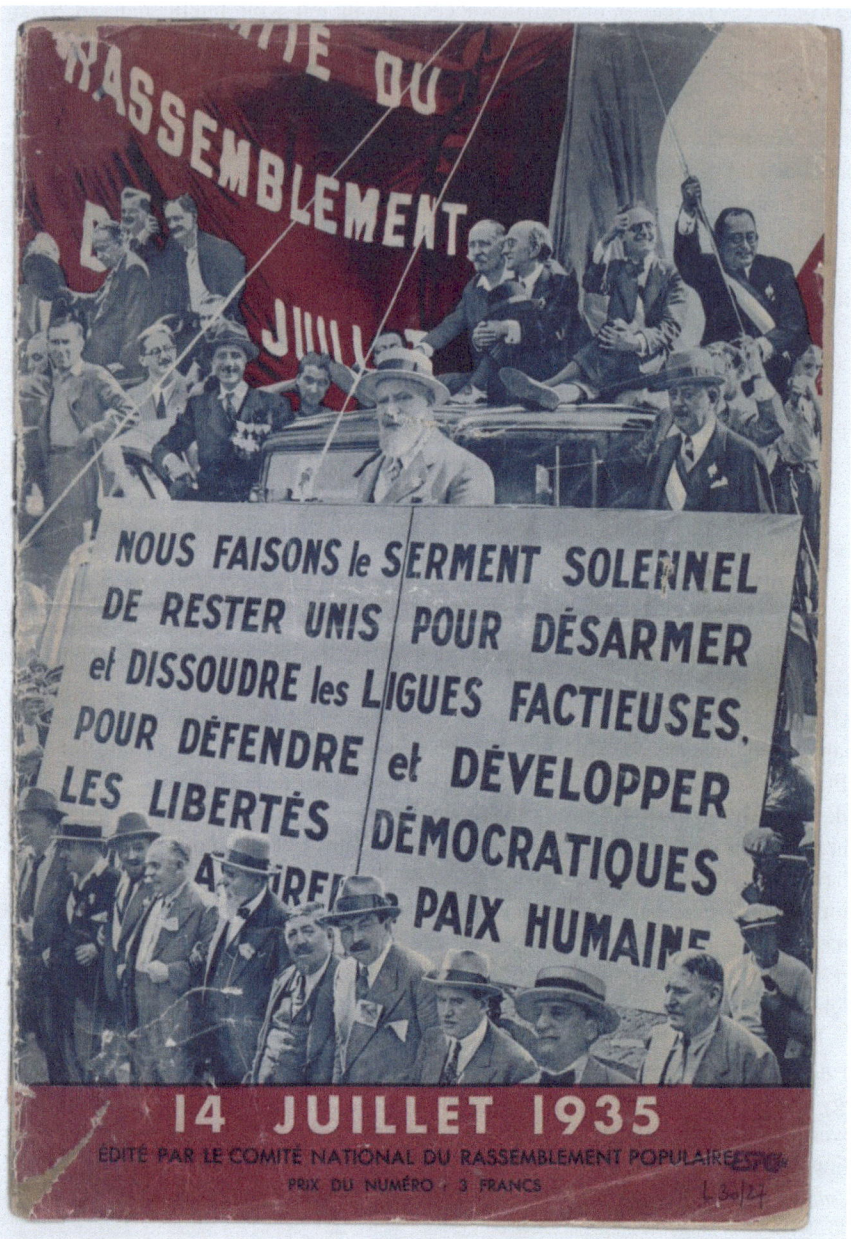

Fig. 13.2 Langevin among members of the *Comité national de rassemblement populaire*, 14 July 1935. (ESPCI, PSL University L030/027)

1937, he had to cancel the next Solvay Physics Council while he relinquished the presidency of the *Société française de pédagogie* to Henri Wallon.

13.2 Declining Scientific Productivity?

Romain Rolland best captured Langevin's profile when he wrote: "[he is] a master of science who leads the popular classes" (Archives L030/044). Langevin certainly deserved the label "Master of Science" for his numerous contributions to physics since 1904, but his research activity inevitably suffered from his commitments in the political sphere. Some of his friends and colleagues complained that his unabated activism diverted him from his laboratory. In an overheard conversation with Joliot-Curie, he said "Was I not wrong in devoting too much of my time to social affairs?" Then a few moments later "After all, I am sure I was right" [2, p. 126].

The question deserves attention because Langevin himself has faced this ethical dilemma. With the benefit of hindsight, how are we to assess his ethical choices? Is it true that after the fruitful pre-war period, he more or less ceased all research activities in favour of social action?

If we use his publication records as a criterion for evaluation—as it is the case today—it is certainly possible distinguish two careers in Langevin's life (Fig. 13.3). Even knowing Langevin's reluctance to publish,[4] we can attempt comparative

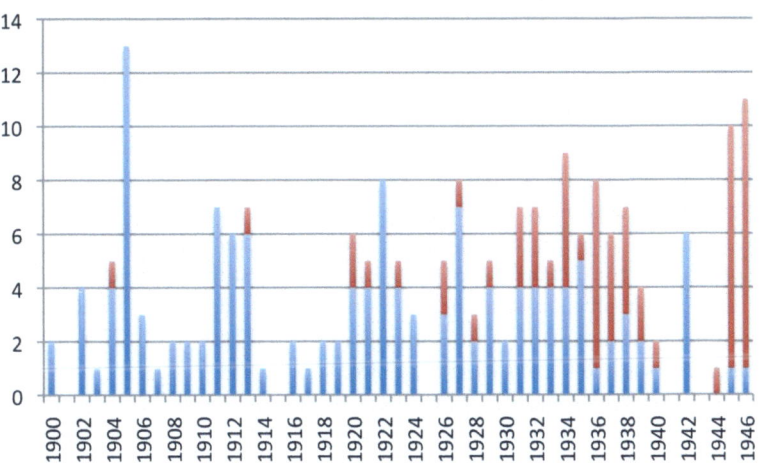

Fig. 13.3 Langevin's scientific (blue) and non-scientific (red) publications, 1900–1945

---

[4] According to Pierre Biquard, Langevin occasionally inserted results of his own personal research into his lectures at the *Collège de France* that have never been published in scientific journals [1, p. 69].

estimates of his production before and after the First World War. For this, we consider not only the quantity of publications, estimated from the bibliography list at the end of the volume, hoping that it is not too incomplete, but also the category they belong to, "scientific" or "non-scientific". As it is not always easy to distinguish them based on their contents, we consider as "scientific" all articles written by Langevin in the exercise of his profession (as a professor or member of a learned society). Within the "scientific publications" category, we then distinguish two types of articles: research articles published in scientific journals (gathered in the volume *Œuvres scientifiques de Paul Langevin*), and more popular writings disseminating new theories to various audiences, or paying homage to colleagues, scattered in multiple journals, often difficult to access. Although this quantitative assessment is imperfect because it does not take into account the length of the articles, the chart provides some interesting data. Overall, Langevin did not slow down his publication activity after the First World War. On the contrary, the annual average is globally increasing for the period 1919–1946. It is the distribution of papers in the categories that changes.

We first observe a spectacular rise in non-scientific publications in the interwar period. While they accounted for less than 4% of the total before 1918, they rise to about 40% after the First World War, with a host of tributes and commemorations, motions and pamphlets, meeting speeches. These short texts have a strong impact on the public.

However, this intense non-scientific publication activity does not imply a spectacular decrease of scientific publications. The average in the category "scientific publications" is stable, around three articles per year between 1919 and 1946. But we observe a noticeable decrease in research articles (Table 13.1). It is even more obvious if we specify that more than half of the results published during this period concern research on ultrasonics, undertaken during the war, which were continued, refined, developed, in the 1920s. It would therefore be less of a decrease in productivity than a decline in basic scientific research. All in all, his scientific publications other than research articles amounted to about one third of his scientific activities in these years that were so rich for atomic physics.

The decline is also confirmed by the number of citations in foreign journals, *Physical Review*, for example. Certainly Langevin is still known among the most renowned French physicists, after the Curies, Joliot, de Broglie and Auger … However, out of seven citations for Langevin, recorded between 1922 and 1939, six refer back to his articles from 1905 [6, p. 88].

The great creative momentum of Langevin's early career therefore seems to have dried up somewhat. Ironically, this is the typical profile of the "great men",

Table 13.1 Langevin's average annual publications

Period	1900–1918	1919–1946
General average	3.3	5.2
Scientific publications	3	3
Non-scientific publications	0.1	2.1
Research	2.5	1.4

13.2 Declining Scientific Productivity?

according to Wilhem Ostwald, the energeticist that Langevin criticized in 1904. Ostwald distinguished the "romantic" and "classical" types of genius. He characterized the romantic genius by intense and early productivity, rapid reaction and a powerful influence on contemporaries. Ostwald added that the romantic genius quickly runs out of steam; he exhausts himself by some considerable expenditure of energy in other activities [5].

In the case of Langevin, can we establish a correlation between the decrease of his research publications and the rising curve of non-scientific publications? The hours spent campaigning in the 1930s might nibble away at the time devoted to physics. This seems all the more likely because, when Langevin was condemned to inaction during his house arrest under the German occupation in the Second World War, he resumed publishing research papers on a new topic, nuclear physics (Langevin 1942b, c, d). Should we therefore conclude that science suffered from the excesses of political action, although Langevin has always denied that they were in antagonism?

The problem is more complex. Despite his social commitments, Langevin maintained an intense scientific activity, even though he no longer was working at the bench. First, Langevin never interrupted his teaching activities, except during a few months in 1931–32 for the League of Nations mission in China, and between 1940 and 1944 because the Vichy government had dismissed him. Throughout this period, his courses at the *Collège de France* remained innovative. After the theory of relativity (1919–1922), he taught ultrasonics in 1923, the structure of atoms and their optical properties (1924–1926), then the structure of light and quanta (1926–1927), exchanges between matter and radiation (1927–1929), recent progress in magnetism (1929–1931), the experimental and theoretical foundations of quantum physics (1931–1932), current ideas and new facts concerning the atom, molecules, electrons and photons (1933–1935), the electromagnetic field, recent works (1935–1936), tensors in pure and applied physics (1936–1938) and the foundations of quantum physics (1938–1939). Langevin always presented cutting-edge research. His lectures were attended not only by his students—among them are Francis Perrin, Frédéric Joliot, Jean Langevin and Henri Grandjouan—but also by a number of colleagues such as the mathematicians Jacques Hadamard and Emile Borel and his assistants René Lucas and Pierre Biquard, or former students such as Léon Brillouin,[5] who were eager to discover and discuss the most recent developments in physics. Some of those attending wished to publish their mimeographed course notes, but Langevin did not let them disseminate their notes [1, p. 69]. It would be some 10 years after he gave the course in ultrasonics that Langevin finally allowed Biquard to publish his notes on this topic.

---

[5] Léon Brillouin (1889–1969), Langevin's student was son of Marcel Brillouin, who was Langevin's professor. He prepared his PhD on the quantum theory of solids under Langevin's supervision and defended it in 1920, the jury included Langevin, Marie Curie and Jean Perrin. He is known for his interpretation of metallic properties in the light of quantum theory, for his book *Science and Information Theory* and for his theoretical study of optical scattering by ultrasound. He moved to the United States in 1940.

Langevin continued to contribute to the advancement of research as director of two productive laboratories: the Laboratory of Electricity at EPCI, which had been previously directed by Pierre Curie, and the laboratory of General and Experimental Physics at the *Collège de France*. They rank second after the Curie laboratory, according to the number of publications in the Journal de physique Journal de Physique between 1920 and 1940 [6, p. 77]. The Curie laboratory is far ahead with 123 articles against only 50 from Langevin's laboratories. The papers published by the Curie laboratory were all focused first on natural radioactivity and then on nuclear fission. By contrast, research conducted under Langevin's supervision was diverse, scattered into a multitude of themes. At the EPCI, René Lucas published not only on the piezoelectricity of quartz and ultrasonics but also on pyroelectricity, magnetic birefringence and amplification processes. The laboratory of the *Collège de France* published on X-ray scattering, atomic spectra, the Raman effect and the properties of ferromagnetic metals; from 1928, when Bauer returned from Strasbourg, theoretical research related to quantum physics also began to develop. The output of Langevin's laboratories reflects the dispersive tendencies of their director, while at the same time they explored several of the paths initiated by Langevin before the war. Obviously this fragmentation does not favour competitiveness, especially in these years when large teams were being formed around big instruments. The members of Langevin's research teams collaborated and occasionally made ground-breaking discoveries, but he remained apart from the new research infrastructures that were emerging in physics in the 1930s, with the cyclotron of Lawrence at Berkeley, later developed in France by Frédéric Joliot-Curie. Thus, Langevin's importance in French scientific productivity between the wars seems weak, when judged by current scientometrics standards.

If quantitative standards suggest a decline, what about the qualitative standards used by his colleagues in the 1930s? Did Langevin keep a high profile in scientific milieu? His personal scientific range was recognized outside France. Fifteen nominations were made in his name to receive a Nobel Prize in Physics, all unsuccessful but reflecting the dispersion of his research. Indeed, the first, in 1910, by his colleague from the Cavendish days, John Townsend, reflected his own respect for Langevin's studies into gas ionization, to which Townsend himself had made his own contributions. Still, the majority of the nominations were made in the inter-war years. On several occasions, he was jointly nominated with Pierre Weiss, whose own studies into the domain theory of ferromagnetism and the "Weiss magneton" were well respected. In 1929, the Austrian physicist Arthur Haas nominated Langevin jointly with Weiss, Louis de Broglie and the American CJ Davisson, De Broglie was awarded the prize individually "for his discovery of the wave nature of electrons". Clinton Davisson shared the 1937 Nobel Prize in Physics for his demonstration of electron diffraction. Perhaps, the closest that Langevin got to the award was in 1933 when he was selected as the first choice, jointly with Robert Wood, whose work on the physical, chemical and biological effects of ultrasound had by then established ultrasonics as a new sphere of scientific investigation. The nomination had been made by the Polish physicist Czeslaw Bialobrzeski, who had been Langevin's student at the *Collége de France* from 1908 to 1910. However, discoveries in acoustics, however interesting, paled into insignificance in comparison with the earthquake enveloping physics at this time. The Nobel Committee over-rode the first selection and awarded the 1933 Physics Prize jointly to Schroedinger and Dirac. Nobel Prize nominations for significant contributions in four different areas of physics, gas ionization, magnetism, ultrasonics and wave-particle duality: Langevin was a prime mover in each but never claimed precedence, leaving others room to claim the prize. And on the one occasion when he himself made a nomination, it was focused and successful: for Albert Einstein in 1921 (awarded in 1922).

13.3 "Scientific Consultant"

Other criteria than the usual peer review are needed to assess Langevin's contribution to science in the interwar period. The testimonies of his colleagues evoking the "flame" and the "radiant heat" of Langevin suggest an action of influence. His students and colleagues presented him as a catalyst, a facilitator, who "never stopped inspiring theoretical and experimental work", who "has awaken beautiful scientific vocations". To describe this diffuse, almost invisible, and not quantifiable action, Pierre Biquard used the phrase "scientific consultant" [1, p. 69].

Langevin's influence on a generation of physicists is especially striking against the background of French physics between the two wars. Experimental research was predominant; but, apart from the Curie-Joliot group, it was not really innovative. French physics was especially weak in theoretical research, still in the hands of mathematicians, while physicists were confined to a role of experimenters [6, pp. 141–144]. Langevin, being one of the few who could bridge the persistent gap between mathematicians and experimentalists, held a key position in this landscape of French physics, which was full of divisions. His major influence consisted precisely in overcoming the divorce between theoretical and experimental traditions. This effect extended beyond the sphere of his laboratories, through his teaching. Langevin emancipated a generation of French physicists from the positivist climate of mistrust for theory. In blurring disciplinary boundaries, and proposing audacious syntheses, he developed a new research style.

In particular, he was keen to bridge the gap between science and the humanities. He did much to engage in dialogue with French philosophers although he did not always have much time to spend with them. In response to a request for an appointment from Emile Meyerson by the end of April 1922, he replied, "I'll be delighted to talk to you. As I'm very busy at the moment, it would be very kind of you to come to the Collège de France on Thursday at five thirty a.m., as you suggested" [4, p. 304]. In a letter to André Metz, Meyerson described him as someone who had a real interest in philosophy:

> My friend Langevin is just as keenly interested in [philosophical issues], but he approaches them in a kind of active way; they are concerns from which it would be easy to extricate oneself (just like ordinary physicists). He's just too intelligent to believe that one can

achieve this by crude negation (as most of the more or less good-natured positivists who make up the vast majority of today's scientists profess) or by a simple pirouette (which is the attitude of the others). [4, pp. 433–434]

Metz was less polite when he noted that Langevin "is so erratic that I'm under no illusion that he'll keep his promise to come and see you" [4, p. 496].

13.4 The "Boss"

In addition to his influence on humanities, Langevin also had a decisive influence on the training of engineers at EPCI. Before he became director of this engineering school, the curriculum was exclusively technology-oriented and trained for scientific careers in industry [10]. Langevin introduced two major changes. On the one hand, he introduced basic sciences in the curricula: the teaching of mathematics was strengthened (16% instead of 9%) and applied mathematics gave way to pure mathematics. Technology and industrial design were reduced in favour of the introduction of new disciplines, such as physical chemistry. On the other hand, Langevin introduced research training in the basic sciences. Most of the students had to devote part of their training to experimental and theoretical investigations on new research fields. Thus the EPCI, which was one of the few top engineering schools dedicated to the link between science and industry became, under Langevin's direction, a centre of excellence in advanced fundamental research. This reorientation, set up by Langevin, had an unintended consequence on the recruitment of students. Before the 1930s, most students came from the working class, like Langevin himself. Gradually a majority of students came from the liberal bourgeoisie [10].

In a less personal style, Langevin also had a direct impact on French research institutions. His students and assistants used to call him "boss": Rightly so. Langevin was a research manager as much as a researcher. At the *Collège de France*, he had to take care of the creation of new laboratories in 1931 and in 1932 he was in charge of the celebrations of the quarter centenary of this institution (Fig. 13.4: Archives L154 and L155). At EPCI, he undertook the construction of new buildings and organized celebrations for the 50th anniversary of the School in 1932 (Archives, L015). Then the French Society of Electricians involved Langevin in the celebration of its 50th anniversary in 1933 and appointed him president in 1934 (Archives, L153). Moreover, Langevin was editor in chief of the *Journal de physique* from 1920 to 1940. With the assistance of Léon Brillouin until 1927, he gave a new impetus to the journal of the French Society of Physics. Half of each issue was devoted to analyses of new books and dissertations published in the most important French and foreign periodicals, and they also wrote overviews and clarifications of important and topical issues, especially quantum mechanics. In 1928, Langevin succeeded Lorentz as president of the Solvay Physics Councils, an important responsibility that was difficult to manage in the context of rising international tensions during the 1930s (Chap. 14).

13.4 The "Boss"

Fig. 13.4 Ceremony for the 400th anniversary of the *Collège de France* (1930). From left to right: front row: Hélène Langevin, Paul Langevin, Fritz Haber, Mrs André Langevin (Luce) and Jacques Solomon; back row: Edmond Bauer, Pierre Auger, André Langevin, Jean Langevin and Madeleine Langevin

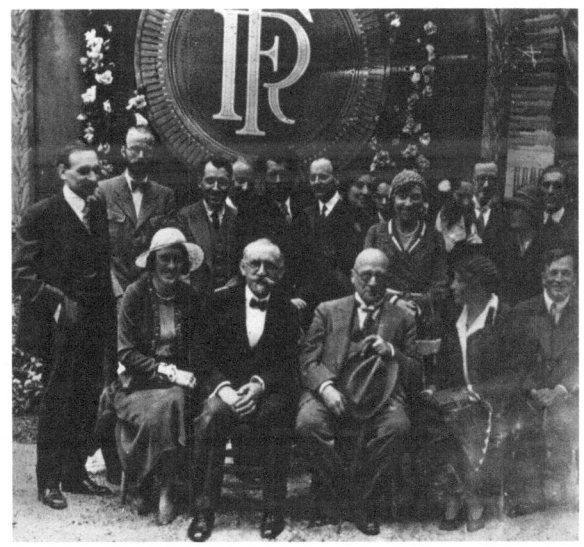

In total, Langevin's career profile reflects the typical profile of many professional scientists at the height of their career, who accumulate institutional functions. The academic system encouraged successful scientists to accumulate responsibilities, entrusting them with heavy administrative burdens and multiple tasks of representation. This phenomenon was particularly accentuated in France: the low incomes of academics combined with the concentration of scientific activities in Paris, especially in the *Quartier Latin*, strongly encouraged the accumulation of duties. This widespread practice became regulated by the end of the 1930s, with a parliamentary law limiting the number of allowed functions for civil servants. In addition, the conditions of scientific researchers was greatly improved following the creation of a national Undersecretary for Research in 1937, and the creation of the National Centre of Scientific Research (*Centre National de la Recherche scientifique*, CNRS), which employed full-time researchers who were independent from education institutions.

But the institutional constraints do not account for everything. The inflection in his scientific productivity is partly due to his will to combine political engagements and professional duties. Like many left-wing intellectuals of his time Langevin considered that his name could influence public opinion. As a result, he was overactive in the interwar period. The survey of his commitments in this period suggests that Langevin had tremendous energy at his disposal. Gone were the days when his friends thought he was always unwell and weak. His career was apparently no longer threatened by poor health and marital circumstances, although he was clearly suffering at times during the 1930s.

If Langevin's research output declined in the 1920s and 1930s, this is partly due to his professional style. Teaching, discussing and disseminating cutting-edge research were his major contributions to physics of this period. He was as much interested in and committed to elite meetings to discuss the advancement of physics, such as the Solvay Councils of Physics, as he was in sharing knowledge with a broader audience.

References

1. Biquard P (1969) Langevin, scientifique, éducateur, citoyen. Seghers, Paris
2. Goldsmith M (1980) Sage, a life of J.D. Bernal. Hutchinson, London
3. Gutierrez L (2010) Paul Langevin: le don d'ubiquité. In: Gutierrez L, Kounelis C (eds) Paul Langevin et la réforme de l'enseignement. Presses universitaires de Grenoble, pp 23–35
4. Meyerson E (2009) Lettres françaises (ed: Bensaude-Vincent B, Telkes-Klein E). éditions CNRS, Paris
5. Ostwald W (1909) Grosse Männer. Akademische Verlagsgesellschaft, Leipzig
6. Pestre D (1984) Physique et physiciens en France, 1918–1940. Archives contemporaines, Paris
7. Prézeau J (2021) Le Mouvement de lutte contre la guerre et le fascisme: Amsterdam-Pleyel (1934–1939). Presses de la Sorbonne, Paris
8. Racine N (1985) Pacifistes et antifascistes. Le Comité de vigilance des intellectuels antifascists. In: Roche A, Tarting C (eds) Des années trente. Groupes et ruptures. éditions du CNRS, Paris
9. Racine N (1995) Le Comité de vigilance des intellectuels antifascists. In: Sirinelli J-F (ed) Dictionnaire historique de la vie politique française. Presses universitaires de France, Paris
10. Shinn T (1981) Des sciences industrielles aux sciences fondamentales, la mutation de l'École Supérieure de Physique et de Chimie. Revue française de Sociologie 22:167–182

Chapter 14
Langevin and the Solvay Physics Councils

Abstract More than any other activity, the Solvay Councils on the international stage demonstrated Langevin's scientific style. His excellence was attributed to a "quite broad, quick and lucid intelligence" that qualified him to guide the developments of physics during his mission as chairman of the international scientific committee. The minutes of the meetings suggest that he did not impress his colleagues by sharp criticisms, as Einstein did. Instead, he adopted a low profile but he was qualified to synthesize the debates on all topics. When he chaired the debates in the 1930s he tried to play the role of a neutral referee although he clearly sided with Einstein. A direct result of Langevin's participation in the physics councils between 1911 and 1939 was the invisible, counted and uncounted friendships, with Einstein in particular.

In June 1911, in the midst of torments in his private life due to the fear of scandal and blackmail pressures, Langevin received an invitation from Ernest Solvay to "an international scientific council to shed light on some topical issues in molecular and kinetic theories" to be held in Brussels at the Hotel Metropole from 30 October to 3 November.

Ernest Solvay, a Belgian chemist, who developed the ammonia-soda process for manufacturing sodium carbonate in large quantities, became a successful industrial entrepreneur who established the successful company Solvay Cie [4]. As he had a love for pure science and was convinced that the progress of science would make mankind happier, he became a generous philanthropist who created several institutes. As in 1910, he had responded positively to a suggestion made by Walther Nernst, director of the Institute of Physical Chemistry in Berlin, to convene a scientific council, because he was convinced that classical theories had to be replaced.[1]

---

[1] Nernst visited Einstein in Zurich in 1910 to discuss whether the quantum hypothesis could be related to the theory of heat that he had proposed in 1906. Nernst's heat theorem states that as absolute zero is approached, the entropy change ΔS for a chemical or physical transformation approaches 0. As he realized that the kinetic molecular theory could not account for the thermal properties of matter, he had the idea to convene a few specialists in a kind of closed "council" for a face-to-face discussion around this crisis in physics.

© The Author(s), under exclusive license to Springer Nature
Switzerland AG 2025
B. Bensaude-Vincent, F. Duck, *Paul Langevin: Physicist and Social Activist*,
Springer Biographies, https://doi.org/10.1007/978-3-031-95260-9_14

He then looked out for an independent sponsor and asked his Belgian assistant Robert Goldschmidt, who was close to Ernest Solvay [6].

Solvay was interested in pure science and had developed a gravito-materialitic theory of the universe. He did not, however, create the first Council of Physics to discuss his theory with eminent scientists. While he pursued his own lines of research, first and foremost Solvay organized the Physics Council to foster international scientific cooperation [6]. Following the foundation of an Institute of Physiology, an Institute of Sociology, and an Institute of Commerce, Solvay wanted to create an Institute of Physics. In this enterprise, he was content to defer to the opinions of his scientific advisors. In particular, he enthusiastically followed the opinion of Hendrik Lorentz, with whom he got along really well.

The invitation to the first Council included a list of eight questions, suggested by Nernst, to be addressed during the conference [2]. They revolved around three major topics: heat, radiation and quantum theory, then named "théorie des degrés" [7, 9]. In 1900, to explain blackbody radiation, Max Planck had ventured the hypothesis that matter can only emit radiant energy in finite quantities proportional to frequency, and determined the proportionality factor with remarkable precision. In 1905, when Einstein was investigating the photoelectric effect, he noted that the energy of the expelled electrons was a function of the frequency of the incident rays, but not of their intensity. This reminded him of Planck's description of blackbody radiation. On the basis of this analogy, Einstein hypothesized that "all monochromatic radiation (of a single colour) is divided into energy grains proportional to frequency according to a proportionality factor equal to h, Planck's constant". So the notion of packets or discrete quantities, sometimes referred as "atoms of action", applied to both heat and light.

Following Lorentz's advice, Solvay finally created two series of Solvay councils, one in physics in 1911 and one in chemistry in 1912, plus two institutes that offered fellowships and grants to support research in physics (ISIP) and chemistry (ISIC). Solvay appointed Lorenz to be President of the Physics Council.[2]

The first physics councils played a central part in the history of science (Fig. 14.1). According to Werner Heisenberg:

> The historical influence of the Solvay Councils is linked to the special style introduced by their founders: a small group of the most eminent specialists from several countries discussing unresolved problems in their field and thereby finding a basis for solving them. [5, p. vii]

In contrast to the style of annual conferences organized by disciplinary scientific societies where scholars present their solutions to well defined puzzles, the Solvay councils aimed to clearly identify and formulate the theoretical problems raised by recent advances in research.

---

[2] Solvay finally rejected Ostwald's proposal for permanent research institutes located in Brussels in favour of virtual institutes.

Fig. 14.1 Brussels, 1911: The Solvay Council brought together the great personalities of pre-war physics. (International Solvay Institutes/ Université Libre de Bruxelles)

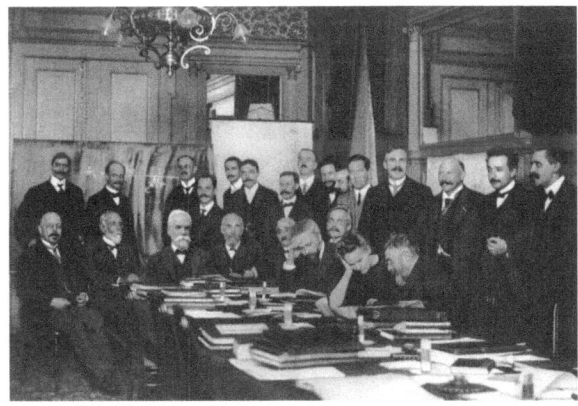

14.1 1911: A "Witches' Sabbath"

This original style is evident from the first meeting in October 1911, which Einstein described in a letter to his friend Michelle Besso as a "Witches' Sabbath" with "enough to satisfy a company of demonic Jesuits" [1].

The company of "demonic Jesuits" was comprised of 24 carefully selected physicists, including one woman. Six French scholars (i.e. one-quarter of the total) were invited to the first council: Marcel Brillouin, Henri Poincaré, Marie Curie, Paul Langevin, Jean Perrin, and Maurice de Broglie. The German delegation included Max Planck, Albert Einstein, Walther Nernst and Arnold Sommerfeld; the British one, James Jeans and Ernest Rutherford, and from other countries Hendrik Lorentz, who presided over the debates, Heike Kamerlingh Onnes, Knut Handsen (secretary) and the Belgian Robert Goldschmidt (intermediary between Solvay and the scientific community). In 1911, Langevin had already extensively discussed theoretical issues with Nernst and Planck, both of whom had been invited to give talks at the *Société française de physique* in 1910. Langevin was also familiar with Lorentz who was a member of the French Physics Society.

There were five hours of meetings on each day, and discussions in the evening giving plenty of opportunity for a free exchange of ideas. A number of participants had prepared a report on a specific field. Langevin spoke on the theory of para- and diamagnetism, based on the assumption that electrons follow closed orbits inside atoms (Fig. 14.2). Agreement with experiment was excellent and his interpretation of diamagnetism was universally accepted. This theory was used by de Haas for obtaining very low temperatures (Joliot 1951). He also suggested a possible relation between Pierre Weiss's hypothesis of the "magneton" and Sommerfeld's principle quantifying the circulation of electrons around atoms [2]. A total of 12 "rapports" were presented during the first council, six of them about radiation and six about matter. This balance suggests that Nernst's initial framework has been displaced for discussing the idea of quanta of energy [6]. Unsurprisingly, Nernst was a bit disappointed at the end of the Council.

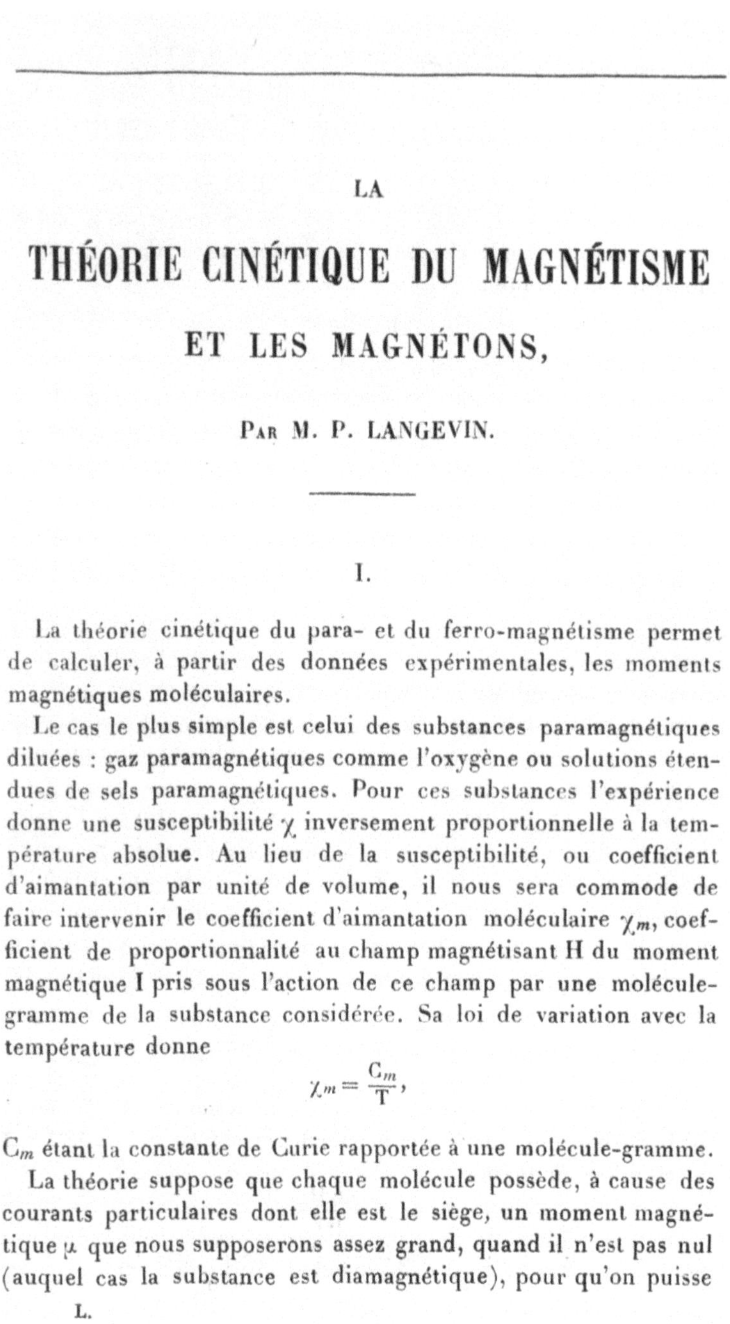

LA

THÉORIE CINÉTIQUE DU MAGNÉTISME
ET LES MAGNÉTONS,

Par M. P. LANGEVIN.

I.

La théorie cinétique du para- et du ferro-magnétisme permet de calculer, à partir des données expérimentales, les moments magnétiques moléculaires.

Le cas le plus simple est celui des substances paramagnétiques diluées : gaz paramagnétiques comme l'oxygène ou solutions étendues de sels paramagnétiques. Pour ces substances l'expérience donne une susceptibilité χ inversement proportionnelle à la température absolue. Au lieu de la susceptibilité, ou coefficient d'aimantation par unité de volume, il nous sera commode de faire intervenir le coefficient d'aimantation moléculaire χ_m, coefficient de proportionnalité au champ magnétisant H du moment magnétique I pris sous l'action de ce champ par une molécule-gramme de la substance considérée. Sa loi de variation avec la température donne

$$\chi_m = \frac{C_m}{T},$$

C_m étant la constante de Curie rapportée à une molécule-gramme.

La théorie suppose que chaque molécule possède, à cause des courants particulaires dont elle est le siège, un moment magnétique μ que nous supposerons assez grand, quand il n'est pas nul (auquel cas la substance est diamagnétique), pour qu'on puisse

L.

Fig. 14.2 Langevin took up Ampère's idea of the existence of molecular currents in connection with magnetic phenomena, and developed a theory of dia- and paramagnetism (*Science et Vigilance*)

14.1 1911: A "Witches' Sabbath"

All later testimonies suggest that Einstein impressed all participants. Lorentz noted: "Einstein is insightful as always, he sees further than all others. Often taking part in the debates, he finds a way each time to contradict his opponents, but in such a charming way that no one would dream of taking offense" (Lorentz letter to his daughter of 28 November 1911, quoted in Lambert and Berend [7, p. 75]). He also noted "Madame Curie was tireless and aware of everything". This council boosted Einstein's career. The remarks of the 32-year-old "scientist from nowhere" so much impressed the views of Nernst and Planck, that they arranged a position for him at the University of Berlin and membership at the Prussian Academy of Science.

The closing speech by Solvay, who had attended all the sessions, shows that he anticipated that it would be a landmark in the history of physics: "You will have fixed the current state of physical science in one of its fundamental directions, in meetings which will occupy a remarkable place in history. The printed reports and discussions will constitute a monument that will be respected for centuries"[3] (ibid., p. 77).

Although Langevin's remarks did not impress Lorentz like Einstein's or Curie's, at the end of the Council he entrusted him with drafting the record of the proceedings, with the help of Maurice de Broglie who had recorded the minutes of the debates (Fig. 14.3). Why was he given this responsibility? Primarily because of his language skills; Solvay had insisted in printing the entire volume in French. Langevin and Lorentz were the only participants with a good command of the three languages used during the sessions (French, German and English). But to take on the onerous task of translating all the reports into French, a good grasp of the recent developments in physics was also required. Apparently, Langevin, combining both linguistic skills and a broad theoretical understanding, was "the man for the job". His understanding of the debates probably benefitted from his continuous attention to early developments in the quantum theory of radiation [3] as well as from the work of his assistant Edmond Bauer, whose PhD dissertation on radiation included a deep analysis of Planck's work and radiation thermodynamics.

The report was published in 1912 with the title *La théorie du rayonnement et les quanta* (there was no mention of molecular theory). It encouraged the introduction of the term "quantum" into both French and English texts. It also proved decisive for the adoption of the quantum theory in the French and British communities: the report of the debates clearly shows that both Henri Poincaré and James Jeans were rather hostile on their arrival in Brussels, but they subsequently became staunch advocates of the quantum theory. On his return to Paris, Poincaré wrote a note explaining that energy quanta had to be accepted as a necessary consequence of Planck's radiation law. The paper arrived in time to be added as a footnote in the volume of the proceedings [6]. Langevin had reviewed all the debates for the publication of the volume and certainly shared Poincaré's conviction. However, in his course at the *Collège de France* for 1912–1913, he pointed out the remaining

---

[3] He nevertheless added. "I hoped to be able to defend Gravito-Materialistic theses in parallel to your theses", suggesting that he didn't want to discuss his views with such eminent theoreticians.

LA

THÉORIE DU RAYONNEMENT

ET LES QUANTA.

RAPPORTS ET DISCUSSIONS

DE LA

Réunion tenue à Bruxelles, du 30 octobre au 3 novembre 1911.

Sous les Auspices de M. E. SOLVAY.

Publiés par MM. P. LANGEVIN et M. de BROGLIE.

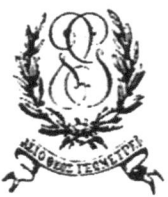

PARIS,

GAUTHIER-VILLARS, IMPRIMEUR-LIBRAIRE

DU BUREAU DES LONGITUDES DE L'ÉCOLE POLYTECHNIQUE.

Quai des Grands-Augustins, 55.

1912

Fig. 14.3 Langevin contributed to the first Solvay Council both as a specialist in magnetism and, with Maurice de Broglie, for publishing the Conference Report (Langevin 1912f) (*Science et Vigilance*)

14.2 A Modest Participation

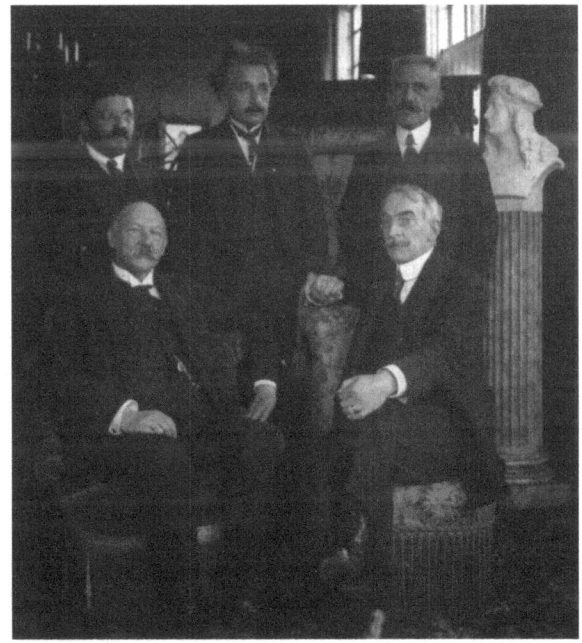

Fig. 14.4 Standing: Paul Erhenfest, Albert Einstein and Paul Langevin; seated: Heike Kamerlingh Onnes and Pierre Weiss, Leiden, The Netherlands, 1912–1913, preparing for the second Solvay Council. (Hebrew University of Jerusalem)

difficulties of the emerging theory of radiation and opened up potential research avenues [3].

If Langevin was called upon to play a role at the first Solvay Congress in 1911 thanks to his individual qualities and his command of the subject at stake, in return, it reinforced his international reputation and authority. The volume of reports co-signed by Langevin and Maurice de Broglie proved decisive in the orientation of promising young physicists. Louis de Broglie, the younger brother of Maurice, then only 19, was so fascinated that he decided to become a physicist, and work on quantum physics [6]. The volume also attracted the attention of Niels Bohr, in Copenhagen, who travelled to Manchester after completing his PhD, to visit Rutherford and worked with him on models of the atom. These models would be discussed during the next council in 1913 (Fig. 14.4). More indirectly, Langevin's report had a wider influence through his course on radiation at the *Collège de France*. In 1912–1913 he attracted a wide audience of young scientists who were thus clearly faced with the theoretical problems at stake [3].

14.2 A Modest Participation

Soon after the first council, an International Scientific Committee was set up. In addition to Solvay and Lorentz, it included Marcel Brillouin, Marie Curie, Warburg, Nernst, Rutherford, Sp. Kamerlingh Onnes, Knudsen, Goldschmidt and two administrative staff. This Committee was in charge of allocating research subsidies, planning topics for the next council and compiling the list of invitees. Langevin was not co-opted as member of this international committee, presumably because of a concern not to over-represent France. Marie Curie clearly enjoyed a higher status, based on her two Nobel Prizes. Yet, when the second meeting of the Scientific Committee took place during the second council in October 1913, Langevin was invited to take part.

The Councils were initially planned to meet every other year. The second Council on "The Structure of Matter" held in October 1913, gathered together 28 scientists who gave eight reports, four in English, three in German and one in French. The second council introduced two novel concepts. First, the structure of the atom, presented by J.J. Thomson, which resulted in a heated debate with Rutherford. Bohr was never mentioned; and second was x-ray diffraction, presented by William Bragg, which impressed the participants by revealing a method to determine crystalline structure. The international scientific committee gathered during the council to discuss the publication of the proceedings, adopting the principle of a multilingual volume in order to speed up the process. Unfortunately, with the onset of the war, publication was delayed until after the armistice. By then, there was no longer a possibility of using German. The entire volume was printed in French.

The planned 2-year periodicity was disrupted by the outbreak of World War One. The third Council in 1921 re-focused on the relationship between classical physics and quantum physics. It was marked by the arrival of Niels Bohr. The 1921 report "Atoms, Electrons, Radiations", extensively discussed his "correspondence principle". Langevin did not co-write the report on magnetism with the Dutch physicist Kamerlingh Onnes, apparently due to poor health. Langevin's relatively low profile at the 1921 Council meeting contrasted with the active participation of Jean Perrin, who made critical comments on Rutherford's atomic model.

Nevertheless, Langevin was unanimously elected as a member of the International Scientific Committee, replacing Augusto Righi, an Italian physicist who specialized in magnetism and electricity. He thus participated in the organization of the 1924 Council on "The Electrical Conductivity of Metals and Related Topics". During this difficult period, due to the boycott of German science, Langevin still kept a low profile on the committee, although he made a name for himself on the French scene by inviting Einstein to Paris in 1922 (Chap. 10). André Langevin claimed that his father strived within an ostracizing, conservative committee to get German scientists admitted and that he was behind the invitation of Abraham Joffe a Russian physicist from Leningrad (André Langevin 2022, p. 98). However, the door remained open for Einstein because he had not signed the appeal of 93 German scientists in 1914 (Chap. 7) and it seems that Einstein was never really considered a German scientist by the Solvay Committee. Yet, in 1921, he declined the invitation to attend the conference presumably because he feared the judgment of his colleagues in Berlin. On the other hand, Langevin intervened in favour of a compatriot as much as for the insertion of foreign scientists. He insisted that Louis de Broglie, who defended his PhD in 1924, be invited to the 1927 board meeting.

14.2 A Modest Participation

On the choice of subjects, Langevin did not take a very firm stance during the preparatory meetings for the 1921 and 1924 councils. According to the minutes, Marie Curie and Rutherford were in the driving seat. Although he took part in all the discussions at these meetings, Langevin remained very much in the background. Still, he reappeared for the planning of the fifth Council. Only a few of members of the Committee attended when they met on 1 and 2 April 1926: Marie Curie, Langevin, Rutherford, Guye and E. van Aubel (the Belgian representative) in addition to Lorentz, the then chairman, and Knudsen, the then secretary. They first elected Einstein as member of the scientific committee to replace Kammerling-Onnes who had died in March. They then unanimously decided to open the council to German scientists, a decision approved by the King of Belgium who acknowledged that "in view of what the Germans had done in physics, it would be hard to work without them". Bohr came first of the list of invitees, which included Max Born, Werner Heisenberg, Louis de Broglie and Erwin Schrödinger. Lorentz broke the balance between French, German and British invitees by adding Paul Dirac and Wolfgang Pauli, with a view to gathering all those who had recently contributed to quantum physics. There were a total of 29 participants, among whom 17 had, or would be, awarded a Nobel Prize.[4]

The fifth council was deliberately planned to be as important for the history of physics as the "Witches' Sabbath" of 1911, according to Lorentz's presentation to the press on the eve of the meeting:

> The subject of the present Council [quanta] is closely related to the one that was discussed sixteen years ago. During this year's meeting, the discussions will focus on the attempts that have recently been made to develop a formalism that one may call "quantum mechanics" and to which de Broglie, Heisenberg, Born, Schrödinger, Dirac and others, have taken part. The proposals of these physicists still constitute an ill-assorted set, for they exhibit some striking divergences, despite their underlying unity. Hence, one may expect that "clashes of opinions" will not be lacking, and that they will lead to a closer approach to the truth. It is precisely under such circumstances that the "Solvay method" is applicable, and that it should accelerate progress through a clarification of ideas ... (Lorentz in *Le Soir* 23 October 1927)

The "clash of opinions" that everyone expected is not reflected in the volume of proceedings. It mentions only one intervention by Einstein during the general discussion, which concluded that, in its present form, quantum mechanics was not a *complete* theory. This is because the well-reported confrontation between Einstein and Bohr about the status of quantum theory took place off session, in the evening conversations.

---

[4] List of participants: H. A. Lorentz, Marie Curie, N. Bohr, M. Born, W. L. Bragg, L. Brillouin, A.H. Compton, L. de Broglie, P. Debye, P. A. M. Dirac, P. Ehrenfest, A. Einstein, R. H. Fowler, Ch.-E. Guye, W. Heisenberg, M. Knudsen, H. A. Kramers, P. Langevin, W. Pauli, M. Planck, O.W. Richardson, E. Schrödinger and C. T. R. Wilson. Secretary of the meeting: J.-E. Verschaffelt. The American Langmuir, travelling in Europe, was added a few days before the conference on a suggestion of Léon Brillouin.

14.3 President of the Scientific Board

As early as 1919, Marcel Brillouin had suggested the name of Langevin to succeed Lorentz as president of the Scientific Board of the Solvay Physics Councils:

> It is useful for you to reflect with Mr. Solvay on the possible presidents after Lorentz. First, it is obvious that we must change generation and move to scientists who are 10 or 15 years younger. Although they are not very numerous, we can find several in France and England, Rutherford, Townsend, Langevin, Perrin, etc. But there is an indispensable condition (...) for the president. He must at least understand English and French very well, and speak both sufficiently. This restricts the choice to Langevin: Rutherford, who has a superior experimental and intuitive genius—but less deep and extensive theoretical knowledge, which is somewhat important—could not, I believe, follow a bilingual discussion down to its details. Among us, Perrin who has a remarkable ingenuity, certainly does not have the experience of English that Langevin possesses. He also has a taste for paradox that is so exaggerated that any discussion with him strays; very amusing in conversation, sometimes very suggestive in the laboratory, this taste would be disastrous for leading an international discussion. Of this generation, it is Langevin who has the deep knowledge, the rapid reading, the solid common sense, tempered with enthusiasm: it is he who provides all his contemporaries with all the precise and profound notions, filtered so to speak, that they utilize for their work. If he has not shown a creative genius of the power of Lorentz, he has an intelligence that is almost as quick and clear. As for diplomatic qualities, he has not had the opportunity to measure them. (Letter of June 1st, 1919, Archives of the Solvay Institute, quoted by André Langevin [8, p. 12])

This recommendation by a senior physicist provides an interesting comparison between the leading figures of the next generation. By February 1928, when Lorentz passed away, Perrin had already left the Physics Councils to concentrate on the Chemistry Councils, which began in 1922. Perrin was a member of the international Scientific Committee of the Institute of Chemistry along with two other French chemists, André Job and Jacques Duclaux.

The appointment of Langevin was made in a climate of consensus. Three reasons qualified him for this function: his fluency in English and German; his quick intelligence; and finally, his familiarity with the Solvay Institute, which he had frequented from the outset. Continuity with the Lorentz "style" is strongly suggested by this letter from Guye to Lefébure, dated 10 March 1928:

> You have kindly told me about the plan to replace Mr Lorentz as Chairman of our Board by Mr Langevin. Allow me to tell you that personally, I would be particularly happy if this choice were confirmed. Not only has Mr. Langevin been a member of the Physics Councils from the outset—he is therefore uniquely placed to take up and continue the fine tradition introduced by Lorentz—but he is also an avant-garde scientist, well aware of the difficulties and problems of modern physics. He also has a remarkably clear, precise and rapid mind, even in the presentation and analysis of the most delicate questions. These are necessary and indispensable qualities for a president. (Letter from Guye quoted by André Langevin [8, p. 18])

Immediately after his appointment, Langevin had to organize the sixth physics council, for 1930, on "Magnetism". As a specialist of this subject, Langevin had already mentioned during the first council of 1911 that the introduction of quanta into atomic physics resonated with the idea of an elementary magnetic moment that would later be named the "magneton". The choice of magnetism was proposed in

14.3 President of the Scientific Board

the early 1920s and it was partially addressed at the 1921 Council. The significant changes brought about during the last eight years by new experimental facts and, above all, by quantum theory, were enough to suggest returning to it in 1930. Langevin himself had dedicated his course at the *Collège de France* to this topic in 1924–1925, a course attended by many physicists from France and abroad.

During the first meeting of the Scientific Committee that he chaired in 1929, Langevin decided on several measures with a view to maximizing exchanges during the sessions of the council. This decision resulted in a heavier workload for him. First, the reports would be drafted and sent to Brussels for circulation among all participants one month before the meeting. They would no longer be read out during the sessions, and participants were required to send the chairman a list of points they wished to discuss, before the meeting. Under Langevin's presidency, the rules governing papers presented during the council changed rapidly. There was a significant decrease in the number of reports, coupled with a gradual increase in the number of invitees. For example, the 1930 Council on Magnetism featured seven papers and 18 invited guests.

In addition, the reports would be drafted in three languages: French, English and German. This solved the language problem that had been debated since 1912 for the publication of reports, and which was brutally resolved following the war, when the reform of the law in 1919 imposed the use of French. Langevin reintroduced German as one of the official languages although the publication of the proceedings still exclusively used French.

All these changes required longer preparation time: the choice of theme and rapporteurs had to be made 18 months in advance, instead of 1 year. The chairman's task of preparation became considerable. Langevin corresponded with each participant, commenting on and guiding his or her contribution. In 1933, he himself translated the French, German and English reports, although he also succeeded in obtaining the assistance of multilingual secretaries. (There were four session secretaries in 1930 and five in 1933.) As a chairman, Langevin could be extremely prescriptive. For example, at the 1930 congress on magnetism, he refused Weiss's request to modify the theme assigned to him by the scientific committee. There was no question of assigning gyromagnetism to Dirac. Langevin did not negotiate and turned out to be much more directive as a chairman than he was as head of his two laboratories. He hesitated to delegate his responsibilities and wanted to control everything, to check everything. Nevertheless, this long preparation time was not in vain, because the 1933 debates were particularly fruitful (Fig. 14.5). One outcome, following the harsh criticism of their report by Lise Meitner, was that Frédéric and Irène Joliot-Curie resumed their experiments from 1932 and discovered artificial radioactivity.[5]

---

[5] In 1933, Irène and Frédéric Joliot-Curie had conducted a decisive experiment of irradiation of an aluminum sheet with a source of polonium. At the Solvay Congress of 1933 they interpret the results of this experiment as an emission of neutrons and positrons. Lise Meitner, who was working on the same subject with Otto Hahn in a competing laboratory in Berlin, criticized this interpretation. The Joliot-Curies, somewhat demoralized, resumed their experiment at the beginning of 1934 to verify their results: they then observed that the emission continues for a few minutes after the polonium source was removed, and discovered that the aluminum sheet had become radioactive.

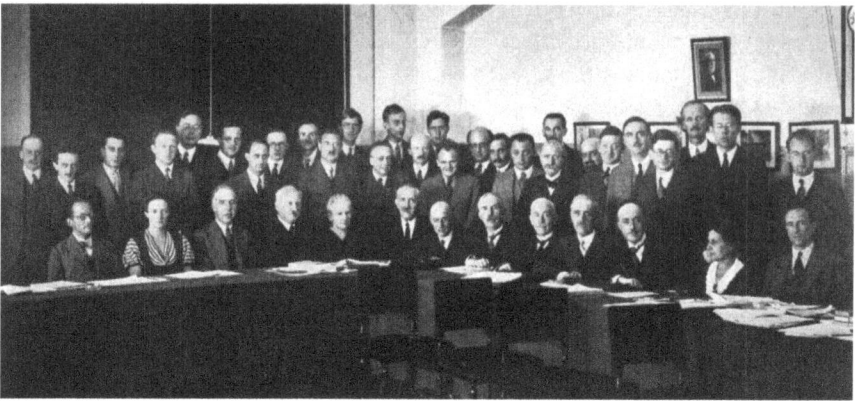

Fig. 14.5 Langevin became president of the Scientific Committee of the Solvay Physics Councils in 1928. This seventh Solvay Council met in 1933, with the theme "structures and properties of nuclei". (International Solvay Institutes/Université Libre de Bruxelles)

If the investment of time was greater for the organizers, it was also more onerous for the participants, who were supposed to have read all the reports a month before the meeting, and to have already prepared their comments. This organization, leaving little room for improvization, never really worked. The Scientific Committee continued to meet a year before the date of the next board meeting, and correspondence shows that many reports were sent out only a few days before the meeting in Brussels.

14.4 Mission Impossible, Given the Circumstances

Only two Councils met under Langevin's chairmanship, in 1930 and 1933. He organized the Council on "Cosmic rays and atomic physics" scheduled for October 1936. The minutes of the preparatory meeting show that the Scientific Committee intended to introduce a dual system of communication. Four "fundamental reports", two theoretical and two experimental, would form the backbone of the Congress. They were to be drafted and sent out before Easter, in preparation for the October meeting. A large number of additional papers, due in June, would revolve around the core reports. This two-tier system introduced a kind of hierarchy between the so-called fundamental reports and the complementary papers, which were more akin to the classic communications in a physics conference, where participants present their own results or those of their group or laboratory. That would have been the end of the "Witches' Sabbath" atmosphere of the early days. Moreover, the system of fundamental reports gave rapporteurs a huge responsibility and considerable power insofar as, through their words, they were able to frame an emerging research field. At a time of intense debate, when rivalry between physics research teams was becoming more and more pronounced, the rapporteur was invested with a kind of halo of neutrality. The choice of rapporteurs by the members of the Scientific Committee therefore became even more strategic than before, and the Chairman's decision to propose a list of themes and names was supposed to be above pressure groups and local research interests.

However, Langevin did not have to exert his diplomatic skills in October 1936, because the council was postponed for two reasons: the first was due to Langevin's own poor health: the second was the international political tension that resulted from the Spanish Civil War.

A new congress was planned on "Elementary particles and interactions" for late October 1939. The final programme was sent to the participants on 11 March 1939. Again, this council could not be held as, by October, the war had already mobilized most of the invited physicists. Neutrinos had to wait until 1948, after Langevin's death (Archives L045).

To sum up, of all the French physicists, Langevin was the most active in the Solvay Physics Councils, as a participant to all councils and as chair of scientific board from 1928 to 1939.

More than any other activity, the Solvay Councils revealed on the international stage the features of Langevin's character that were remembered by his colleagues. His excellence was attributed to a "quite broad, quick and lucid intelligence" that qualified him to guide the developments of physics during his mission as chairman of the international scientific committee. The minutes of the meetings suggest that he did not impress his colleagues by sharp criticisms, as Einstein did. Instead, he adopted a low profile. When he chaired the debates in the 1930s he tried to play the role of a neutral referee that Lorentz, still attached to classical physics, had been able to adopt in the debates of the first congresses. However, he could not position himself as a neutral judge in the debates between Bohr and Einstein that continued during the 1933 council on "Structure and properties of atomic nucleus". Perhaps the most notable outcome was the invisible, counted and uncounted friendships, with Einstein in particular, that Langevin developed between 1911 and 1939 as a direct result of participating in the Solvay Councils.

References

1. Barkan D (1993) The Witches Sabbath: the first international Solvay congress in physics. Science in Context 6:59–82
2. Bustamante MC (2011) Paul Langevin et le conseil Solvay de 1911: au cœur de l'histoire de la physique du XXe siècle. Images de la physique
3. Bustamante MC (2021) A l'aube de la théorie des quanta. Notes inédites d' Emile Borel sur un cours de Paul Langevin (1912) 1913. Brepols, Bruxelles
4. Despy-Meyer A, Devriese D (eds) (1997) Ernest Solvay et son temps. Archives de l'ULB, Brussels
5. Heisenberg W (1975) Preface in Mehra, Jagdish. In: The Solvay conferences on physics. Aspects of the Development of Physics since 1911. Reidel, Dordrecht
6. Lambert F (2010) Internationalisme scientifique et révolution quantique. Revue germanique internationale 12:159–173

7. Lambert F, Berends F (2021) Einstein Witches' Sabbath and the Early Solvay Councils. The untold story. EDP Sciences, Les Ulis
8. Langevin A (1966) Paul Langevin et les congrès de physique Solvay. La Pensée 129:89–104
9. Marage P, Wallenborn G (1995) Les Conseils Solvay et les débuts de la physique moderne. éditions de l'Université libre de Bruxelles, Brussels

Chapter 15
Sharing Knowledge as a Duty

Abstract Langevin was convinced that science cannot advance if it is confiscated by a minority. It is a common good, to be shared. He accordingly spent much time in outreach activities which count as 20% of his scientific publications. But how did he disseminate his broad scientific culture? Did he just bring science to the people in a top-down manner as most science popularisers used to do in the 1930s or did he engage in dialogue with specific audiences? He was engaged in the big official cultural enterprises of 1930s such as the *Encyclopédie française, the Palais de la découverte*, and the *Centre international de synthèse*. But above all he treasured cross-disciplinary exchanges such as the Semaines internationales de synthèse that gathered natural scientists and humanities scholars each year to discuss a specific topic. We argue that these exchanges helped him consolidate his own position in the on-going controversies in theoretical physics.

In cutting-edge research, on technical subjects such as electron physics, magnetism and relativity, we have seen that Langevin developed broad views with historical panoramas scattered with philosophical reflections. This inclination, visible from the earliest lectures, qualified him for a specialist in the dissemination of new physical theories. This activity represents around 20% of the publications that we have placed under the category "scientific publications" (Chap. 13). For Langevin, sharing knowledge was as important as producing new knowledge.

> We must join the effort to build science with that of making it accessible so that mankind continues its march in tight formation without a lost vanguard or a trailing rearguard. We must maintain contact, and I am, for my part, fully convinced of the possibility of fulfilling this duty of disseminating true science which is imposed on us as one of the aspects of our social action. (Langevin 1946a, p. 20)

He was convinced that science cannot advance if it is confiscated by a minority. It is a common good, to be shared. This is a corollary of the social function he assigned to science (Chap. 12). Given that science is the driver of human progress, it must percolate through the entire society instead of being the exclusive property of an elite. It is therefore the duty of the happy few who have been fed "on the good milk of science, also full of human tenderness" (Langevin 1932a, p. 239) to share this precious food with others.

But how did Langevin disseminate his broad scientific culture? Did he just bring science to the people in a top-down manner as most science popularisers used to do in the 1930s or did he try to engage in dialogue with specific audiences?

15.1 Public Outreach

Judging by his correspondence, Langevin reached a variety of the lay public. For instance, the writer J.-H. Rosny senior took him as a scientific advisor and submitted to him "riddles" on relativity (Letter February 1924, Archives, L076/034). We also discovered a letter from a 13-year-old high school student asking for his opinion on a matter of physics (31 May 1934, Archives L085/049). A mutilated worker from Cherbourg discussed his interpretation of the crisis of determinism (4 August 1934. Archives L085). How did Langevin gain such an audience?

Far from shunning modern means of communication, he invested in the new world of radio (Fig. 15.1). In 1934, Langevin was part of a Radio Commission linked to the preparation of the international exhibition of 1937. He was also the president, alongside Vaillant-Couturier, of the Administrative Committee of *Radio-Liberté*, an association of listeners for the defence of impartiality of information, the improvement of programmes and the enhancement of heritage (Archives, L044). Langevin himself became used to the microphone: he participated in a series of "Philosophical conversations" on Radio-Paris (Langevin 1936a) and in a series of talks on "What Modern Civilization Owes to Disinterested Research" (Langevin 1936b, c), that prepared the opening of the Palais de la découverte (Langevin 1937e).

Fig. 15.1 Broadcasting. (ESPCI)

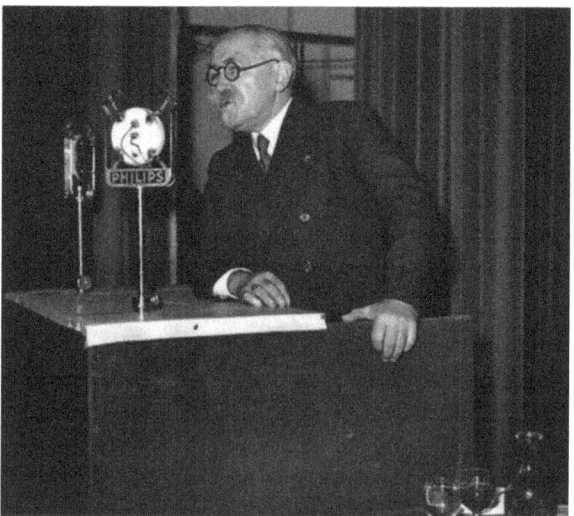

Langevin thus fully participated in the grand offensive of the French scientific community that aimed to restore public trust in science, after "the prostitution of science"[1] during the Great War. A plethora of big projects were launched in the 1930s, including an imposing series of books, encyclopaedias, popular universities, exhibitions and museums [2].

However, the French champions of popular science displayed competing views of the value of science. On one side, Charles Andler, a colleague of Langevin at the *Collège de France*, who translated into French a number of Karl Marx's works, advocated "Labour Humanism" (*L'humanisme travailliste*). This essay of social pedagogy recommended that the socialist party develop a modern high-level education for the working class in Work Institutes (*Instituts du travail*), whose major goal was to bridge the gap between workers and engineers. He recommended a rational organization of social life inspired by the management theory of Frederick Taylor [1, p. 50]. By contrast, the *Université ouvrière* (Labour University), founded in 1932, aimed instead to emancipate the masses through culture and scientific education and mobilized the leaders of peace movement, like Langevin, Barbusse, Alain and Rolland.

During the 1930s the model of the Labour University prevailed. Its advocates—Alain, Langevin and Perrin—had political alliances and personal links dating back to their student years at the *Ecole Normale Supérieure* (ENS) in the 1890s. These included politicians who were in power during the 1920s and 1930s, such as Edouard Herriot, historian and politician from the *Parti radical* who served three times as Prime Minister (1924–1925; 1926; 1932) and twice as President of the Chamber of deputies, and Léon Blum, politician from the socialist party, three-time prime minister and leader of the Popular Front in 1936–1937.

15.2 Three Big Cultural Enterprises in the 1930s

As a result of this network of associates, Langevin was involved in creating the *Encyclopédie française*, an extensive cultural enterprise initiated by the French minister of Education Anatole de Monzie and Lucien Febvre, in 1932.[2] The project, launched at the Congress of the International League for New Education in Nice (Langevin 1932a), was meant to counter the *Italian Encyclopaedia* that was supported by Mussolini's fascist regime. It proceeded from a desire to conduct "an intellectual self-examination" after the shock of the First World War ([4]. Archives L040/003). The *Encyclopédie française* was neither a dictionary in alphabetic order,

---

[1] Langevin's phrase in 1925, see Chap. 12.
[2] Anatole de Monzie, a republican socialist politician, served ten times as minister in the Third Republic. He later supported the Vichy Regime during the German occupation. Lucien Febvre, a historian, co-founder with Marc Bloch of the journal *Annales* around which a research school formed. He was elected professor at the *Collège de France* in 1933 and collaborated with Langevin on several projects, including the *Encyclopédie française* [4].

nor a collection of disciplinary volumes. To avoid a fixed or completed compilation of knowledge, it was designed in the form of booklets that would be constantly updated and could be bound into several volumes. The initial plan outlined by Febvre included ten volumes, and was later extended to 18 volumes and even 21. As a member of the Steering Committee, Langevin was responsible for the first volumes dealing with "Matter: Its Constitution, Energy, the Earth and the Universe" (Archives, L041/064).

Yet, the philosophy of the enterprise was very close to Langevin's ideas on science and culture. Febvre shared with Langevin the cult of a living science, and wished to highlight unsolved problems as much as established knowledge [7]. Febvre demanded from his collaborators human testimonies from active researchers rather than popular treaties. He wanted "to reach a wide public—but not to win it by lowering oneself" and "to create understanding by awakening a critical sense").

How did Langevin rise to this challenge in the volumes he supervised? We cannot, alas, judge from the result. The project was interrupted by the war, and the physics volumes published in 1956 were edited by de Broglie, who completely revised them. We know, however, from Febvre's account in the Foreword of volume II, that Langevin led his project at a brisk pace, as a "conductor":

> I will never forget, me the incompetent, me the ignorant, that afternoon around 1938 when, in my office on rue du Four, all the army of French physics of the time assembled (…): the two Perrins, and the two de Broglies, and the two Joliot-Curies and a few others of the same stature. Langevin presented his plan, assigned a subject area to each of his collaborators and even the most critical could only bow before the power, logic, strength, let's say the mastery of such work that mobilized with such a singular force all the ideas, all the hypotheses that the men, so simple in appearance, who surrounded the leader of this orchestra of creators, used to imagine and establish a new reality.[3]

One can get an idea of the plan conceived by Langevin from the outlines he wrote in 1937 and 1938 (Archives L041). Volume II was supposed to include two sections: a first section organized around the concept of "configuration changes" and the second around the concept of "structures". The first was to start with energy, then deal with mechanics, thermodynamics and morphogenesis. The second was to present the structure of matter, of light and of crystals. Finally, wave mechanics and quantum mechanics were to be treated separately in a third part, titled *The Quanta*. The few documents available in the archives do not allow us to understand why quantum theory should have been treated separately. The purpose might be to respond to Febvre's urge to put the emphasis on unsolved problems. Langevin personally took charge of an introduction on the method and history of physics, where he intended to address a host of philosophical themes, like the relationships between

---

[3] Among the collaborators chosen by Langevin, there were senior scholars—Marcel Brillouin, Georges Bruhat, Aimé Cotton and Jean Perrin, for physics and the chemist Georges Urbain. He also involved young scholars who sometimes paired with their elders on a chapter: Francis Perrin, Louis de Broglie, Frédéric Joliot, Pierre Auger who was starting in the study of cosmic rays, Edmond Bauer and Jacques Solomon who came from medicine to nuclear physics and would later become Langevin's son-in-law.

concrete and abstract, between subject and object, or between positivism and realism.

Langevin's inclination towards an epistemological approach to physics is also visible in his collaboration with another big cultural enterprise of the 1930s. Marie Lahy-Hollebecque, editor of a massive collective multivolume project entitled *The Evolution of Mankind from the Origins to Today (L'Évolution humaine, des origines à nos jours, étude biologique, psychologique et sociologique de l'homme)*, entrusted Langevin with the task of writing the preface. Why choose a physicist, rather than a biologist or an anthropologist, to introduce a collection dedicated to mankind? Clearly, she did not want the point of view of an expert and instead expected someone who could outline the philosophy of the project. Langevin dutifully responded to her expectation in authoring a little text, repeatedly reprinted, on "The Human Value of Science" (Langevin 1934a). It is written as a manifesto, explicitly aimed at replying to those who doubt "the services, both material, spiritual and moral" that science provides to humans (ibid. vii). To convince them, Langevin masterfully develops his familiar conviction that science is one factor in the adaptation and liberation of mankind (Chap. 12). It is worth noticing that Langevin did not target the wave of criticism against science and technology that developed among French intellectuals during the 1920s and 1930s in his campaign for science [6]. Instead, he criticized the rising technocratic wave which valued technological progress more than the spiritual liberation of mankind. Langevin did not just claim that material progress matters less than spiritual liberation by invoking the ancient figure of Epicurus as a pioneer of spiritual liberation (ibid., p. 46). He deplored the "technological intoxication" of our civilization which he held responsible for the economic crisis. Furthermore, he assumed that "by its moral and spiritual value", science "can help us fight the dangers resulting from its too great or too premature utilitarian value" (ibid., pp. 44–45).

The campaign for pure science, the living source of all technological applications, culminated in the project of the *Palais de la découverte* (Palace of Discovery) opened in 1937 for the World Exhibition *Les arts et les techniques dans la vie moderne*.

The project, initiated in 1932, included a section on "Manifestations of Thought" divided up into three groups: expression, formation and dissemination of thought. The whole project was supervised by the *Commission de synthèse et de coopération intellectuelle*, directed by the politician Henry de Jouvenel. The *Palais de la découverte* was included in Group 1 "expression of thought", whose promoters shared the republican concern for education and the transnational ideal underlying the Confederation of Intellectual Workers (*Confédération des travailleurs intellectuels*) [3]. However, they did not have exactly the same view of intellectual work. Paul Valéry, a poet and essayist, imagined a Society of Minds (*Société des esprits*), based on international solidarity created by intelligence and culture. Georges Duhamel, a novelist and peace activist like Langevin, proposed a *Palais de l'esprit,* a sanctuary of the mind enriched with a library. Perrin wanted to celebrate pure science (Fig. 15.2). Over the course of the preliminary projects, the *Palais de l'esprit* turned into the *Palais de la découverte*, exclusively dedicated to science. This spectacular,

Fig. 15.2 Jean Perrin in 1935, director of the project of the *Palais de le Découverte*. (*Science et Vigilance*)

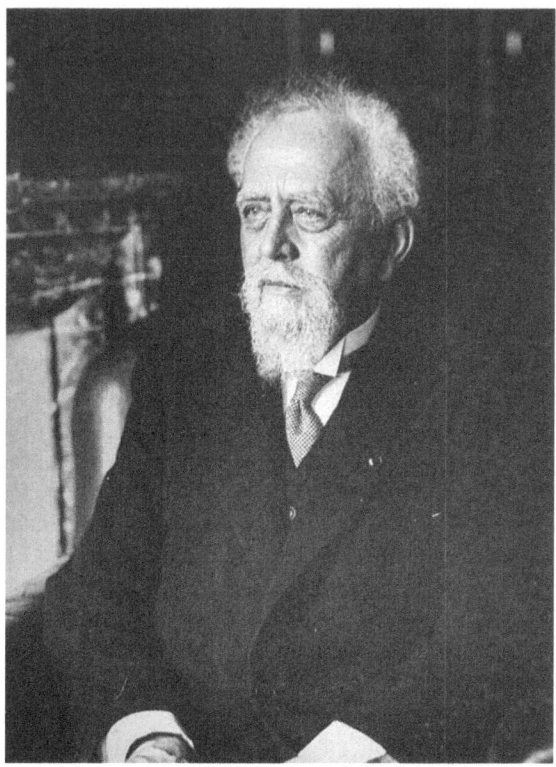

lively and wonderful staging of the power of science has been described as a "cathedral for science" [8]. It displayed a number of discoveries made without practical purpose that nevertheless became sources of technological progress.

> The Palace of Discovery (…) must make this origin manifest and make the public understand that, in the past, but also in the future, we can hope for nothing really new, nothing that changes the Destiny that seemed imposed on men, except through scientific research and discovery. [10, p. 6]

This monumental work, entirely entrusted to professional scientists, was led by Jean Perrin. If Langevin was not deeply involved in the design of the exhibitions—he is only mentioned in relation to two rooms on oscillating phenomena—he participated in the preliminary stage that defined the objectives of the Palace, as noted by Perrin:

> Langevin, myself and a few friends defended these ideas in front of Henry de Jouvenel, […] We noted that an Exhibition of Technicians, in which the role of Discovery would not be highlighted, would be like a beautiful statue without a head and we asked if it would be possible to erect in this spirit a Palace of Discovery. [10, p. 5]

The priority of disinterested research is a theme that had been largely developed by Langevin in his talks since 1928. In his public presentation of the *Palais de la découverte*, Perrin occasionally used Langevin's words, always punctuated with the

15.2 Three Big Cultural Enterprises in the 1930s

same example of Michael Faraday, the modest bookbinder turned scientist, committed to pure and disinterested research, who enabled the electrification of the world. Perrin's concept of the exhibition also reveals a strong community of views. The Palace of Discovery should not be a conservatory displaying established results. It rather would display science in action. It would be a real "working laboratory", emphasizing current trends of research. In short, a kind of "popular university" capable of awakening research callings among youngsters.

The Palace of Discovery was not unrelated to Perrin's campaign to the government to obtain employment for full-time researchers by creating a state agency of scientific research [12]. The opening of the Palace, a few months before the establishment of the CNRS and also a state Undersecretary for Research, can be seen as a propaganda gesture in support of political action to secure the status of scientific research [5]. This corporatist dimension did not go unnoticed by those who had alternative projects for displaying the "Expression of Thought" at the World Exhibition. The frenzy of communication in the group of physicists raised some concern in the world of humanities. Duhamel suggested it was unethical. In his fiction *Chronique des Pasquier*, one of the characters Nicolas Rohner is a modern scientist, efficient, a media star, but he is inhuman and satanic. Valéry also considered that the "fever" of communication was a phenomenon of civilization, "a real disease of culture", a threat of destruction of the mind by the mind. "Life ends by devouring life" ([13], p. 279).

Despite these criticisms, the Palace was a big success. It attracted many visitors during the international exhibition and effectively contributed to awaken scientific interests among younger generation once it was had been transferred and transformed into a permanent museum.

The participation of Langevin in these three major outreach projects, *L'Encyclopédie française*, *L'Évolution humaine* and *the Palais de la découverte*, during the interwar period confirms that he was a key figure in the milieu of intellectual workers who promoted an aggressive policy of scientific culture, based on transnational and democratic ideals. Langevin and Perrin were key players in the cultural policy implemented under the *Front Populaire* [9]. Langevin's outreach activities allow us to better understand who he was for his contemporaries, how they perceived him. He was undoubtedly recognized as an international scientific authority, but he did not embody the figure of an expert in physical sciences. Instead, he embodied the figure of a transnational intellectual promoting the values of peace and solidarity through the practice of science.

Yet, there is a dissonance between Langevin's words and his deeds. How can we accept the exhortations to disseminate knowledge from a man who failed to publish much of his own work? Why should we accept this advice from someone who hid his technical achievements in secret patents? And how does a man who is steeped in education never write a textbook?

There is need to understand his purpose for sharing knowledge. He has no interest in laying out his personal scientific advances for future historians to inspect. There is no intent to leave a legacy in publications so as to claim personal precedents. His method of dissemination is closer to the forums and academies of the

Ancients than to the formalized academic journals of the nineteenth century. The ways he chose for sharing knowledge are intimately connected to his view of science as an active, dynamic expression of life. It has to be shared, in the present, accepting all its challenging messiness and uncertainty because it is part of the collective effort of humans to adapt to their environment. Even his use of patents can make sense, viewed as a means to create a secure commercial environment now, and not to be owned and filed away to prevent others from using them.

Viewed in this light, science communicated as a shared dynamic human endeavour in the present and not as a ledger in which to record the detailed step by step of scientific advancement, it is possible to reconcile Langevin's views on sharing knowledge with his method of doing so and the audiences of his activities of communication.

15.3 Actor in Cross-Disciplinary Exchanges

In particular, Langevin played a central role in the emergence of a special kind of science popularization in France in the interwar period: a high culture dissemination of science through exchanges between educated people. The public curiosity for physics aroused from the aura of a few star scientists, Marie Curie for radioactivity, Einstein for relativity, and Louis de Broglie's Nobel Prize for quantum physics in 1929. This interest was nurtured by an extensive series of booklets *Actualités scientifiques et industrielles*, created by the publishing house Hermann in 1929. It was based on a series of lectures that started in 1927 at the National Conservatory of Arts and Crafts (Conservatoire national des arts et métiers).[4] The purpose of this series as described in the first volume was to inform the regular audience of the *Conservatoire national des Arts and Métiers*, and those who are fond of "scientific culture". Nearly 900 small booklets, each 50 to 100 pages long, were published between 1929 and 1940, each one written by a specialist. The "General Physics" series, which was divided into subsections on relativity, atomic physics, quantum theory and nuclear physics, supported a resurgence of interest in theoretical physics from French physicists, who became aware of the most recent advances ([11], pp. 119–126).[5] In the beginning, the volumes were almost exclusively dedicated to physics; then the horizon gradually expanded to include mathematics, other natural sciences and the

---

[4] The *Conservatoire national des arts et métiers* is a life-long learning centre located in Paris created in 1794. It includes a museum of arts and crafts.

[5] Marie Curie was in charge of the series radioactivity and nuclear physics, Léon Brillouin of the series *Exposés sur la théorie des quanta* in which Jacques Solomon published a volume on *The Theory of the Passage of Cosmic Rays Through Matter*" in 1936. Brillouin himself contributed the second volume, on light diffraction by ultrasound, in 1933. Brillouin also managed the series on acoustics, for which the first volume by Rytov was again on ultrasonic diffraction (1938). Néda Marinesco was editor of a series of *Exposés sur le rayonnement et la biophysique*, himself contributing the first two volumes, on the chemical, physical and biological effects of ultrasound in 1937 and 1938.

humanities. In 1933, a "Philosophy of Sciences" series was created, with Louis de Broglie as chief editor, which published Meyerson's essay *Réel et déterminisme dans la physique quantique* (Chap. 16) and many other volumes related to quantum mechanics.

Langevin's personal action was oriented both towards the disciplines neighbouring physics and towards humanities. He presented the new theories of physics to astronomers, engineers and chemists. Far from making a standard and generic summary, he cared about highlighting their consequences on the discipline of the readers, even if it means embarking on a lengthy preliminary tutorial. In particular, Langevin strived to develop cross-disciplinary fields, like astrophysics, for example, where "the observatory is a laboratory that has the entire universe as field of experience" (Langevin 1927h). He so much favoured cross-boundaries fields that he was invited to present the inaugural lecture at the International Congress of Chemical Physics held in Paris in 1933.[6]

This attitude can be seen as a sign of continuity in Langevin's work. After working in his youth to replace classical mechanics with a new synthesis of all branches of physics, he set up to build bridges between various natural sciences. On a different scale, he pursued the same dream of unity by highlighting that astronomy and chemistry were both connected to the new physics. However, a noticeable change in style can be seen in Langevin's popular lectures on the theory of relativity. It is no longer presented as a product of the human mind in its effort to adapt to the outside world in the 1930s, but as the work of one man, Einstein. As he personalized relativity physics, Langevin emphasized the contrast between Einstein and Poincaré:

> Poincaré had adopted a somewhat eclectic attitude: since there is no difference between the logical values of the various geometries, one can indifferently take one or the other, even modifying the physical laws, when passing from one to the other. He had not foreseen that by resorting to Riemannian geometry, in which the curvature properties of space-time are determined by its content, Einstein would succeed in shedding new light on the old mystery of gravitation. (Langevin 1922b, p. 11)

He even described Einstein physically and morally, calling him the "flower of Israel" and paying tribute to the intellectual wealth of the Jewish people (Langevin 1931a, p. 278). He paid new attention to the human realities of scientific activity, encouraged in the case of Einstein, by the threats weighing on German Jews. We must recognize, however, that this tendency to "humanize" physics did not much favour a rapprochement with French philosophers, who were more inclined to describe the advancement of science as "the progress of reason" (Brunschvicg) or the deployment of "latent possibilities of a pre-existing human reason" (Meyerson). We can fear that Langevin did not find more response among those who shook up classical rationalism. Bachelard, for example, assumed the autonomy of the scientific spirit and even argued that it is formed from a rupture with common sense.

Did this discourage Langevin from continuing to engage in discussions with philosophers? Not at all. Just as he had turned to the philosophy community in 1911

---

[6] Jean Perrin was the leader of this new branch of science in France.

and 1922 to discuss relativity theory, he brought quantum theory to philosophical circles after the 1927 Solvay Council of Physics. His first presentation of quantum mechanics was to philosophy graduates whom he addresses in 1929, during a series of lectures on the current orientation of science, organized by Léon Brunschvicg at the *Ecole normale supérieure* ENS. (Langevin 1930a). Brunschvicg's introduction underlines the historical importance of these exchanges. He describes the nineteenth century as a period of "divorce" between science and philosophy, of closing both philosophical and scientific systems, and contrasts it with a twentieth century of rediscoveries, where, under the effect of the crises in physics, "scientific knowledge and philosophical reflection become contemporary again". Langevin again met Brunschvicg at the "Summer Talks" of the abbey of Pontigny, which gathered personalities from all walks of life, philosophers, poets, essayists, scientists and industrialists. In 1929, he rubbed shoulders with Gaston Bachelard, Alexandre Koyré and Martin Buber.[7] Langevin was so immersed in French philosophical circles that, in 1937, he was quite naturally asked to contribute to the International Congress of Philosophy, organized by Emile Bréhier, to celebrate the anniversary of Descartes's *Discours de la méthode*, as if he belonged by right to the community of philosophers.

15.4 At the *Centre international de synthèse*

Finally, Langevin contributed above all to the rapprochement with humanities through his attendance at a high table of interdisciplinarity, the *Centre international de synthèse*. This organization, created in 1925 by the historian Henri Berr linked to the *Institut international de coopération intellectuelle*, had at first an essentially historical purpose, with a clear focus on the history of sciences. Around 1930, when the *Revue de synthèse historique* was renamed *Revue de synthèse*, the field widened to meet the objectives of two sections, "Natural Sciences", directed by Langevin, and "General Synthesis", directed by the philosopher Abel Rey. The unity of natural and human sciences was assumed as a postulate and not as a problem. This credo was the very foundation of the project (*Revue de synthèse*, Oct. 1931, pp. 6–7) and inspired all activities of the Centre de synthèse, in particular, the organization of International Synthesis Weeks, major annual conferences where current issues in the sciences of the mind and nature were debated.

---

[7] Gaston Bachelard (1884–1962) had a profound influence on French intellectual life, not only through his work in epistemology and the history of the exact sciences—mathematics, physics and chemistry—but also through his work of literary and philosophical analysis of poetry, of dreaming and symbolism. Alexandre Koyré (1892–1964), a historian and philosopher of sciences, had a more international career. Born in Russia, he studied in Germany and then in Paris, where he taught as well as in American universities. He is particularly famous for his *Galilean Studies* and his *Newtonian Studies*. Finally, Martin Buber (1869–1965) was a philosopher of religions: his doctrine is centred on the concepts of encounter, dialogue and reciprocity.

Langevin presided over the Synthesis Week of 1930 dedicated to "Relativity" (Langevin 1932b). In 1931, during a Week on "The Theory of Quanta" (alas, not published), he gave a lecture on "The Philosophical Consequences of Quantum Theory". In 1933, he participated in the debates of the Week on "Science and Law". In 1935, he gave an important lecture on "Statistics and Determinism" (Langevin 1935e). He also participated in a Synthesis Week dedicated to "Invention" in 1937, and to that of 1938 on "Sensitivity in Man and in Nature" (Langevin 1938c). Not only was Langevin a regular at the Hôtel de Nevers, but he also brought with him young physicists, like Edmond Bauer and Jacques Solomon, who also became artisans of dialogue. Moreover, Langevin did not just attend the debates. The reports of these Weeks show that he often intervened. During the fifth Week on "Science and Law", for example, he constantly made contributions. He mostly developed his interpretation of "the crisis of science", without evoking the polemical context from which it originated. With the seductive formulae he had a knack for, he had no trouble imposing his views. So much so that in his preface to the volume, Henri Berr took up Langevin's words as the official interpretation of the crisis in quantum theory.

In these multiple presentations to an audience of the educated public, Langevin did not always choose a neutral or impersonal discourse. He presented relativity as a fully established theory that is no longer discussed but simply used (Langevin 1931a, p. 278). When it comes to quantum physics, as we will see in the next chapter, he adopted a partisan attitude on the crisis of determinism. Each of these exposés was for him a way to deepen the problems at stake in the crisis of determinism and to take an increasingly firm position in the debates. Thus Langevin appeared less and less as an anonymous spokesman for the physics community, and more and more as an influential interpreter of the new theories of physics.

References

1. Andler C (1927) L'Humanisme travailliste. Essais de pédagogie sociale. éditions civilisation française, Paris
2. Bensaude-Vincent B (2010) Popular science and politics in interwar France. In: Workshop 20th century science communication in Europe: the political and cultural context. Max Planck Institut fur Wissenschaftgeschichte, Berlin, 6–8 May 2010
3. Bergeron A, Bigg C (2015) D'ombres et de lumières. L'exposition de 1937 et les premières années du palais de la découverte au prisme du transnational. Revue germanique internationale 21:187–206
4. De Monzie A (1933) Pour une encyclopédie française. Booklet Archives L040/003
5. Eidelmann J (1986) The cathedral of French scinece: The early years of the palis de la découverte, in Shinn T,Whitley R eds, Expository science. Forms and functions of popularisation, Sociology of the Sciences, vol. 9, p. 195–208
6. Hardy Q (2022) Les philosophies du progrès à l'épreuve du machinisme dans les années 1920–1939. Ph.D. Dissertation, University of Paris 1 Panthéon-Sorbonne
7. Müller B (2002) L'Encyclopédie française dans l'oeuvre de Lucien Febvre. Cahiers Jaurès 163–164:33–63

8. Ory P (1991) Une cathédrale pour les temps nouveaux? Le palais de la Découverte (1934–1940). In: Régine R (ed) Masses et culture de masses dans les années 30. éditions ouvrières, Paris, pp 180–204
9. Ory P (1994) La belle illusion. Culture et politique sous le signe du Front Populaire (1935–1938). Plon, Paris
10. Perrin J (1948) La science et l'espérance. Presses universitaires de France, Paris
11. Pestre D (1984) Physique et physiciens en France 1918-1940, Archives contemporaines, Paris
12. Picard J-F (1990) La République des savants. La recherche française et le CNRS. Flammarion, Paris
13. Valéry P. (1945) La liberté de l'esprit in Regards sur le monde actuel, Gallimard, Paris, p. 285-292.

Chapter 16
Langevin in the Debates on Quantum Mechanics

Abstract The quantum emerged at about the same time as Langevin entered the physics community, in 1900. He followed the development of this new theory from the very outset, attending Marcel Brillouin's course at the Collège de France on "Thermodynamics and Radiation" and through the first Solvay Council in 1911 that really brought quantum theory to the core of physics. In 1912–1913 he devoted his annual course at the *Collège de France* to "The difficulties of the theory of radiation" and he felt deeply upset by the crisis of determinism at the 1927 Solvay Council. In the 1930s he forged a personal interpretation, arguing that it was a crisis of mechanics rather than a crisis of determinism.

16.1 The First Quantum Theory[1]

Planck introduced the notion of the quantum of action in 1900 to account for the discontinuities observed in exchanges of energy. This notion was extended to the specific heat of solids and to light by Einstein in 1905. In 1911, Planck elucidated the puzzle of the thermal radiation emitted by a black-body in his lecture "Energy and temperature" at the *Société française de physique*. He stated that the emission of energy is discontinuous while its absorption is a continuous phenomenon that follows Maxwell's electrodynamics laws.

Fortunately, Langevin's survey of the first quantum theory is accessible thanks to the publication of the notes taken by Emile Borel during Langevin's course in 1912–1913 [4]. Langevin acknowledged that Planck's and Einstein's contributions were spectacular achievements that solved a number of local puzzles. However, he insisted on "The difficulties of the theory of radiation" (the title of the course) and struggled to make sense of them. He clearly pointed out the unknowns: what are the laws ruling these quanta of radiation? What kind of mathematics can be used, given that differential and integral calculus are inadequate for expressing discontinuous

---
[1] The second quantum theory, based on the works of Bohr, Heisenberg, Schrödinger and de Broglie, was the one discussed at the Fifth Solvay Physics Council in 1927.

phenomena? In 1913, Langevin gave a lecture on "The physics of the discontinuous" (Langevin 1913d) at the *Société française de physique*. Here, instead, he emphasized the limitations of the classical theory of physics, "which is only suitable for the study of systems accessible to our senses, and which are generally composed of a large number of elements [...] That's the task we're currently facing: to establish the link between the background and the surface, between the principles of the grain and those of the aggregate, in order to explain the overall facts". And the metaphor of the "new world" that he had used in 1904 for the "the physics of electrons" resurfaced to describe the physics of quanta:

> A new world is revealed to us, whose laws dominate all physics. We must try to trace them back, and we may hope to find them simpler than their distant consequences, than the average or statistical results to which we are accustomed. (Ibid., p. 3)

The physics of the discontinuous opens up a research programme that is presented with great optimism. In Langevin's view, quanta do not have the same disruptive potential as the theory of relativity. According to Louis de Broglie, Langevin would have claimed that the "quanta of light", or photons, could not threaten the electromagnetic theory of light. In 1922, he even discouraged one of his students from working on the photon hypothesis [7, pp. 262–263]. Nevertheless, he still taught Bohr and Sommerfeld's quantization methods in greater depth at the *Collège de France* in 1919.

16.2 Louis de Broglie "Lifted a Corner of the Great Veil"

Louis de Broglie (Fig. 16.1) studied physics thanks to his brother Maurice de Broglie, who had the use of a private laboratory. His doctoral thesis, submitted in 1924, developed a wave theory of electrons. It seems that Langevin's interest in quantum physics was revived by de Broglie's PhD thesis in November 1924, an important work establishing wave mechanics that would be rewarded by a Physics Nobel prize in 1929. His report, as a member of the jury, suggests that de Broglie's hypothesis opened the way to a new synthesis of physics:

> The work of Mr. Louis de Broglie represents an important effort towards the solution of the most important problem of current physics, the synthesis of the two optical theories of waves and quanta, hitherto contradictory at least in appearance, each of which is based on a whole set of facts and remarkable experimental confirmations and whose opposition has unexpectedly renewed the old conflict of emission and waves.
>
> The general connection thus established between the movement of a particle, whether electrified or not, and the propagation of a periodic phenomenon is linked by the author to general principles in a very profound way through a series of remarks such that the paradoxical hypothesis appears at first glance more and more in line with the nature of things. He shows in particular that the movement of a grain of energy and the propagation of the accompanying periodic phenomenon are exactly of the same nature as those introduced by Lord Rayleigh and Gouy between the movement of a wave group and the propagation of the phase of an exactly periodic wave.

16.2 Louis de Broglie "Lifted a Corner of the Great Veil"

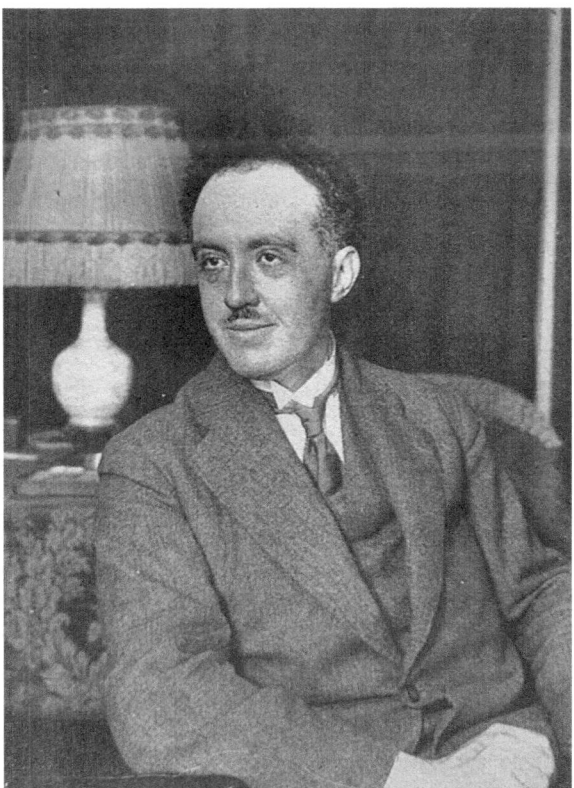

Fig. 16.1 Louis de Broglie (1892–1987)

On the other hand, and this is perhaps the most interesting aspect of Mr. de Broglie's ideas, this connection seems to correspond to the analogy, purely formal until now, but perhaps very profound, between on one hand the statements of stationary integrals that are at the basis of dynamics with Hamilton's and Maupertuis' principles and the wave theory, and on the other hand with Fermat's principle as introduced and justified by the concepts of Huyghens and Fresnel.

The paradoxes that had to be introduced by the theory of quanta are themselves of two orders that correspond to what can be called the dynamic aspect on one side and that of the "quanta of light" on the other. To account for the composition of black-body radiation and the structure of emission and absorption spectra it was necessary, with Planck, Bohr, Sommerfeld, to admit that among all the movements of electrified centres compatible with the laws of classical dynamics, only those for which the electronic orbits satisfy certain simple numerical relations are possible. On the other hand, Einstein ("and J. J. Thomson" added in Langevin's hand writing) has shown that the so-called photoelectric effects, where the absorption of radiation is accompanied by the emission of cathode particles as well as fluctuations in black radiation, seem to impose the idea that the energy of the radiation itself is not distributed continuously in space but is composed of grains of energy proportional to the frequency.

De Broglie's fundamental idea is to unify the two types of statements about quanta by associating with each electrified particle, considered as an independent grain of energy, a periodic frequency phenomenon proportional to the energy of the grain, exactly as the hypothesis of light quanta associates with periodic light waves non-electrified grains in which their energy is concentrated.

Just as the principles of the dynamics from the material point of view take their simplest expression through the introduction of a four-dimensional vector, the momentum of the universe (*l'impulsion d'univers*), whose space component is the quantity of movement and the time component is the energy of movement, the author shows that Fermat's principle and all the kinematics of waves lead to the introduction of a "wave vector" of the universe whose space component is directed along the radius and whose time component is frequency.

The introduction of these two vectors first leads to generalizing the quantum relation in an intrinsic form valid for all Galilean reference systems, and to specify the relationship between the movement of a particle and the associated periodic phenomenon, by assuming the identity of the two vectors, of the momentum of the universe of the particle and the wave vector for the periodic phenomenon (or rather, due to the choice of units, the constancy of the ratio equal to h, the Planck constant). The relationship of the quantum, considered so far only for the components of time, energy and frequency, is thus extended in a sense entirely in line with the spirit of the theory of relativity to the four components of each vector.

Under these conditions, the principles of Hamilton and Fermat merge and represent two aspects of the same principle, one concerning the movement of the particle, the other of the associated wave. Perhaps here is the origin of a wave interpretation of the principles of dynamics. (Langevin 1924d)

The young de Broglie reactivated the aspiration for a synthesis in the senior physicist. The promise of an imminent synthesis of physics rests on the unification of two aspects of the quantum, Bohr's stationary states and the "grains of energy" of Planck and Einstein. Langevin especially retained de Broglie's attempt to elucidate the unresolved puzzle of the formal analogy between the principles of Hamilton and Fermat. He shared with de Broglie the hope that this formal analogy would take on a physical meaning. In short, Langevin and de Broglie shared a concern with realism and unity.

Langevin immediately sent the PhD thesis to Einstein, who responded, on 16 December 1924: "Louis de Broglie's work made a great impression on me; it lifted a corner of the great veil" (Archives, L072/029). Einstein then made this work known to the Berlin Academy of sciences in January 1925.[2] For his part, Langevin dedicated his entire 1926–1927 course to "The Structure of Light and Quanta", before attending the Fifth Solvay Council on "Electrons and Photons" at the end of 1927. Unfortunately it is impossible to determine how de Broglie influenced Langevin's exposition of the theory of quanta because no record of this course remains.

---

[2] Langevin had few opportunities to discuss with Einstein about the crisis of determinism. In 1932, Langevin met Einstein in Antwerp, just before his departure for California, but according to later letters they discussed instead the international situation. The correspondence of the following years contains only one reference to quantum mechanics: in a letter of 3 October 1935, Einstein states that it cannot become "a usable foundation for all physics" and that "instinct revolts against it" (Archives, L072/035).

16.3 The Crisis of Determinism

At the Fifth Solvay Physics Council in 1927, quantum mechanics appeared for the first time as a constituted theory, breaking with classical ideas about matter and light. Experimental data on atomic spectra were explained and nothing remained beyond its reach. It had its special mathematical tools, in fact two mathematical formalisms: the wave formalism of Erwin Schrödinger, still compatible with mechanical images, and the more abstract matrix formalism invented by Heisenberg. Each one had its own followers, depending on their interest in visualizing physical phenomena.

However, this completely new theory raised a number of paradoxes, which generated a crisis in the foundations of physics. They stem primarily from Bohr's principle of complementarity. This principle, formulated in a previous 1927 Congress in Italy, provides a non-contradictory representation of phenomena at the microscopic level [6]. To the term "complementarity" Bohr attaches less the idea of an association of certain features in the description of objects than their mutual exclusion. Three essential ideas are contained in this notion: (1) several descriptions of the same phenomenon are necessary; (2) there are pairs of descriptions that cannot be applied at the same time without implying contradiction; (3) neither of these mutually exclusive descriptions is sufficient to give an exhaustive description of the phenomenon in question. The notion of complementarity thus challenged the physicists' habits of thought.

This first paradox is enhanced by the principle of indeterminacy presented by Max Born and Werner Heisenberg at the 1927 Solvay Council (Fig. 16.2). They presented their mathematical formalism, stressing that no sensible physical image could correspond to it. They then added that, since these calculations are based on average values, they are statistical in nature. They do not consequently allow the prediction of an isolated event. This claim would have been trivial, had it not been for their assertion that this incapacity is essential, "deeply rooted in the nature of our power to know", and calls into question the postulate of determinism hitherto accepted as the basis of all natural sciences.

A debate ensued between Bohr and Einstein: Bohr assumed the indeterminacy of electrons as well as the wave-particle duality, considering these as two aspects that are mutually exclusive or complementary. Einstein rejected Bohr's notion of complementarity and refused to elevate indeterminacy to a principle.

Upon returning from Brussels, Louis de Broglie seemed convinced by Bohr and for a few years supported the Copenhagen interpretation (Langevin 1937a; [8]). How did Langevin respond to the crisis? Which camp will he join, Bohr or Einstein? (Fig. 16.3).

Just as he did in 1911 in his response to Einstein's theory of special relativity, he articulated his first response to the crisis of determinism to an audience of philosophers. He was invited by Brunschvicg to give a lecture for philosophy students at the *École normale supérieure* in 1929 (Langevin 1930a). Once again, Langevin's exposé reveals his intellectual capacity to metabolize new ideas, because he

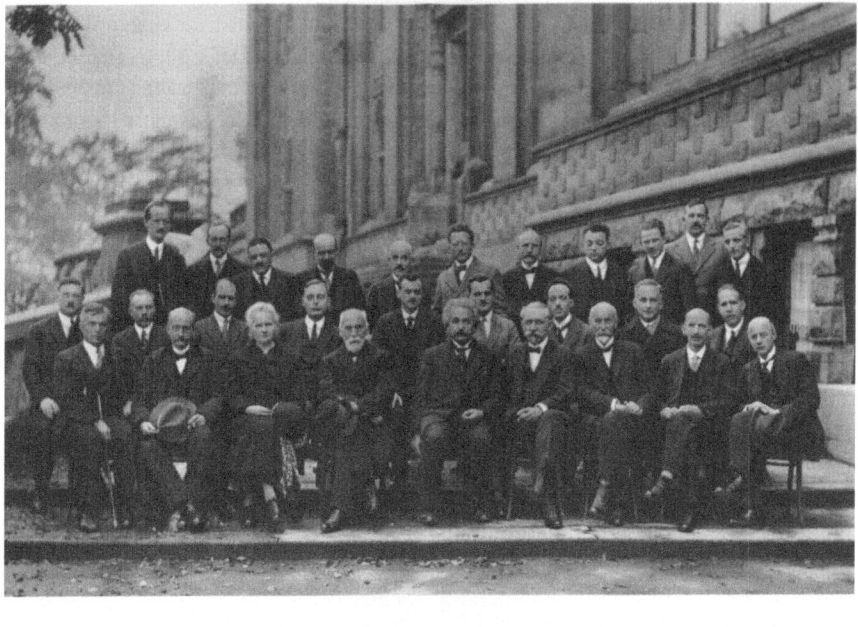

Fig. 16.2 The Fifth Solvay Council, 1927, on the theme "Electrons and Photons", marked the beginning of the theory of quantum mechanics and the start of a long debate between the supporters and opponents of determinism. (International Solvay Institutes/Université Libre de Bruxelles)

provides a broad historical survey of theoretical physics leading to the recent crisis. However, in 1929, Langevin struggles with the views of the Copenhagen school and does not clearly take sides in the controversy between Bohr and Einstein. Whereas, in 1904, Langevin seemed impermeable to the atmosphere of crisis when he considered vast syntheses, he now seems to be permeated by it.

In his 1929 lecture he focuses on the notion of contradiction presented as a driving force bringing historical changes in physics. He finds contradictions everywhere: a contradiction between experience and theory characterizes the method of physicists; the contradiction between matter and radiation is at the core of the theory of physics; last but not least, the contradiction between continuity and discontinuity is the major obstacle to make sense of quantum mechanics from a physical point of view.

This exposé, bringing the idea of contradiction in the foreground, is itself woven with contradictions. Langevin hammers a revolutionary, scathing message: the only way out of the crisis lies in the critical examination of the notions of classical physics and the invention of new concepts that suit the new situation. In this respect, Langevin expresses his admiration for Heisenberg who, according to him, resumes Einstein's constructive approach by introducing new notions derived from

16.3 The Crisis of Determinism

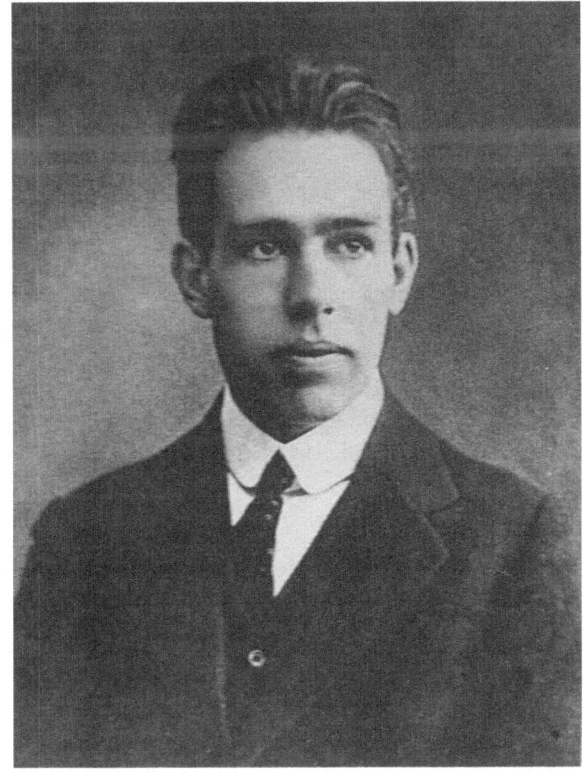

Fig. 16.3 Niels Bohr (1875–1962), winner of the Nobel Prize for Physics in 1922, leader of the "Copenhagen School" and author of the theory of complementarity

experimental reality. He perceives Heisenberg's contribution as "a return to a tendency that is more phenomenological than explanatory" (ibid., p. 56). But the praise is ambivalent, as Heisenberg finds himself confined in the phenomenological tradition that limits the scope of his conclusions to the descriptive level. Langevin emphasizes that the matrices proposed by Heisenberg are a powerful instrument of description and prediction, but he does not hide his preference for the equivalent formalism of Schrödinger which he considers easier, less abstract and closer to the Hamiltonian conception of the theory of mechanics. Schrödinger is "more in line with the habits of mind and conceptions of physicists, who for a long time have been familiar with the handling of the image of a wave" (ibid., p. 59). On the one hand, Langevin recommends a thorough revision of classical notions and, on the other hand, he values the physicists' familiar habits of thought. He is not ready to maintain a critical attitude to the end. He considers the statistical nature of quantum theory to be "provisional" and only mentions Heisenberg's so-called indeterminacy principle in the very last lines. While presenting it as the culmination of the critical spirit of the Copenhagen school, he strives to keep it in the margins:

> Heisenberg's critique of the notion of observation currently raises the question of the limits of determinism and reaches to the very foundations on which we believe it is possible to

construct a science of reality. The fact mentioned earlier as a consequence of the existence of quanta, that it is impossible to follow the movement of an individual particle without profoundly disturbing it, led Heisenberg to state a so-called indeterminacy principle, from which would result the experimental impossibility of reaching anything other than statistical laws. (…) It is appropriate to wait before making a judgment on such a serious subject, and to trust, once again, in critical reflection on the exact meaning of words and ideas. The search for determinism is so much the essential driving force of all efforts in scientific construction, that one must ask oneself, when nature leaves a question unanswered, whether it is not appropriate to consider the question as poorly posed and to abandon the representation that provoked it. (Ibid., p. 62)

For the first time, Langevin concludes a physics lecture on an expectant note without promising a bright future. He is reluctant to abandon determinism while admitting the need for a radical reassessment of the fundamental concepts of physics theory. But, unlike Einstein, Langevin does not multiply thought experiments to prove that the problem has been ill defined and that quantum mechanics is incomplete. He will take an alternative pathway.

16.4 It's a Crisis in the Theory of Mechanics

After the disarray that followed the 1927 Solvay Council, Langevin regained control of the situation. The secret of his recovery lies in a diagnosis: it is not determinism that is in crisis but there is a crisis in the theory of mechanics.

First outlined in a short article in a non-specialized journal, *Le Mois* (Langevin 1931f), this interpretation was further developed in a lecture given in 1932 at the International Conference of the Society of Physical Chemistry. For this conference, celebrating the twentieth anniversary of the Society created by Perrin, Langevin chose a broad topic "The notion of particle and atom" (Langevin 1933a). As usual, he adopts a historical approach, but this time his survey does not cover the *longue durée*. He begins with the introduction of atoms in nineteenth-century chemistry and focuses on "experimental preliminaries". Here we rediscover another face of Langevin, almost fascinated by the prowess of visualization techniques that he complacently enumerates. As if reacting against the tendencies towards abstraction and formalization of the younger generation of Heisenbergs, Paulis and Diracs, Langevin rereads the whole construction of atomic physics from the point of view of experimental evidence. Concerning electricity, for instance, he focuses on the experimental demonstration of the granular structure of electric charge, on the measurement of the size of the grain of electricity. When he turns to the investigation of the structure of atoms, he describes in great details the beautiful images obtained using the Wilson cloud chamber. These snapshots are presented as the pinnacle of corpuscular physics.

The second, more theoretical, part of the lecture is, by Langevin's own admission, more tentative but also the most promising for the future. He begins with Bohr's planetary atom, which introduced discontinuity where classical (electromagnetic) theory knew only continuity, then moves on to quantum dynamics, with scant

16.4 It's a Crisis in the Theory of Mechanics

reference to Heisenberg's matrix. Langevin prefers to dwell on de Broglie's wave mechanics and its experimental basis. Langevin progresses to Bohr's principle of complementarity and Heisenberg's principle of indeterminacy. He refers to remarks by Dirac, Eddington and Bohr, and clearly concludes that it is premature to declare the bankruptcy of determinism.

He does not minimize the scope of the crisis in quantum physics. On the contrary, he quickly argues that it requires the sacrifice of a fundamental notion for physics to resume a normal course. But he finds in history a margin of freedom for the choice of the victim. On the altar of sacrifice, Langevin therefore substitutes the notion of the individual particle for that of determinism. This position, close to the one adopted by Max Planck in 1932, finds deep roots in Langevin's earlier work and shows the continuity in his views.

What is wrong with the idea of "corpuscle"? For Langevin, this notion owes its success to the fact that it has always been conceived as having material individuality analogous to human individuals. It is an anthropomorphic notion. The conservation of particles has been modelled on the permanence of the self. It is not surprising therefore that quantum physicists end up attributing a will to particles. Langevin targets the "daring spirits who proclaim the bankruptcy of determinism to lend a free will to electrons". For Langevin, this anthropomorphism is not a fanciful, marginal hypothesis or a deviant interpretation. It is in the direct line of classical mechanics. Langevin acknowledges that Bohr is opposed to such "fantasies", but he rages against his notion of complementarity. He describes it as "ingenious", and praises Bohr's "judicious exploitation" of it in biology, in psychology or sociology. But he finds that this notion is ineffective for overcoming the crisis. Bohr settles into contradiction instead of resolving it. More precisely, he translates the puzzle raised by quantum particles into a more classical difficulty, familiar to philosophers for discerning the subject from the object or the observer from the object under observation. Ultimately, Bohr's principle of complementarity leads to the sacrifice of determinism while preserving the simplistic image of an identifiable and locatable particle.

Langevin does not spare Bohr. Already, in 1929, he presented him as a dilettante who achieved enormous success with an atomic model that was manifestly contradictory (Langevin 1930a, pp. 53–54). The only credit he gives to Bohr is to have brought to light the contradictions that undermine physics. But, for Langevin, the true founder of quantum mechanics, the worthy successor of Einstein, is Heisenberg. To conclude, Langevin ironically notes that the so-called indeterminacy measured by a quantity as precise as h, Planck's constant, is in fact highly determined.

Following all these criticisms of the Copenhagen school, Langevin articulates his own diagnosis of the situation—a crisis of mechanics and not of determinism—in three steps. He first assumes that concepts working at the macroscopic scale are inappropriate at the microscopic level. "It is not possible to represent the intra-atomic world by extrapolating to the extreme limit our macroscopic conception of movement" (Langevin 1933a, p. 35). The notion of the individual corpuscle, forged on the macroscopic scale, has been abusively extended to the microscopic and sub-microscopic world, investigated thanks to new instruments. However, it is not legitimate to apply this anthropomorphic concept, which belongs to the superficial and ancestral level of our experience, to the atomic scale. The macroscopic and the microscopic scales are not of the same order, of the same nature. This criticism can be seen as an instantiation of the "law of exaggeration" in the history of physics that he presented in 1926 (Chap. 12). It is the tendency to extend a well-established explanatory scheme beyond its domain in order to explain "the unknown by the known", in the expectation of a unitary synthesis.

The second argument, rather semantic, concerns the very notion of a particle: Langevin highlights a kind of paradox between the idea of an infinitely small, simple, indiscernible atomic particle and that of individuality which implies a certain complexity, a differentiation and therefore a substrate for differences. In his view, indeterminacy is but the apparent effect of this antinomy between the notions of a particle and individuality. Here, Langevin develops an interesting analysis of the concept of the individual, revealing the ambiguity between the notion of ultimate principle—which presupposes an indivisible whole—and the notion of individual—which presupposes a complex, multiple structure. An organism is individual, but not its components, which nevertheless maintain the individuality of the whole. "An analogous consideration applied to physics would allow individuality to be attributed to the molecule, and denied to its components."

As a third argument in support of his interpretation, Langevin mentions the new quantum statistics developed by Bose-Einstein and Fermi-Dirac. In his course at the *Collège de France*, he clearly argued that these statistics individualize the states of corpuscles rather than the corpuscles themselves, which are considered as indistinguishable. He therefore concludes that this is the right direction: thinking in statistical terms is not burying determinism but relinquishing the substance of the individual particle.

Sacrifice the particle to rescue determinism, Langevin's interpretation of the crisis of quantum physics may be deeply rooted in his previous criticism of classical mechanics, but to what extent did he manage to convince his audience? Did he assemble followers in the controversy that was shaking up the international community of physicists?

16.5 Langevin in the Bohr-Einstein Controversy

Although Langevin's interpretation is ultimately controversial, it was not immediately perceived as such. Between 1933 and 1935, when the battle raged between Bohr and Einstein, Langevin was not officially siding with either camp. As chair of the Solvay Physics Councils he had to stay above the fray. During the Sixth Council, he did not support Einstein's attack on the indeterminacy relations with a new thought experiment nor Bohr's devastating response. Later in 1935 he remained outside the debates raised by the Einstein-Podolski-Rosen paradox aimed at demonstrating that the quantum theory was incomplete. Between 1935 and 1940 Bohr and

16.5 Langevin in the Bohr-Einstein Controversy

the Copenhagen group grew in stature and influence and Bohr's position was considered to be the orthodoxy. Bohr had the strong support of the Vienna Circle, a group of early twentieth-century scientifically trained philosophers established in Vienna until 1936. Their programme was to make philosophy scientific with the help of logic. They took a radically anti-metaphysical stance and advocated a form of logical positivism. They held their Second International Congress in Copenhagen in 1936, on "The Problem of Causality with Special Consideration to Physics and Biology". Bohr participated in the congress and, from then on, the Copenhagen interpretation was labelled as positivist while Einstein's position was labelled as realist.

How did Bohr and his group react to Langevin's interpretation? It is likely that it was disseminated, but it did not apparently elicit any response from Copenhagen. Maybe it seemed less critical than it actually was, for three possible reasons.

The main argument, the inadequacy of the concepts of classical physics at the level of sub-atomic processes, could not shock Bohr and Heisenberg who had themselves developed a similar argument. It is true that, for Bohr and Heisenberg, this inadequacy concerns all the notions of classical physics, including those of determinism and observation. It is, on the contrary, very selective of Langevin, who emphasized the inadequacy of the particle to rescue determinism.

Second, a semantic problem might have prevented a real debate. Langevin condemned the particle through a critical analysis of the notion of individuality. But it is precisely the term that Bohr used to characterize phenomena at the quantum scale: "Every atomic process contains a trait of discontinuity or rather of individuality that is totally lacking in classical theories and which is characterized by Planck's quantum of action" [2, p. 216]. In fact, Bohr and Langevin did not agree on the meaning of the term "individuality". For Bohr, it is a strictly quantum notion; for Langevin, on the contrary, it characterizes classical mechanics; it is recent for Bohr and outdated for Langevin.

Finally, Langevin's position may have been assimilated into de Broglie's position. In the various essays he published on quantum mechanics during the 1930s, de Broglie presented himself as a supporter of the Copenhagen interpretation, although his views were close to those of Langevin. Like his senior colleague, he insisted on the failure of mechanics and of the Cartesian ideal (Langevin 1937b, p. 274).

In France, by contrast, Langevin's interpretation generated a debate in the series of *Actualités scientifiques et industrielles.* Langevin's lecture was published a year after a publication by the philosopher Meyerson in the same series. Meyerson's *Réel et déterminisme dans la physique quantique* was, in fact, a response to Langevin's outline of his position in *Le Mois* (Langevin 1931f). Meyerson begins cautiously by evoking the "high authority" of Langevin and his conversations with him. He nonetheless expresses his radical disagreement. To make a long nuanced and complex argument short, let's say that Meyerson adopts, on the problem of determinism, a symmetrical and opposite position to that of Langevin. He refuses to sacrifice the individuality of the particle but he is ready to negotiate determinism. Like Langevin, Meyerson is aware that the crisis demands a radical revision of the foundations of physics. The quantum theory "was not only evolution, but revolution". Physicists can no longer form an image of reality and must be content with an abstract mathematical framework, whereas before, they could link thought to an image, even though they were aware of its inadequacy [11, pp. 47–48]. Yet, for Meyerson, questioning determinism does not undermine the foundations of physics, because scientific knowledge inevitably has to confront irrationals. The crisis raised by quanta is therefore not entirely new. By placing us before indeterminacy, before a reality opaque to reason, quantum physics confirms in a certain way Kant's transcendental realism (ibid., p. 45). Meyerson even suspects that denying indeterminacy is a vestige of positivism which has always overestimated the principle of legality (ibid., pp. 9–10, 39–40). On the other hand, he denies that physics could pretend to represent reality without admitting individuality, which is, for Meyerson, the necessary condition of the permanence of reality and the only way to rationalize the world out there. All physicists spontaneously assume the existence of an individual reality, even if they ignore its essence. Thus Meyerson remained faithful to the realism he professed in his work on the theory of relativity. Ironically, this realistic credo which had created the rapprochement between Meyerson, Langevin, and Einstein became the source of their conflict on quantum physics. Meyerson blamed Langevin for sacrificing reality to rescue determinism.

Unfortunately, the "corpuscle war", or rather the dialogue between Langevin and Meyerson, never took place. Meyerson who was already sick and ageing, passed away in 1933. The only response to Meyerson's last work came from Gaston Bachelard in 1934, in *Le Nouvel esprit scientifique*. He criticized Meyerson for rejecting quantum physics, in the name of a common sense realism, hostile to epistemological novelties. Bachelard, on the contrary, celebrated this novelty which he described as the advent of a "new scientific spirit" educated in mathematical physics. He therefore seemed to side with Langevin. Bachelard makes an allusion to Planck and Langevin when he argues that individuality must be sacrificed. But the reference is indirect and the argument quite different. Bachelard claims that the loss of individuality results from the appearance of elementary individuals in a class. He invokes Langevin's argument in support of his own critique of Meyerson's physical realism and in defence of his own mathematical realism:

> What seems to give M. Langevin's position all its philosophical strength, is that it is a postulated reality. So it is a methodological necessity to refuse individuality in this postulated reality. We have no more right than the means to inscribe individual qualities to elements that we will define by integration into a set. Elementary realism is therefore a mistake. In the microphysical domain, realistic mindset must therefore be fought with vigilance. ([1], p. 134)

Bachelard, like Meyerson, saw in Langevin's interpretation a renouncement to the realism of physics. And they were not the only ones. This interpretation has been favoured by Langevin's comments in the Fifth *Semaine de synthèse* [5, p. 221]. Langevin was extremely critical of Arthur Eddington who argued in a conference recently published in French that determinism needed to be proven and that, far from being a scandal for science, indeterminism seemed more plausible, less miraculous than determinism. Eddington concluded that, "by freeing us from determinism, [quantum theory] marks a great step forward. I would even venture to say that in the current theory we have arrived at something that a reasonable man could believe" [9, p. 24]. Langevin claimed that with such a "scalp dance" around the old determinism, Eddington was deluding himself. He firmly stated that physicists cannot dispense with causality, the postulate of determinism, which will always persist (*Centre international de Synthèse*, 120). At the end of the debates, Stephan Lupesco classified the speakers into two categories: on one hand, the "realists", including the astronomer Henri Mineur and the psychologist Henri Piéron and, on the other hand, the "dialecticians" including Langevin and the philosopher Abel Rey.

More explicitly the young Alexandre Koyré, a philosopher and historian of science, disciple of Meyerson, cast doubt on Langevin's realism in a review of his lecture *La notion de corpuscules et d'atomes*:

> M. Langevin's solution seems to us to be, like the identity postulate, an attempt to hypostasize a rule of calculation, to transform an operative rule into a judgment about the real [...].
> A non-individual real being is something perfectly unintelligible. A non-individual being is, necessarily, an abstract being. [10, pp. 436–437]

Finally, Marcel Boll, a physicist and popular writer, who played an important role in the dissemination of the quantum theory in France as well as the ideas of the Vienna Circle, interpreted Langevin's proposals as a renunciation of the notion of object and thing [3].[3]

Such a convergence of views about the idealism of Langevin's interpretation helps to better understand why he was not considered as a supporter of Einstein's camp despite his commitment to the deterministic cause. But it also sheds light on the subsequent evolution of Langevin's positions.

References

1. Bachelard G (1934) Le nouvel esprit scientifique, Félix Alcan, Paris.
2. Bohr N (1927) Le postulat des quanta et le nouveau développement de l'atomistique. In: *Électrons et photons*, rapports et discussions du cinquième Conseil de Physique Solvay. Gauthier-Villars, Paris, p 215 (1928)
3. Boll M (1939) Les quatre forces de la physique. Explications concrètes. Reider, Paris
4. Bustamante MC (2021) A l'aube de la théorie des quanta. Notes inédites d' Emile Borel sur un cours de Paul Langevin (1912)1913. Brepols, Bruxelles
5. Centre international de synthèse (1934) Science et loi, 5th Semaine internationale de synthèse. Félix Alcan, Paris
6. Chevalley C (1992) Physique quantique et philosophie. Le Débat 5(72):61–71

---

[3] Jacques Solomon criticized Boll's interpretation for misunderstanding Langevin's position. He himself denounced Boll's idealistic prejudice: "We recognize there", he writes, "the classic process: because we modify the conception we have of things external to us, it means we renounce the existence of these things themselves independently of us" (*La Pensée* 1939, 1(2), 156–157).

7. De Broglie L (1951) Les premiers Congrès Solvay. Albin Michel, Paris
8. De Broglie (1976) recherches d'un demi-siècle, Albin Michel, Paris.
9. Eddington A (1934) Sur le problème du déterminisme. Hermann, Actualités scientifiques et industrielles, Paris
10. Koyré A (1934) Recherches philosophiques 4:436–437
11. Meyerson E (1933) Réel et déterminisme dans la physique quantique. Hermann, Paris

Chapter 17
Langevin Marxist?

Abstract In the late 1930s, Langevin often claimed that dialectical materialism allowed him to better understand his own discipline. This chapter discusses this claim through a close examination of what he meant by dialectical materialism. Langevin was initiated to dialectical materialism through the *Cercle de la Russie neuve* and his family environment. Langevin was Marxist in the sense that he adopted a specific view of dialectical materialism as the heritage of the French Enlightenment and the triumph of rationalism. While he contributed to spreading this *Marxisme à la française*, Langevin nevertheless remained convinced that scientific ideas were the driving force of history.

Did Langevin feel betrayed by the consensus of philosophers that pulled his interpretation of quantum physics towards idealism? Did he decide to react, to make a point? In any case, a clear shift in his positions on quantum mechanics can be observed from 1935 onwards. Langevin changed his mind and ended up claiming in December 1938 that dialectical materialism allowed him to better understand his own discipline: "In this great doctrine, illustrated by Marx, Engels and Lenin, I have found clarification of things I would never have understood in my own science" (Langevin 1938e). This personal confession is confirmed by one of Langevin's close friends, Georges Cogniot, who claimed that Langevin "achieved full mastery of the Marxist way of thinking", at the end of "a long ascent" towards enlightenment.

> Paul Langevin, who in 1926 called on science to resolve its contradictions "on the Hegelian rhythm", has gone down in the history of French thought as the first scientist in the full glory of the term to have grasped, after a long effort, the dialectical unity of identity and difference in physical phenomena, and to proclaim the truth and necessity of Marxism based on the approaches and results of physics. (Quoted in Labérenne [11, p. 19])

Cogniot's claims are echoed by Labérenne's conviction that "every day he [Langevin] saw more of what help dialectical materialism could be to him in his own scientific research" (ibid., p. 292).

How could Langevin change his expert opinion on quantum physics on the basis of a philosophical-political doctrine? The goal of this chapter is twofold. We will try to understand how Langevin became a Marxist in an attempt to retrace the process of learning that led him to embrace this doctrine. We will also critically examine his version of Marxism and try to assess to what extent he actually converted to dialectical materialism. To begin with, it is important to stress that the controversy raised by quantum physics acted as a driving force in his intellectual evolution.

17.1 Quantum Physics as a Prompt Towards Marxism

The first signs of Langevin's shifting opinion about the crisis raised by quantum physics can be noticed during the *Semaine de synthèse* on "Statistics" (Langevin 1935e). He gave a talk after Max Born and was supposed, in principle, to draw the philosophical consequences of the directions that Born outlined (ibid., p. 240). A delicate situation, as Born was on the side of the principle of indeterminacy, even if he took care, in concluding his presentation, to clearly distinguish determinism from "laws" which, themselves, were not affected by quantum mechanics:

> Modern mechanics believes that everything in nature happens according to exact laws. It only denies that the knowledge of these laws is sufficient to predict the future with certainty or even to direct it. (Ibid., p. 241)

Indeed, Langevin seems to outbid Born by venturing a new philosophical formulation of the problem of determinism:

> Just as the theory of relativity has substituted the classic idols of space and time with conceptions relative to the observer, the theory of quanta has led us to give determinism a more subjective and therefore more human character, without diminishing in any way, it must be emphasized, its scientific rigour and its value of action, which on the contrary is enhanced. (Ibid., pp. 246–247)

Langevin no longer sought to rescue determinism. Without adhering to the indeterminacy principle, he accepted a revision of the notion of determinism by admitting that it is "more subjective and more human". What exactly did he mean? It is, at first glance, a very personal way of translating the discovery of a non-negligible and inevitable interaction between the observed system and the measurement instruments. It is as if Langevin, being obsessed by his ideas about the human value of science, projected humans everywhere, at the risk of distorting the problem.

In fact, it seems that quantum mechanics poured new wine into old bottles. It reactivated Langevin's longstanding project, first articulated in 1904, to build a non-mechanistic theory of matter. In 1935, Langevin envisaged reconceptualizing the notion of particle on the basis of Fermi-Dirac statistics and probably also to consider a new space.[1] This programme required a revision of Laplace's principle of

---

[1] Fermi–Dirac statistics is a type of quantum statistics that applies to the physics of a system consisting of many non-interacting particles that allows determination of the distribution of particles over energy states. The assumptions are that (1) none of the states of the particles can hold more than one particle (Pauli exclusion principle); and (2) exchanging one particle for another similar particle will not lead to a new state, but will give the same state (principle of identical particles).

17.1 Quantum Physics as a Prompt Towards Marxism

determinism, which allows the prediction of any event from any state of a system. In Langevin's view, this principle ruled the abstract idealized world of classical mechanics, a world detached from humans. He therefore claimed that to understand the real world, to extract all the meaning of Planck's constant, we must reintroduce a human factor into the world.

In 1938, Langevin further elaborated his position in a conference on the "The positivist and realist currents of physics" in Warsaw. There, he presented his new version of determinism-with-a-human-factor to Bohr, the leader of the Copenhagen school.

He took the floor just after Bohr's lecture, who developed an epistemological analysis of the notion of causality without addressing the question of what is real [1]. Langevin decided to argue on the grounds of philosophy, explaining that it is the recent evolution of physics that forced him to change his views:

> The profound changes that have accompanied these crises have forced physicists to think more precisely about the way they work and the philosophy of their science, to reflect on how the structure of their theory evolves in contact with facts, to take into account the answers given by nature to the questions posed by our theories […] The difficulties we are currently experiencing in constituting this language, force us to examine its structure and the rules it obeys. We must remake this grammar of science that represents epistemology and, like Mr. Jourdain, think about the way we speak, although we have been doing this for a long time. (Langevin 1938b, pp. 231–232)

So far Bohr, who had seriously questioned the relation between ordinary (i.e. unformalized) language and physical objects, could not disagree with Langevin [4]. For Bohr as for Langevin, at the atomic scale one can no longer assume the continuity between physical objects and our representation of them in space and time. Bohr opposed Einstein precisely on the entanglement or non-separability of systems [9]. And Langevin equally questioned the individuation of particles (Chap. 16). So Bohr and Langevin were in agreement on the necessity of relinquishing the concepts of classical mechanics.

But Langevin opens fire on another battlefield, on the basis of a tacit identification of the Copenhagen interpretation with positivism. He directly attacks the positivism of the Vienna Circle that he hastily defined as an operational empiricism: "Any statement about the natural sciences or of man must be expressible in the language of experiments or operations to be performed" (ibid., p. 233). He acknowledges that positivism is a very useful and precious critical attitude, in a period of crisis, to highlight contradictions. He brings two examples to illustrate his point: Einstein's approach in establishing special relativity and Heisenberg's 1927 paper on the impossibility of knowing precisely both the position and momentum of a given particle. Then, he deplores that the success of this attitude generated a philosophical doctrine, that he names "physicalism". He blames the Vienna Circle for denying the historicity of science and for closing the future. His major reproach lies here: they close the future because they deprive physics from the ambition to describe the outside reality. They are content with idealistic subjective, at best intersubjective, statements (ibid., pp. 236–237):

This attitude is therefore essentially critical, analytical and static. [...] It allows the elimination of notions or theories, the denunciation of problems and meaningless affirmations, but it does not allow the formulation of indications for the construction of new notions or theories. (Ibid., p. 237)

In short, for Langevin, positivism turns into negativism. It is useless to build a new physics because of its agnosticism about reality. It must be surpassed in favour of a more constructive attitude, formulated as a credo.

I *believe* that physicists would bind themselves in a very tight and uncomfortable way if they renounced the word reality and you would feel then, that personally, I am a realist; I believe that it is difficult to be an experimental physicist without believing in reality, not only of other physicists but also of the world. (Ibid., p. 236)

To support his realism, Langevin embarks in a long critical examination of the notion of object. It is a complex notion, built step by step through the synthesis of successive sensations, until invariants are identified that are independent of experience and observation. And it is the set of these invariants that compose an external reality (ibid., p. 239). In this process of constructing the object, Langevin notes, we move from the abstract to the concrete by gradually familiarizing ourselves with the invariants that have been identified. Thus relativistic time or Dirac's positive electron can be said to be "concrete" when physicists have become accustomed to manipulating them.

Next, Langevin attempts to develop a "realistic" concept of determinism. Contrary to the positivists who claim determinism to have been abolished by Heisenberg, Langevin claims that it is renewed and more robust. He concedes the failure of the old concept of determinism used in classical mechanics. Laplace's determinism was a metaphysical and almost fatalistic concept, triply inhuman: it assumes information that exceeds human possibilities; it assumes a contemplation of reality without interaction with it; finally "it separates the mind from the matter it seeks to penetrate" (ibid., p. 241). On the contrary, the determinism suggested by quantum physics makes our predictions depend on our information and the behaviour of the observed system on the observer:

There is, in opposition to the absolute determinism of everything at the moment, which leads to fatalism, a doctrine of action that teaches us that we must first act on ourselves and transform our representation of nature in order to act on it and transform the world. This is therefore an active and realistic attitude. (Ibid., p. 242)

Determinism is no longer a postulate of absolute necessity, it is an invitation to act, to intervene on the outside world. To conclude Langevin returns to the failure of mechanics and its classical notion of the corpuscle-projectile, which is the source of apparent indeterminacy, and he suggests building a new notion through Dirac's formalism.

In 1938, Langevin has therefore taken sides in the on-going controversy raised by quantum physics between two philosophical interpretations of its paradoxes, positivism versus realism. One would therefore expect a rather heated debate between Bohr and Langevin. In fact, the discussion was very courteous, full of nuance and reverence. Instead of a clash of ideas, the two protagonists did their utmost to highlight the points of agreement: Bohr insisted on the rational, non-mystical side of the quantum physics; Langevin noted their agreement on the necessity to reconsider the language of physics (1938b, p. 246). The disagreements were mentioned with many euphemisms. On the critique of positivism, Bohr said nothing—perhaps because he too was trying to distance himself from the Vienna Circle. But he challenged Langevin's realism: pretending to avoid any misunderstanding on the meaning of the word "indeterminism", he emphasized that objects do not behave independently of measuring instruments (1938b, p. 246). And concerning the notion of the corpuscle, he made a clear distinction between the photon, a quantum entity that cannot be individualized, and the electron, which he judged, despite Louis de Broglie's contribution, susceptible to a classical description (1938b, p. 247).

Langevin could easily shift from realism to materialism because the two notions were more or less identical in the Marxist doctrine then prevailing in France. In this respect, Langevin adopted the interpretation of materialism developed by his son-in-law Jacques Solomon, who was instrumental in introducing him to Marxism (Fig. 17.1).

Born in 1908, Solomon married Hélène Langevin in 1929 while he was completing his medical studies [2]. Interested by the new theory of quantum physics after attending Langevin's course at the *Collège de France*, he left medicine to start

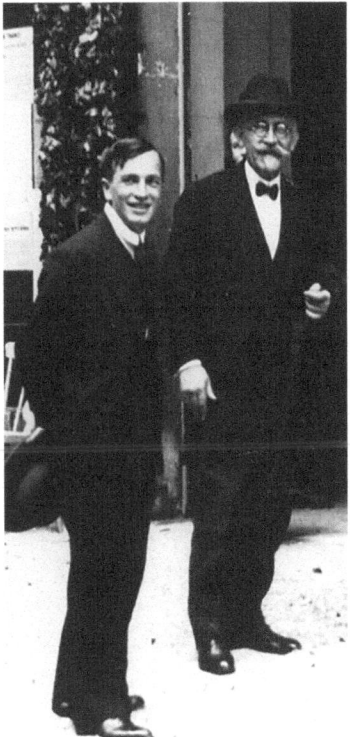

Fig. 17.1 Langevin with his son-in-law Jacques Solomon (1930) (*Science et Vigilance*)

doctoral research on Dirac's quantum field theory under the supervision of Léon Brillouin: Brillouin had himself been supervised by Langevin ten years earlier. In the course of his research, Solomon spent a few months in Copenhagen where he worked with Bohr and Léon Rosenfeld. His PhD dissertation reformulated Pauli's quantum field theory in more general and more abstract terms and, in 1933, he collaborated with Wolfgang Pauli in an attempt to reconcile Dirac's equation with the general theory of relativity. He was apparently driven by an ambition to unify physics, presumably not unrelated to Langevin's influence on this brilliant and creative scholar [5].

However, as a philosopher, Solomon had a no less significant influence on Langevin. For this young doctor, who joined the French Communist Party (PCF) in March 1934, was fascinated by German philosophy, by Hegel's dialectics and, in particular, Marx's materialism. Solomon struck up a close friendship with the Marxist philosopher Georges Politzer, who did his utmost to discredit Bergson's position on the theory of relativity in the 1920s. Both Politzer and Solomon embraced the view that Marxism was a science based on political economy (Fig. 17.2) (Bustamante [2], chapter 6). Together they translated German Marxist texts into French and taught courses at the *Université ouvrière*. They co-authored a number of papers in journals close to the Communist Party or to the *Union rationaliste*. They were both concerned with the relation between dialectical materialism and science and eager to treat idealism as a form of irrationalism or obscurantism. Nevertheless, Solomon fully endorsed Bohr's principle of complementarity while sharing Langevin's belief in the realism of physics theories. He endorsed Meyerson's

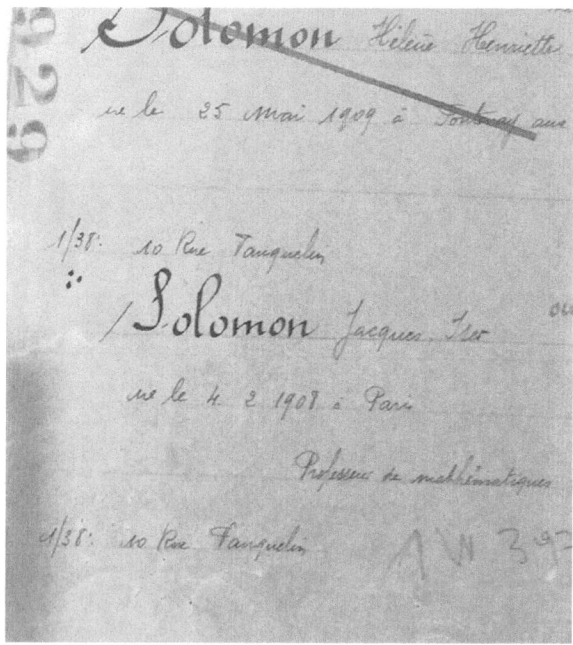

Fig. 17.2 Solomon's police record. (B. Bensaude-Vincent)

realism and argued that it was close to Marx's dialectical materialism [16]. For him, Meyerson was a materialist because he insisted that every physicist believes in the material reality of electrons, atoms and molecules. And this is, in Solomon's view, a form of dialectical materialism since reason, for Meyerson, constantly strives to resolve contradictions to assimilate identity and reality. Without siding with Meyerson's critique of Langevin's interpretation of the crisis of determinism as a crisis of classical mechanics, Solomon clearly adhered to the critique of positivism that runs through Meyerson's work and supported his realist postulate.

17.2 Marxist Initiation Through the *Cercle de la Russie neuve*

Langevin assimilated Marxism through his son-in-law, who himself reflected a French intellectual movement. Without going into the details of the reception of Marxism in France, we may note that Marxism had been a constant reference for French left-wing thinkers since 1900, although they were not all enthusiastic [8]. Ironically, in France, Marxism had been more widely disseminated by its opponents than by its supporters [14]. In any case, both supporters and opponents had access to a large part of Marx's work in French translation, thanks to an intense academic publishing activity from 1890 to 1905 [7]. After the Bolshevik revolution, Langevin, like many left-wing intellectuals, showed sympathy and curiosity for the implementation of Marxist ideas. But Langevin was far too busy with his professional and social activism to spend time reading Marx's original works.

His introduction to Marxism took place in the Cercle de la Russie neuve, a group founded in 1933 on the initiative of Gabrielle Duchêne, a feminist, pacifist activist and fellow PCF supporter.[2] This group aimed to oppose anti-Bolshevik propaganda "with authentic documents and information". Solomon and Jean Langevin were the organizers of meetings of this group that took place at the EPCI. These meetings brought together scientists, such as Langevin and Henri Wallon, a child psychologist and Langevin's colleague at the *Collège de France*, philosophers such as Félicien Challaye and René Maublanc, and artists such as the Autan-Lara couple [3, 12]. After a period of discovery of Soviet culture—cinema, science and poetry—the *Cercle* turned to the study of Marxism in a series of more theoretical lectures. It was organized into groups of specialist scientists who conducted comparisons between the situation of sciences and technology in the USSR and in France ([17], p. 11). The lectures were published in 1935 in a collective volume entitled *A la lumière du marxisme* ("In the Light of Marxism") which sold thousands of copies. Wallon, the volume editor, pointed out that "each specialist had to say how he felt about Marxism in his particular field", without concern for orthodoxy. Langevin was not only

---

[2] The group was renamed the *Société d'étude pour la culture soviétique* in 1934 and the *Association d'étude pour la culture soviétique* in 1936 [2].

content to attend the *Cercle de la Russie neuve*'s public lectures. Encouraged by his son-in-law and his son Jean, he presided over another initiative of collective analysis of dialectical materialism. The *Académie matérialiste*, founded in 1933 by Jean-Maurice Lahy, head of the Laboratory of Applied Psychology at the *Ecole pratique des hautes études*, met from 1934 to 1939 at Langevin's invitation in the EPCI library and took the name *Groupe d'études matérialistes* [3].

In the course of this collective and mutual learning process, Langevin was especially attracted by the dialectic relation between knowledge and action that emerged as a major characteristic of Marxism.

This is the topic he chose to develop in 1945 in a paper entitled *La pensée et l'action* which has often been presented as his philosophical testament (Labérenne 1964). He declared on 10 June 1945:

> I am aware that I only really understood the history of physics from the moment I became aware of the fundamental ideas of dialectical materialism (…) On the level of action where doctrine must be translated into method, dialectical materialism seems to be as fruitful as on the level of explanation and understanding. It seems to allow an extension of the experimental method itself. (Langevin 1945f, pp. 174–175)

What attracted Langevin in Marxism was above all the rationalist approach to the world ("an extension of the experimental method") and the close interaction between action and the mind.

This version of Marxism as a rationalist worldview, inherited from the French Enlightenment, was actively promoted by Georges Cogniot, a member of the Central Committee of the PCF that he represented on the Komintern Executive Committee in 1936–1937, while serving as deputy for the 11th arrondissement of Paris from 1936 to 1940 [6]. In the 1930s, he was the architect of the PCF policy of reaching out to intellectuals, based on the invention of a French-style Marxism, *marxisme à la française* [8, 14]. He forged, from scratch, a version of dialectical materialism rooted in the tradition of eighteenth-century French materialists, presenting Marx, Engels and Lenin as heirs to the philosophy of the Enlightenment and the French Revolution. Georges Politzer, in his course at the *Université ouvrière*, developed a positivist interpretation of Marxism inspired by Auguste Comte's law of three stages in the evolution of human societies: religious, metaphysical, and positive. He described dialectical materialism as the positive or scientific stage of materialism while the mechanistic materialism of eighteenth-century philosophers was characteristic of the metaphysical age.

This view was reinforced by intellectuals who claimed that Marxism was a scientific doctrine. Marcel Prenant, for example, a communist biologist who was active in the Amsterdam-Pleyel movement and in the CVIA, considered Marxism to be the result of scientific investigation [13]. Whereas Charles Andler's critical analysis, in the preface to his 1901 translation of the *Communist Manifesto*, tended to reduce Marxism to a compilation of nineteenth-century French socialists, Cogniot and Politzer leaped over the nineteenth century to establish a direct connection between Marxism and the Enlightenment, invoking figures such as Pierre Bayle, Diderot and Voltaire. They equated Marxism with rationalism and materialism with scientific realism, both converging to subvert religion and superstition. They diluted Marxism into a vast universal movement aimed at human emancipation through science and towards democracy.

17.3 Marxist "à la française"

Langevin was comfortable with this French-style version of Marxism. Dialectical materialism appeared to him as the current stage in the progress of universal Reason, expressed in the scientific vision of the world. The dialectics between action and the mind resonated with his own interpretation of the history of science (Chap. 12). Did he truly revise his idealistic vision of history "in the light of Marxism"? Apparently, he quickly took advantage of Hegel's dialectics in his reflections on quantum physics. In his lecture *La notion de corpuscule et d'atome* delivered at the ENS in 1932 he vaguely identified dialectics and contradiction in his comment on Bohr's notion of complementarity:

> Bohr calls these two aspects [wave and particle] "complementary"; he even formulates a "principle of complementarity" for them. Should we accept living in this kind of contradiction, in a kind of Hegelian, dialectical situation, where we observe oppositions without yet having achieved a synthesis? It seems to me desirable that we should not accept this solution too easily, that we should not settle into the contradiction when the profound tendency of our science is, on the contrary, to increasingly achieve comprehensive syntheses by extending old concepts or creating the necessary new ones. (Langevin 1933a, p. 284)

And in 1935, the wave/particle duality seems to lead him from Hegel's dialectic to dialectical materialism:

> The history of science is dialectical, to borrow Hegel's expression, and it is perhaps historical materialism that best accounts for this evolution of science which takes place under the pressure of experience through the synthetic solutions of conflicts. (Langevin 1935e, p. 224)

It remains a vague hint. Hegel is poorly distinguished from historical materialism. Twelve years later, Langevin did not show a better understanding of the history of physics through dialectical materialism when he points out contradictions and syntheses everywhere: a synthesis of physics and geometry in the space-time of relativity theory; a synthesis of matter and light in the notion of energy; of wave and particle in quantum theory, a synthesis of science and technology, of theory and experiment (Langevin 1945f, pp. 172–173).[3] This inflated notion of dialectics has only a faint resemblance to Hegel's *aufhebung*. It basically refers to the unification of two competing concepts or theories to which the young physicist Langevin aspired in 1904. The few themes with dialectical resonance that are introduced, like "not to eliminate" one of the two terms, or "overcome" the contradiction, do not demonstrate an enlightened rereading of the history of physics through the lens of

---

[3] Unlike Langevin, Solomon resisted the temptation to identify the wave-particle theory with dialectics. He firmly opposed de Broglie and always remained faithful to Bohr's view of complementarity as mutual exclusion (Colin 2015).

dialectical materialism. Langevin found in dialectical materialism a post-rationalisation of his long-term aspiration to a unified theory of physics.

At the very moment when he publicly declared that he only understood the history of physics thanks to dialectical materialism, his words suggest that he was above all seduced by the emphasis on synthesis. Langevin's alleged conversion to Marxism rather reflects his adhesion to the *marxisme à la française* forged by Cogniot and the PCF.

> This doctrine (dialectical materialism), which extends the great line of human philosophical thought, is itself the result of a synthesis begun a century ago by Karl Marx and Friedrich Engels between the mechanistic materialism of our French philosophers of the eighteenth century and the idealistic dialectic of Hegel. (Ibid., p. 174)

Throughout his life, Langevin boldly attempted to reconcile rival theories. Dialectical materialism produced no revelation. It did not subvert Langevin's philosophy of history. It rather somewhat reinforced it. Encouraged by the French-style Marxism that he discovered in the sessions of the *Cercle de la Russie neuve*, Langevin "digested" Hegel and Marx and quickly metabolized them into his own mental framework. He thus favoured murky amalgams between Marxism and physics, as represented in an article titled "Paul Langevin, incomparable master".

> He showed that the logic of contradiction, a fundamental element of this dialectic, illuminated the entire theory of quanta, and that the famous principle of uncertainty was only a particular case of this fact on which Marx always insisted, that there is no observer who is only an observer. (Georges Teissier, *L'Humanité*, 30 December 1946)

If it was relatively easy for Langevin to graft Hegel's dialectic onto his unabated quest for synthesis, historical materialism radically disrupted his view of history. Had he not written that "the domination of the world by the mind is the necessary means and the final goal of the emancipation of mankind from the animal state" (Langevin 1927f)? Langevin's philosophy of history driven by the emancipation of the human mind from nature strikes one as essentially mind-centred. His idealism has been pointed out by his admirers. For instance, in 1931, a Mr Pivert thanked him for his speech to the Fraternal Group of Education:

> And to conclude I will say again, my dear Master, how much we are happy to be able to support our daily action with these penetrating reflections that have enriched our view of reality. Certainly, it is possible that in the explanation of things, other hypotheses, other interpretations may take place. It is evident that the interpretation of social transformations could be discussed. You have asserted that Newton was, in sum, the initiator of the French Revolution, almost as Ronald claimed that the French Revolution was the last volume of the *Encyclopédie*, this idealistic interpretation of history is certainly not the only possible one. (Langevin 1931c, p. 26)

To adopt a materialist philosophy of history, Langevin had therefore to radically change his views of science and its history described in Chap. 12. There are signs of his gradual conversion to a materialist perspective. Ironically it is in his defence of pure and disinterested science, that he attacked head-on the dualism of matter and spirit:

17.3 Marxist "à la française"

> The lessons of life have revealed and gradually formed a human reason that is increasingly rich, comprehensive, self-aware and subject to its own laws, to the point of coming to believe itself independent of any external reality and capable by its own forces of reconstructing the world. The scholasticism in the Middle Ages and more recently the philosophy of Hegel are examples of this youthful intoxication where the human reason's intellectual superstructure of the world believes it can detach itself from its support and fly with its own wings in a realm of the spirit entirely distinct from matter. (Langevin 1936b, p. 5)

The change is more pronounced in Langevin's last lecture *La pensée et l'action* delivered in 1946 within a series dedicated to a French science policy (Langevin 1946a). Here he develops historical examples of the interactions between science and technology and of the influence of action on thinking. He clearly acknowledges a causal link between dualism and social organization:

> This dualistic conception of soul and body, mind and matter, the world of ideas and that of sensible appearances, was probably itself no more than a reflection of the social structure in which the free man was opposed to the slave, intellectual activities to manual ones, thought to action. (Ibid., p. 339)

However, Langevin, unlike Solomon, never paid attention to political economy. His socio-historical analyses rather suggest the influence of Henri Wallon's psychology focused on the interaction of hands and brain, and possibly of the anthropologist André Leroi-Gourhan who insisted on the coevolution of technology and language [15].

> The *homo faber* and the *homo sapiens* are one. Science, born from the needs of action and only capable of fertilizing it, can only grow itself by calling on action through experience and using the increasingly large means of action made available by technology. We know that the hand of man through handling tools has created the brain and that thought, born from action, must, according to the old myth of Antaeus, to remain strong and fertile, return to action by inspiring it with forms that are increasingly rich and increasingly elevated. (Langevin 1945f, p. 167)

Although he sprinkled his remarks on fascism and the crisis with vague references to "an unjust economic regime" (Langevin 1938g), until the end of his life he firmly assumed that there is an "instinct that today pushes nations towards peace" and forces them to "unite or die" (ibid., p. 53). Nothing is more alien to Langevin's thinking than the role of the class struggle in social evolution: he kept saying with the same unshakeable faith that there is only progress through mutual aid, that science is the driving force of human evolution and that it determines the organization of society.

Very revealing in this respect is the article where Langevin translated the introduction of a book by John Desmond Bernal (Langevin 1939b). An Irish scientist who introduced the use of x-ray crystallography into molecular biology, Bernal was a Marxist and member of the British Communist Party. Langevin admired him a great deal and decided to translate into French his book *The Social Function of Science*, a pioneering essay on the social history of science. But Langevin completely changed the meaning of Bernal's socio-historical account of scientific advances. He entitled his translation as *Science as a Factor of Moral and Social Evolution*. Langevin remained impervious to Bernal's explicit attempt to consider current and past science as an institution that is dependent on social order and imbued with the spirit of the ruling classes (ibid., p. 132). He only retained from Bernal's book the message that comforted his own views: that the history of science and technology was intimately connected with society, and above all the defence of science against its detractors.

It is therefore fair to say that Langevin never truly endorsed a Marxist interpretation of the world and rather assimilated Marxism with his own cult of rationalism and his concern with synthesis. This is how he was perceived by Frédéric Joliot-Curie when he presented his mentor in his obituary: "Langevin, great philosopher, spoke to us about dialectical materialism which he defined as being scientific rationalism" [10, p. 58]. Marxism was a late graft onto Langevin's already established rationalist framework. Far from being isolated, Langevin followed the orthodoxy of the French Communist Party who forged a *marxisme à la française* in a vast campaign of propaganda among intellectuals in the inter-war period.

References

1. Bohr N (1938) Le problème causal en physique atomique, in Les Nouvelles théories de la physique, Institut international de coopération intellectuelle, 1939.
2. Bustamante M-C (in print) Jacques Solomon (1908-1942). Physicien, militant fusillé. Et sa valise de manuscrits dans la clandestinité. Brepols, Brussels
3. Carlino F (2015) Sur l'introduction du matérialisme scientifique en France: le programme du Cercle de la Russie neuve dans le processus de formation du rationalisme moderne. Actuel Marx 57:142–155
4. Chevalley C (1985) Complémentarité et langage dans l'interprétation de Copenhague. Revue d'histoire des sciences 38(2–4):251–292
5. Colin C (2010) Jacques Solomon et l'interprétation de la théorie quantique. Rev Hist Sci 63:221–246
6. Courtois S (1996) Georges Cogniot. In: Julliard J, Winok M (eds) Dictionnaire des intellectuels français. Seuil, Paris, pp 279–280
7. Ducange J-N (2011) Introduction. Réceptions de Marx en Europe avant 1914. Cah Hist Rev Hist Crit 114:11–17. http://journals.openedition.org/chrhc/2214, https://doi.org/10.4000/chrhc.2214
8. Gouarné I (2013) L'Introduction du marxisme en France. Philosoviétisme et sciences humaines, 1920–1939. Presses universitaires de Rennes
9. Howard D (2009) Revisiting Eisntein-Bohr dialogue. https://www.science20.com/don_howard/revisiting_einsteinbohr_dialogue
10. Joliot-Curie F (1947) Paul Langevin Rationaliste. La Pensée 12:57–58
11. Labérenne P (1964) La Pensée et l'action. Éditions Sociales, Paris
12. Labérenne P (1979) Le Cercle de la Russie Neuve (1928-1936) et l'Association pour l'étude de la culture soviétique (1936-1939). La Pensée 205:10–25
13. Prenant M (1935) Biologie et marxisme. Éditions Sociales Internationales, Paris
14. Prochasson C (2004) L'invention du marxisme français. In: Becker J-J, Candar G (eds) Histoire des gauches en France, vol 1. Éditions La Découverte, Paris, pp 427–443
15. Schlanger N (2023) L'invention de la technologie. Une histoire intellectuelle avec André Leroi-Gourhan. Presses universitaires de Rennes, Rennes
16. Solomon J (n.d.) "Marx et Meyerson", unpublished manuscript found in the archives of the *Cercle de Russie Neuve*, published by Fabrizio Carlino in *La Pensée*, 374, 2013, pp 157–180
17. Wallon H (1935) Introduction in A la lumière du marxisme, éditions sociales internationales, Paris, p. 9–16.

Chapter 18
Langevin and the French Communist Party

Abstract How are we to understand that Langevin, who has been a fellow traveller of the PCF since its creation in 1920, who worked shoulder to shoulder with PCF members in several movements, and who frequented Communist circles, only joined the Party in his late career, when he was over 70? It was neither a lack of courage that prevented him from joining earlier, because he has taken many other risks. It is not a lack of contacts either, as there were already many communist activists among his children. Finally, it is not out of mistrust for the Soviet Union, since he has never formulated the slightest criticism of this regime. Against the testimony of close friends who claimed that Langevin was convinced long before his membership of the validity of the PCF political line, we argue that despite years of fighting side by side, Langevin kept a distance and did not always follow the line of the Party. We conclude that it is equally simplistic to label Langevin as a communist scientist as to argue that he has been instrumentalized by the PCF. His relations with the PCF were complex.

On 26 September 1944, Langevin, back in Paris after 4 years of "exile", came to the headquarters of the French Communist Party (PCF) in Paris and requested party membership [10, pp. 186–188]. Indeed, he was already well known to members of the Central Bureau. Many of his friends, colleagues and relatives had already joined the PCF in the 1930s. And Langevin himself had officially expressed his sympathy at the Seventh Regional Conference of the Party in Gennevilliers in 28 December 1938:

> It is the honour of your Party to closely unite thought and action. It has been said that a communist should always be educated, but I will tell: "Your party is the only one to have clear ideas: it is a kind of expansion of the French Revolution as the doctrine of Marx-Engels-Lenin is an expansion of the thought of the great French thinkers of the 18th century". (Langevin 1938e)

18.1 A Vignette

This statement, which sheds light on Langevin's adhesion to the *Marxisme à la française* (Chap. 17), has often been cited by his friends and disciples as evidence of Langevin's adhesion to communism [2, p. 114, 8, pp. 291–292]. As they were themselves deeply involved in the PCF, they were quick to label him a communist after his death. Pierre Biquard, in his biography of Langevin, *Paul Langevin, scientifique, éducateur et citoyen*, added: "Langevin was convinced of the rightness of the PCF's political theses long before he joined" [2, p. 114]. Georges Cogniot was keen to use Langevin's fame as a flagship to attract more and more intellectuals into the PCF. He portrayed Langevin as a physicist who rebelled against academic orthodoxy and "achieved full mastery of the Marxist way of thinking", at the end of "a long ascent" into the light.

> Paul Langevin, who in 1926 called on science to resolve its contradictions "on the Hegelian rhythm", entered the history of French thought as the first scientist in the full glory of the term to have grasped, after a long effort, the dialectical unity of identity and difference in physical phenomena, and to proclaim the truth and necessity of Marxism based on the approaches and results of physics. (Cogniot in Labérenne [8, p. 23])

Indeed, Cogniot's assertion is based on a number of statements made by Langevin, as well as his real efforts to assimilate into Marxism. Still, as we have seen in the previous chapter, Langevin's "full mastery of the Marxist way of thinking" is questionable. Even if they stem from a noble and generous feeling of camaraderie and solidarity, these testimonies tell us as much about the PCF's strategy in the mid-twentieth century as they do about Langevin's convictions. They have established Langevin as a communist scientist in the national memory, a label reinforced by the communist municipalities that have named schools after him in the 1950s and 1960s. The vignette of communist scientist may have enhanced Langevin's fame in the aftermath of his death but they contributed to tarnish his image in the next decades.

It is therefore important to adopt a historian's perspective, freed from the traps of vivid memory to clarify Langevin's relations with the French Communist Party. How are we to understand that Langevin, who has been a fellow traveller of the PCF since its creation in 1920, who has worked shoulder to shoulder with PCF members in several movements, and who has frequented Communist circles such as the *Cercle de la Russie neuve*, only joined the Party in his late career, when he was over 70? It is not a lack of courage that prevented him from joining earlier, because he has taken many other risks. It is not a lack of contacts either as there were already many communist activists among his children: his daughter-in-law Luce Langevin, his daughter Hélène Solomon and his son-in-law Jacques Solomon. Finally, it is not out of mistrust for the Soviet Union, since he has never formulated the slightest criticism of this regime.

How are we to understand that he who could have justified his membership in 1944 on political grounds put forward a very personal reason? He said that he joined the Party to take the place of Jacques Solomon, his son-in-law, who had been shot by the Nazis in 1942, "without pretending to be able to fill the great void left by him" [10, pp. 186–188]. A beautiful tribute, certainly, to this young communist and promising physicist. But why give a personal and emotional tone to a political gesture that has long been predictable and perhaps eagerly awaited?[1]

---

[1] The same half-political, half-emotional gesture is repeated 2–3 years later. André Langevin, Paul Langevin's second son, gives his support to the French Communist Party a few days after his father's death.

18.2 The PCF and the Intellectuals

Let us briefly mention the main lines of the evolution of the relationship between the French Communist Party (PCF) and the intellectuals. The PCF, created at the *Congrès de Tours* in 1920, remained relatively isolated in French political life until 1924 [4, 5]. However, a number of intellectuals, like Langevin, expressed their solidarity with the PCF, when it was the victim of government repression after it had protested against the occupation of the German industrial region Ruhr in 1923. In 1925, the Party was reorganized along the lines dictated by Moscow during the World Congress of the Communist Internationale in 1924. The repression by the French troops of Moroccan movements in the Rif war triggered the conversion *en masse* of the Surrealist movement. However, the number of party members drastically dropped in the next few years from 60,000 members in 1925 to about 20,000–25,000 in 1933 [7].

Consequently, the PCF launched a big campaign to attract left-wing intellectuals. The party opened up the columns of its newspapers and offered generous trips in the Soviet Union to many French intellectuals. Most of them came back admiring and enthusiastic about the Soviet education system and were convinced that the Soviet regime was a kind of enlightened despotism in the hands of fervent educators [5, p. 301]. This idyllic period was soon followed by an era of suspicion. From 1928 to 1935, the Stalinization of western communist parties was accompanied by a wave of anti-intellectualism in the wake of the deportation of Trotsky. Distrust and suspicion, however, declined in 1935 in the face of the urgency of a response to fascist threats. The membership increased from about 88,000 in December 1935 to 320,000 in December 1937. Left-wing intellectuals aligned themselves with the PCF because they were alarmed by the international situation and the Party presented itself as a powerful and effective organization. Often the rapprochement resulted less from a philosophical conversion than from a pragmatic concern for action.

A similar "principle of utility" prevailed in the Central Committee of the PCF, which sought to secure the cooperation of prestigious intellectuals with a fluent style who could influence the masses [4, pp. 38–39]. They approved and advertised the initiatives of scientists like Langevin and Perrin, of artists like Le Corbusier and Fernand Léger, of writers like André Gide, Julien Benda or Jean-Richard Bloch, as symbols of the struggle against oppression. Their works were widely circulated in the Soviet Union. As a result, some ended up being as popular there as in France. In 1937, Paul Vaillant-Couturier, a member of the Political Bureau of the PCF, published *Au service de l'esprit* (*In the Service of the Mind*), which pampered and flattered intellectuals. Shortly afterwards, Cogniot launched an aggressive campaign to try to attract intellectuals through an attempt to assimilate the Marxist doctrine, in the form a *Marxisme à la française* (see Chap. 17). This exchange of mutual support between intellectuals and the PCF was not really diminished by the revolt of a few of the intellectuals, notably Gide, who criticized the Soviet regime in *Retour de l'URSS* [6]. Gide's defection did not undermine the consensus. Those who tried to intervene on behalf of Soviet intellectuals condemned by Stalin, like Romain Rolland, chose to keep silent, although in his private journal he noted that "it is the regime of the most uncontrolled and absolute arbitrariness ..." [5, p. 163]. The watchword of defending the USSR against its enemies still prevailed, even after the liquidation of German and Italian communists. As the PCF was the only party that had become well established outside the USSR, it was invested with a kind of international responsibility and, as such, deserved to be supported at all costs. It was out of question to harm the Party's brand image. This alliance between intellectuals and the PCF reached a climax in 1938, in the joint denunciation of the Munich agreements.

18.3 A Fellow Traveller

To what extent is Langevin's personal evolution an exemplar of this general trajectory? From the outset, he appeared as a fellow traveller. Even before the campaign to attract intellectuals in 1924, in 1920, he stood alongside the PCF, protesting against the "blockade" of the USSR and against the use of students as strike breakers, in his defence of the mutineers of the Black Sea. His first political words appeared in *L'Humanité* (Langevin 1920e, 1920f). Not content to express his admiration for the Russian revolution and the hope it inspired, Langevin actively developed solidarity with the Soviet Union: first at the scientific level, and at the association of *Les amitiés franco-russes*, created in 1924.

Like many left-wing intellectuals, Langevin was invited to visit the Soviet Union. His first trip, in May 1928, was organized by the PCF. The second occasion, in 1929, was to receive a distinction from the Academy of Sciences (Fig. 18.1). He also made a brief third visit to Moscow, in 1932, on his return journey from China. Like most of the visitors of this period, Langevin marvelled at the progress and accomplishments in the Soviet Union. He wrote a few lines in *Pravda*, the official newspaper of the Central Committee of the Communist Party of the Soviet Union, on 24 May 1928, to acknowledge "the excellent scientific work being done here in all areas, as well as the favourable conditions for work" of Soviet scientists [10, p. 93]. While there is no reason to doubt his sincerity, Langevin managed to keep his distance. He was not dazzled to the point of taking the USSR as a model of scientific or educational organization, maybe because he did not agree that the plans for scientific research be subordinated to technological needs. Wallon by contrast promoted this model at the International Congress of Nice in 1932, and at the *Cercle de la Russie neuve* in 1933–1934 [11, pp. 11–14].

Like many other intellectuals in the 1930s, Langevin loyally supported the PCF and publicly expressed his sympathy with it. For instance, at the opening of the Annual Congress of the PCF in Villeurbanne in January 1936, two messages of support were presented, one from Perrin and one from Langevin [3, p. 132]. As much as through messages of sympathy, Langevin supported the PCF by his silence. As vice-president of the League of Human Rights, he could (or should) have denounced

18.3 A Fellow Traveller

Fig. 18.1 Langevin during his visit to the USSR in 1929. (ESPCI)

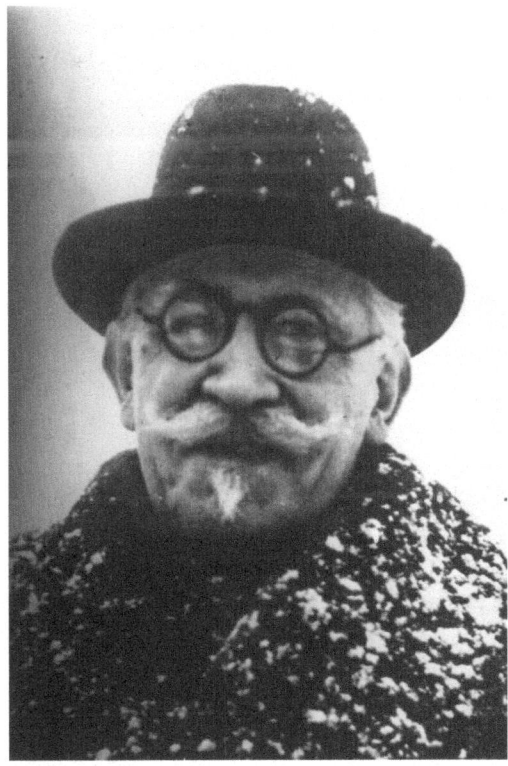

the violations of human rights in the Soviet Union. He did not respond to the rumours about purges, trials and imprisonments that were circulating. He kept silent during the campaigns of the communists against the anarchists and Trotskyists, in Barcelona in May 1937, while Paul Rivet, leader of the CVIA publicly protested with Gide [4]. However, unlike Rivet, Langevin resisted pressures from his family to take up political responsibilities. In 1934, Solomon and Langevin's daughter Hélène, both members of the communist party cell of the fifth arrondissement, pressed him to be the candidate for the left wing parties at the municipal elections. He refused, leaving Rivet to be the candidate [3, p. 132].

But still, Langevin was considered close enough to the communist party to stand as its spokesman in the triumvirate who led the CVIA, alongside with Paul Rivet for the socialist party and Alain for the radical party (Chap. 13). In common with many French intellectuals, Langevin developed stronger links with the PCF within this specifically antifascist movement. In 1934, at the express request of Barbusse, the communists of the Amsterdam-Pleyel Committee joined the CVIA *en masse*. On 14 July 1935, Langevin led the parade, side by side with Maurice Thorez, leader of the Communist Party (Fig. 18.2). The coalition of the three left-wing parties—named *rassemblement populaire* –allowed the formation of the Front Populaire and its subsequent electoral victory in 1936.

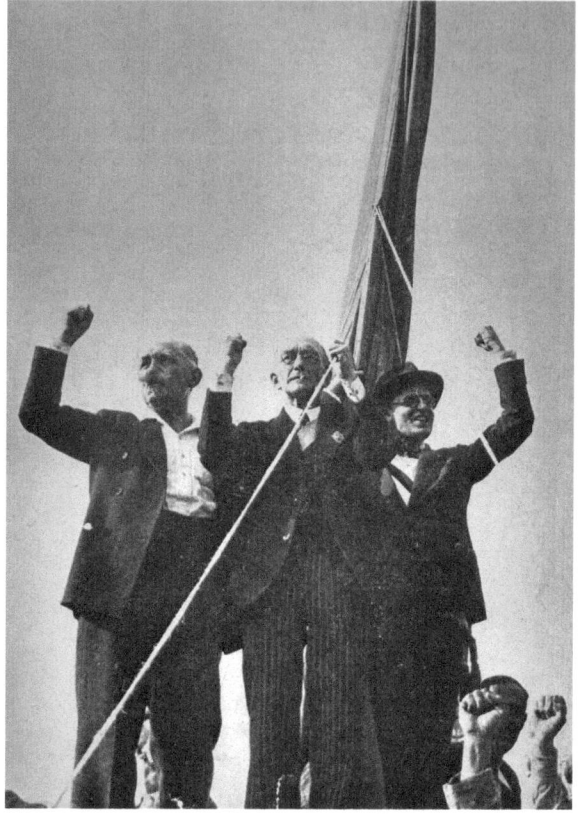

Fig. 18.2 Langevin during the National parade at the Bastille on 14 July 1935 alongside Paul Rivet and Pierre Cot, co-founders of the *Comité de vigilance des intellectuels antifascistes*. (ESPCI)

But the time of this idyllic alliance was soon followed by inner divisions in the antifascist movement. In June 1936, a schism occurred within the CVIA about the Spanish civil war. Langevin was concerned about the danger of a non-intervention policy and distanced himself from the pacifism of *Vigilance*. He left the leadership of the CVIA with a minority of members and created a new campaign "Peace and Freedom" to clearly mark his new orientation that was more in line with the PCF: no longer championing the unconditional defence of peace but now supporting the liberation of oppressed peoples. Langevin and Rolland launched a vibrant call for an international united front against fascism: "all united to defend peace and freedom". Their main arguments were "the Spanish war threatens not only freedom but also the treasure of our culture", "Today it's Spain; tomorrow it will be Czechoslovakia; it will be France; it will be Europe", which was to prove terribly prescient (Archives, L032/042) (Fig. 18.3). In November 1936, Langevin was one of seven members of a French left-wing delegation, visiting London to meet various members of British liberal and pacifist organizations. They shared views with a group of 20 MPs in the House of Commons, possibly including Winston Churchill, and met notable pacifists including H.G. Wells and Sir Walter Citrine.

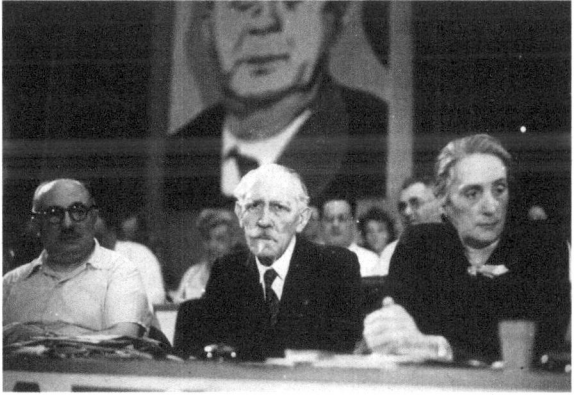

Fig. 18.3 Langevin, Jacques Duclos and *la Pasionaria* during a meeting in support of the Republicans during the Spanish Civil War. (ESPCI)

18.4 One Step Forward…

In 1938, Langevin publicly broke with "total pacifism" and condemned nonviolence not for circumstantial reasons, but as being wrong in principle. "It is elementary common sense, and moreover confirmed by history, that bowing to force can only lead to an ever more brutal reign of force" (Langevin 1938g, p. 11). However, he refrained from mocking pacifism or giving it a political label. He was caught in a "tragic contradiction" between the horror of war and the love of justice and freedom. He explained his conversion by a kind of disillusionment:

> The action against war, the search for causes and the denunciation of past or possible horrors, may have seemed sufficient as long as we believed it possible to convince all peoples and bring them to the necessary union. (Ibid., pp. 12–13)

Langevin also politicized his interpretation of the fascist phenomenon. If he still used phrases such as "regression to barbarism", or "liberation of selfish instincts", he assumed that fascism resulted from an "unjust and outdated economic regime" that seeks to maintain its caste domination, invoking the pretext of race, by "widespread violence and stupefaction". He attributed two essential characteristics to fascism: the destruction of men and goods and the stifling of free thought and science (ibid., p. 13). Finally, bitterly noting the spread of fascism in several parts of the planet, Langevin called for international solidarity. He added that if our ancestors had given in to blackmail like the democratic nations of today, our species and our civilization would not exist. He finally concluded:

> Solidarity with our ancestors and descendants implies solidarity with those who are currently dying in Spain and China. Just as our ancestors, to defend themselves against both the cold and the great beasts, surrounded their women, their children and their most precious possessions with a belt of flames, we must place between war, fascism and ourselves the ever-higher flame of our faith in a human ideal of freedom, justice and peace. (Ibid., p. 15)

After so many pathetic calls for international mobilization against fascism, what could be Langevin's attitude in front of the Munich agreement signed by Nazi

Germany, the United Kingdom, the French Republic and Fascist Italy in September 1938? He was not afraid to shout his indignation. Although he was old and worn out by so many campaigns, he did not capitulate and founded a new movement: Peace and Democracy, on the basis of the League of Human Rights since it was cofounded with Victor Basch and Albert Bayet (Fig. 18.4). He brought together around 30 anti-Munich intellectuals—including Jean-Richard Bloch, Joliot-Curie, Cotton and Maublanc—to try to obtain the creation of an anti-fascist front, an Anglo-French-Soviet alliance). Together with Joliot, Perrin, Solomon, the poet Aragon and others, Langevin created the *Union des intellectuels pour la justice, la liberté et la paix* (UDIF). This new collective of committed scientists and intellectuals supposedly "above party divisions" protested against "the Munich Diktat, the shameful dismemberment of Czechoslovak democracy, Italian fascism's designs on the Mediterranean, Spain's threatened independence" [9].

Langevin nevertheless complacently supported an initiative taken by Solomon and Politzer with the support of the PCF, who got the permission from Moscow to create a new journal *La Pensée* subtitled *Revue du rationalisme moderne* (Fig. 18.5) [3, pp. 182–195]. The purpose was to create a Marxist journal targeting a wide readership. Solomon, Politzer and Cogniot invited Langevin to a dinner with his favourite wine (*vin d'Arbois*) because they needed a prestigious name on the front page. In addition to appearing as the editor-in-chief, Langevin also contributed an article in the first issue on *La physique moderne et le déterminisme*. However, his participation soon increased due to the political circumstances. Three issues were prepared by Solomon and his associate Jean Bruhat, all scheduled for 1939. The first issue included scientific papers such as the one written by Langevin and a paper by J.B.S. Haldane on hemophilia in the royal families, together with more controversial papers like Politzer's *La philosophie et ses mythes* about the 1937 Conference on Descartes. The second issue came out in Spring 1939 as scheduled but the third issue, dated October, November, December 1939, was prepared by Langevin because Solomon, Politzer and Cogniot had been mobilized in September.

Thus, we see that the response to Munich, after his break from the CVIA, brought Langevin ever closer to the line of Communist Party (Fig. 18.6). The summer of 1938 was the climax of his cooperation with PCF initiatives. And it was a matter of

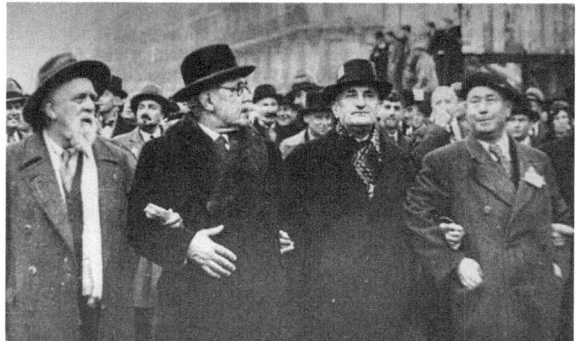

Fig. 18.4 Langevin during an antifascist demonstration, linking arms with Jean Perrin and Victor Basch, president of the League of Human Rights (*Ligue des Droits de l'Homme*) (*Science et Vigilance*)

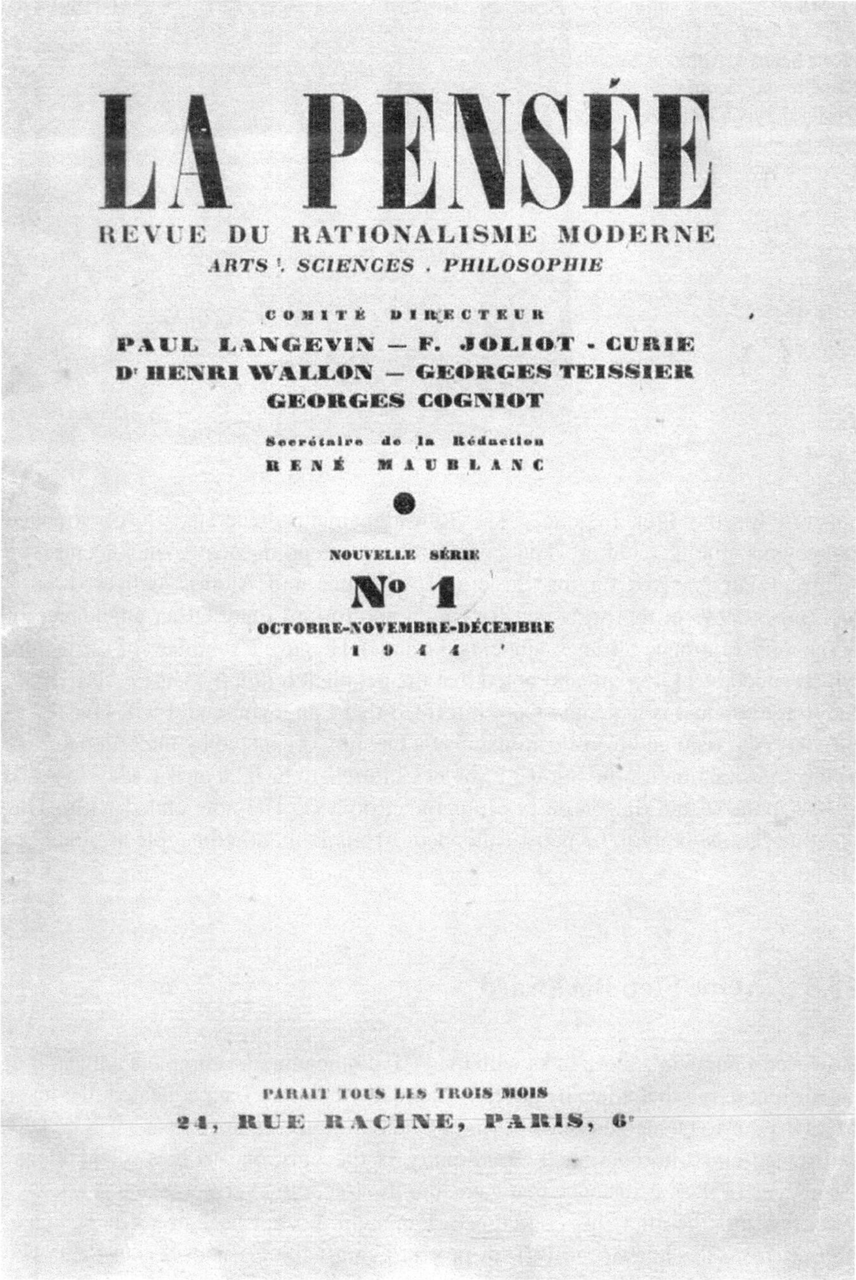

LA PENSÉE

REVUE DU RATIONALISME MODERNE

ARTS . SCIENCES . PHILOSOPHIE

COMITÉ DIRECTEUR

PAUL LANGEVIN — F. JOLIOT - CURIE

Dr HENRI WALLON — GEORGES TEISSIER

GEORGES COGNIOT

Secrétaire de la Rédaction

RENÉ MAUBLANC

NOUVELLE SÉRIE

N° 1

OCTOBRE-NOVEMBRE-DÉCEMBRE

1944

PARAIT TOUS LES TROIS MOIS

24, RUE RACINE, PARIS, 6e

Fig. 18.5 La Pensée No.1. This magazine, founded by Langevin in 1939, renewed its publication, interrupted by the war, starting a New Series in 1944

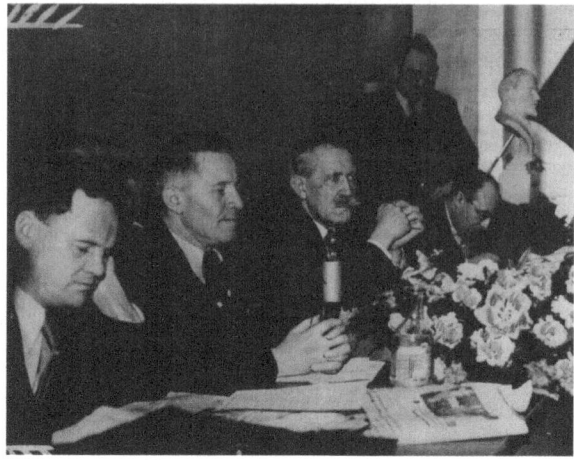

Fig. 18.6 Langevin sitting between Maurice Thorez, Pierre Semard, Arthur Ramette and Jacques Duclos during a national meeting of the French Communist Party. (ESPCI)

concern for the French police. The Renseignements généraux closely tracked Langevin's public lectures. The police officer attending Langevin's lecture on "Current Perspectives on the Structure of Matter and Atoms" delivered on 9 December 1938 in the Sorbonne Richelieu auditorium reported an attendance of 300 people (entrance 5 francs, students 3 francs). He gave a summary of the lecture which ended at 11.15 p.m. and noted that the people left quietly. On 17 April 1939, the Renseignements généraux were informed that Langevin would will give a lecture on "Marxism and Neo-Positivism" at a meeting organized by the group known as the "Association for the Study of Soviet Culture", to be held on Tuesday 18 April at 8.45 p.m. at the Maison de la Mutualité, Room G. The note ended with "This meeting seems likely to be poorly attended. Around a hundred people are likely to attend."

18.5 ...One Step Backward

However, Langevin's close links with the PCF did not entail a complete adhesion. It is worth noticing that when he publicly claimed "the more I am educated, the more I feel myself to be a communist" at the PCF conference in November 1938 he kept a distance since he continued "*Your* party is the only one to have clear ideas" (Langevin 1938e): A distance that gave him the freedom to criticize.

A few months after this conference, Langevin did not hesitate to disassociate himself from the line of the PCF in protest against the German-Soviet Pact. The intellectuals of the Party, including Jacques Solomon, Langevin's son-in-law, maintained an embarrassed silence, with the exception of Paul Nizan. On 29 August 1939, Langevin joined Joliot-Curie, Jean Perrin, Aimé Cotton, Victor Basch and Albert Bayet in publishing a manifesto in the name of the Union of French Intellectuals expressing indignation about a gesture that was so unexpected at a time when the Nazis threatened Poland and all free countries [4].

Conversely, when the PCF was the victim of governmental measures, Langevin supported his members. In 1940, the French government took advantage of the revival of anti-Bolshevism to dissolve newspapers and communist groups, and to bring to military court 44 communist deputies accused of treason. Their political trial, behind closed doors, was too great a reminder of the Dreyfus Affair. Langevin testified in favour of the deputies on 29 March 1940 with J.-R. Bloch, Maublanc and Wallon [10, pp. 141–145]. His deposition clearly confirmed his version of the Marxist doctrine:

> I met them to discuss ideas, sharing their ideal of social justice and their desire to implement this ideal through a human effort to transform the world materially and morally. To achieve this, they put their trust in the possibility of an unlimited enhancement of science and human awareness (…). Reaching justice through science seems to me to be the formula that best summarizes their doctrine. [10, pp. 142–143]

We can see that despite some complacent silences, Langevin followed his conscience rather than the party line. He did not want to "oppose tactics to truth". These are the words used by Aragon, a Communist French poet and novelist in his novel *Les Communistes*. Aragon noted that in those years "when history was heard creaking", the prestige and aura of the small group of intellectuals such as Rolland and Langevin, "embodied world peace and gave these mad hopes that men had all over the earth that by pronouncing it one would avoid massacre and death" [1, p. 230]. Aragon emphasizes the admiration and respect these white-haired men inspired in young communist activists like him. But the signing of the manifesto against the Pact suddenly created a fracture, a misunderstanding. For the young communists, it was a betrayal.

Thus, Langevin's relations with the PCF seem to us more complex than the testimonies of his comrades, Labérenne, Cogniot and Biquard. It is impossible to assume with them that Langevin was convinced long before his membership of the validity of the PCF political line. Langevin's political evolution was less "an ascent" towards the light of Marxism than a wavering march with a few steps forward, followed by a step backwards.

However, it would be equally simplistic to conclude that the PCF used Langevin's prestige to attract intellectuals, as suggested by one report of the Renseignements généraux. The confidential note of March 1936 reporting that Langevin had health problems that would keep him away from Paris for two months added: "The Communist leaders were very upset by this news; they had intended to make extensive use of the professor's support for the election campaign, but this was now proving impossible" (Police archives file 4929, 31 March 1936).

Langevin was not instrumentalized by the PCF. He rather sincerely tried to assimilate the Marxist ideal under the influence of his son-in-law, daughter and friends in the 1930s. For a younger communist like Aragon, despite years of fighting side by side, despite his late adhesion to the PCF, Langevin remained an idealist, a man of another generation, living in a different world.

References

1. Aragon L (1949) Les communistes, vol I. (1949) reprint. Livre Club Diderot, Paris, 1973–74, T.1
2. Biquard P (1969) Paul Langevin, scientifique, éducateur, citoyen. Seghers, Paris
3. Bustamante M-C (in print) Jacques Solomon (1908-1942) Physicien militant fusillé. Brepols, Bruxelles
4. Caute D (1964) Communism and the French intellectuals (1914–1960). Deutsch, London
5. Caute D (1979) Les compagnons de route. Laffont, Paris
6. Gide A (1936) Retour de l'URSS. Reprint Culturea (2022)
7. Kriegel A (1985) Les Communistes français. Historiographie. Le Seuil, Paris
8. Labérenne P (1964) La Pensée et l'action. Éditions Sociales, Paris
9. Lacaze Y (1991) L'opinion publique française et la crise de Munich. P. Lang, Berne
10. Langevin A (2022) Paul Langevin my father. EDP Sciences, Paris. English edition: Duck F
11. Wallon H (ed) (1935) A la lumière du marxisme. Éditions Sociales Internationales, Paris

Chapter 19
Through the Hardships of World War Two

Abstract In 1940, Langevin was dismissed from his professorship at the *Collège de France* and arrested by the Gestapo in October. This arrest raised a wave of protests from students and colleagues. Langevin endured the torments and humiliation of jail for two months before being placed under house arrest in Troyes. He spent more than three years in this exile, deprived of his freedom of action and from his daily contacts with friends and family. He used this mandatory vacation to conduct further theoretical research, notably in the emerging field of nuclear physics. Frédéric Joliot organized his escape from Troyes in 1944 and Langevin was celebrated as a hero when he returned to Paris, especially on the occasion of his 73rd birthday in January 1945. Caught up in the enthusiasm of the tasks of reconstruction, Langevin did not feel the shock of Hiroshima with the gravity he had given to the deadly applications of science in World War One. The chapter ends with a discussion of his optimistic response to Hiroshima against the background of the emerging French nuclear power.

May 1940, Langevin, like other research directors, received the order to evacuate his laboratories, which formed group IV of the recent CNRS, far away from Paris. In June 1940, as France surrenders to Nazi Germany; Langevin retreated to Toulouse in the South of France. In early July, highly agitated, amid hasty departures abroad of many colleagues, Langevin returned to Paris by train and begun to quietly prepare the next academic year at EPCI. Why didn't he decide to settle in the United States like his friend Perrin, and try to act against fascism from there? Langevin did not consider this option for long. The idea of leaving the homeland in distress, in the hands of invaders, seemed to him not very brave. Like Joliot, who sent his assistants Hans von Halban and Lev Kowarski to England with a stock of heavy water necessary for nuclear chain reaction, he preferred to stay in Paris [7]. They both assumed that they had to stay in their post to face the danger.

On 3 October, Langevin was dismissed from his duties at the *Collège de France*. A letter of 11 October 1940 from the Military Commandant to the Delegate of the French Government to the Military Command in France stated that:

The activity of Professors Ernest Tonnelat, Paul Langevin and Henri Wallon at the *Collège de France* is incompatible with the interests and prestige of the occupying authorities. I ask you to do what is necessary and inform me of the measures you have taken in this regard …

On 30 October 1940, at 14:45 after a lunch that brought the whole family together in Langevin's apartment, two cars of the Gestapo entered the courtyard of the EPCI, rue Vauquelin and blocked all exits [2]. Hélène Langevin-Solomon reported that a German officer accompanied by a soldier asked for professor Langevin, exchanged a few words with him in his study. Langevin came out very pale and asked his wife to pack his suitcase as he had to leave. He then followed the officer in silence, handcuffs on wrists, to an unknown destination. Workers on the roof watched the scene in horror and anger. Langevin's wife immediately called the Dean of Paris University to inform him about the arrest of the EPCI director. It will be known, many hours later, that Langevin was incarcerated in the Santé prison (named after its location on the Rue de la Santé in the 11th arrondissement of Paris). Opened since 1867, this prison had both VIP and maximum-security sections.

The official reasons for the arrest remain opaque. And Jeanne Langevin's requests for an explanation remained unanswered. There is no mention of this arrest conducted by the Gestapo in the files of French police. Langevin was certainly suspected of anti-fascist activities, but many activists and intellectuals who fought with him were not arrested.

19.1 Humiliated, Honoured

Then begun long days of trials and torments. Nothing was spared for this illustrious professor, who, in a few hours, became a common law prisoner. He was left destitute in a cell with sagging trousers and unfastened shoes, without belt or laces, without a book, without paper, without a pencil. Visits were forbidden for weeks.

It often happens that a brief stay in an extreme environment reveals, better than years of daily life, someone's personality. Such was the effect produced by the 40 days that Langevin spent at La Santé from 30 October to 7 December 1940. Far from being discouraged, this almost septuagenarian man, already worn out by a busy life, immediately pulled himself together. Two days after his incarceration, he started working to keep his spirits up, and to recover his dignity. He begun long calculations on toilet paper with spent matches picked up from the ground and dipped in a solution of activated charcoal that he used as a medicine for digestive disorders (Fig. 19.1). Thus, keeping himself occupied, he managed to overcome humiliations and loneliness.

Ironically, the sessions of interrogation by the Gestapo afforded an opportunity to regain some pride. The list of accusations clearly demonstrated that in 20 years of struggle for peace and against fascism, Langevin has acquired more than a personal reputation, he embodied an ideal. "An individual as dangerous for National Socialism as the philosophers of the eighteenth century for the *Ancien Régime*", said the colonel who interrogated him on 2 November [5, p. 147]. In his response,

19.1 Humiliated, Honoured

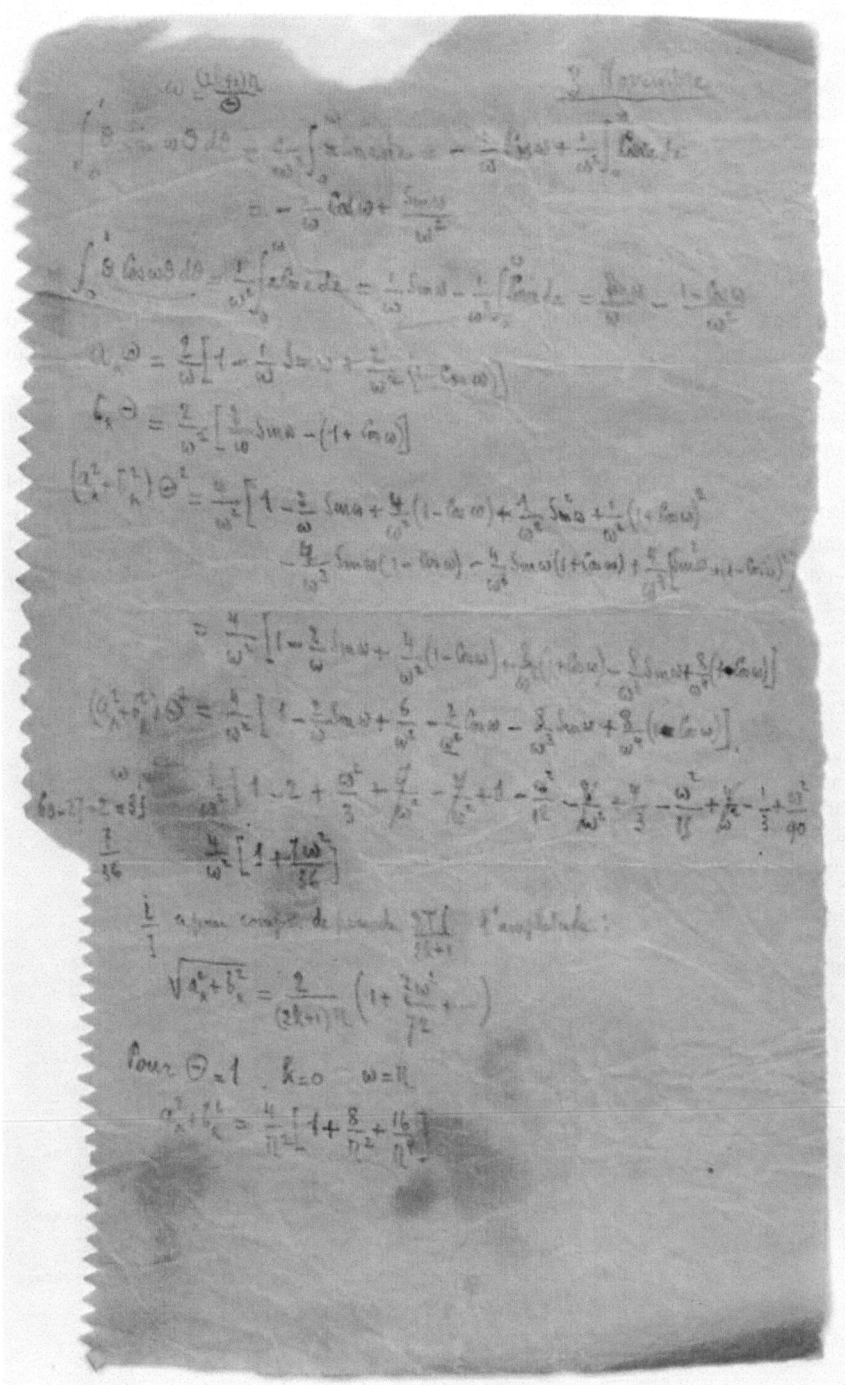

Fig. 19.1 During his stay in prison, Langevin carried out calculations using charcoal on toilet paper. (ESPCI, PSL University L048/001)

Langevin fully endorsed the comparison and reiterated his attachment to the Enlightenment values.

> My action has always been: 1) only on the human level; I do not place myself in any race sect or political party. 2) only in the realm of ideas, for the defence of those who are dear to me: for individual and collective justice, freedom and peace. (…) I have never at any moment, said or written a word in the sense of a provocation to war. 3) absolutely in the open, on the basis of public presentation and discussion of ideas and facts. I have never participated in any covert action of any kind. 4) absolutely disinterested: I have devoted almost all I had and have no assets or other resources than my salary or possible retirement pension (Ibid., p. 148: Archives L048/02)

Langevin's arrest raised many protests abroad. They came from both the United States and the USSR and always from scientific colleagues. With the help of an American diplomat, Einstein tried to release him and at the same time to find him a position in the United States (Fig. 19.2). Piotr Kapitza ensured that the Academy of Sciences would invite Langevin to Moscow.

His British scientific friends also gave support, with the strength of official and formal endorsement. The Royal Society of London awarded him its most prestigious award, the Copley Medal; the announcement was made public in *Nature* on 7 December, just 2 days before his release from the imprisonment. On 1 January 1941, Sir Henry Dale, the President of the Royal Society, broadcast to French scientists on the BBC's *Demi heure française matin* in which, speaking in French, he

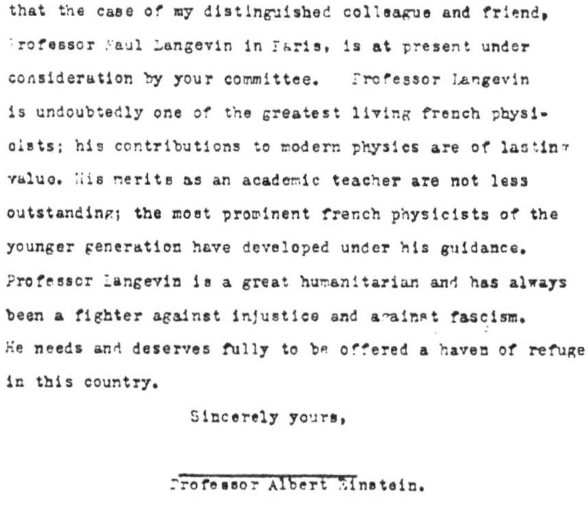

Fig. 19.2 Einstein's letter, from Princeton, to George Warren of the President's Advisory Committee for Political Refugees in the USA, asking that Langevin should be given refugee status. (ESPCI, PSL University L072/042)

```
                                        January 28, 1941

Mr. George Warren
President's Advisory Committee
for Political Refugees
122 East 22nd Str.
New York City

Dear Mr. Warren:
        Ambassador William C. Bullitt has informed me
that the case of my distinguished colleague and friend,
Professor Paul Langevin in Paris, is at present under
consideration by your committee.  Professor Langevin
is undoubtedly one of the greatest living french physi-
cists; his contributions to modern physics are of lasting
value. His merits as an academic teacher are not less
outstanding; the most prominent french physicists of the
younger generation have developed under his guidance.
Professor Langevin is a great humanitarian and has always
been a fighter against injustice and against fascism.
He needs and deserves fully to be offered a haven of refuge
in this country.
                        Sincerely yours,

                        Professor Albert Einstein.
```

announced the award to Langevin and offered fraternal greetings to his French colleagues, "united by the common idea of scientific freedom".

In France, Langevin's arrest also triggered a surge of solidarity. As a sign of protest, Frédéric Joliot refused to go to his laboratory.[1] There were many who, at the risk of compromising themselves, sent letters to prison: Letters of support as much as of protest, clearly intended to be read by the authorities as they complacently listed Langevin's titles and expressed their indignation at the treatment to which he was being subjected (Archives L048).

Beyond the circle of friends and collaborators, Langevin's incarceration has caused a stir among the communist students who were operating underground. They immediately circulated a leaflet entitled "The arrest of Professor Langevin signals the open battle of the obscurantist powers against culture and free thought" [4]. They set up a defence committee calling for his immediate release. On 8 November, about 50 students demonstrated in front of the *Collège de France* at the time of Langevin's weekly lecture with the intention to get into the room where he used to teach for one hour and a half. But they found the gates closed, as were all the nearby cafés. So they retreated on the Boulevard St Michel singing the national anthem, *La Marseillaise*. On 11 November, another demonstration gathered a thousand students to the *Place de l'Etoile* in front of the tomb of the unknown soldier. It was repressed by the German troops and caused 143 temporary arrests. The Vichy government retaliated by closing the University of Paris and dismissing its rector Gustave Roussy. Solomon and Politzer organized a resistance network, the National University Front, which launched an underground journal titled *l'Université libre*.

On 19 November, Langevin was formally dismissed from his post at EPCI. A statement by the Secretary of State for Public Education at Vichy announces that "Mr. Langevin (Paul), professor at the *Collège de France*, director of the *Ecole Pratique des Hautes Etudes* (sic.)" is dismissed from both positions, under laws passed earlier in the year.

The French police tend to minimize the importance of the students protests. A note dated 21 November 1940 reported:

> Following the arrest of Professor Langevin and the announcement on the radio and in the press that he had been relieved of his duties at the same time as Mr Rivet, a professor at the Musée National d'Histoire Naturelle, surveys were carried out among the students of these two professors to find out how they felt about these measures. Generally speaking, there was no reaction. The arrest of the Professor Langevin, in particular, had caused real surprise among left-wing students, which resulted in a demonstration project at the Collège de France that was not followed up. Since then, there has been no outburst and it seems that, apart from about thirty of Pr Langevin's students, the whole student body is rather indiffer-

---

[1] Frédéric Joliot (1900–1958) studied at EPCI under Langevin's direction. Langevin then pointed him towards the Radium Institute, directed by Marie Curie. He married her daughter Irène. They both discovered artificial radioactivity in 1934 and were awarded the Nobel Prize for Chemistry in 1935. Joliot joined the fight against fascism and joined the French Communist Party during the Resistance, in 1942. In 1945, General de Gaulle appointed him as the head of the Commission for Atomic Energy; however, in 1950, he was dismissed from the post for political reasons.

ent. In any case, we have not heard any recriminations or criticisms from the schools concerned. (Police Archives file 4929)

Emile Picard, Perpetual Secretary of the Academy of Science wrote a very cautious and respectful letter to a French army chief general asking for the reasons of Langevin's arrest (Police Archives file 4929). By contrast, Henri Wallon protested in the name of the French Society of Pedagogy, recently dissolved by the Vichy Government, against the tactics of intimidation:

> Without a shadow of a pretext, this is the arrest of a scientist who was among the most illustrious physicists of his time, an eminent thinker, a democrat full of prestige. In the person of Paul Langevin, what is being targeted is the whole tradition of science and progress of which our country has been and remains the home, the prestige of culture in the world. The aim is to intimidate, to reduce French intellectuals to mercy. [9]

Thus, Langevin's arrest catalyzed academic resistance. While he was himself forced into inactivity by his age and his arrest, he triggered multiple gestures of resistance among French academics. By the end of 1940, he was above all a symbol of intelligence and freedom, a flagship of resistance. Younger academics already saw him only as an icon—too old to be active any more.

19.2 Mandatory Vacation

Yet Langevin was firmly attached to life. He was released from *La Santé* in December and then placed under house arrest. On 9 December 1940, he settled into a requisitioned apartment in Troyes, a small medieval city about 180 km upstream from Paris on the river Seine in Champagne. He would stay there for nearly 4 years, prohibited from leaving the city, signing in with the Commandant every four days. He started a new lifestyle, provincial and quiet, with enforced rest, the first that Langevin allowed himself since his military service!

During these years of forced retirement, Langevin dedicated himself to physics and tried to keep up his professional activities. He continued to award a number of prizes at the Academy of Sciences. He even took advantage of his enforced rest to deal with his "wicker trunk of remorses". He used this phrase to refer to the tasks that had been pending for years and that he used to take on vacation in a large wicker trunk, hoping to find the time to get rid of them [5, p. 203]. At last, he could read and comment on his son André's PhD dissertation, which had been waiting for ten years in a trunk. He also wrote, for the Academy, a secret report on Joliot in support of his candidature in 1943 (Archives, L073/011). Langevin even found ways to continue teaching. In 1941, he gave a course on atomic physics, at the *Ecole normale d'instructrices de l'Aube* (Aube training college for female primary school teachers). In his course, he retraced the adventure of atomic physics from Becquerel's discovery to Joliot's recent work, but omitting quantum mechanics and indeterminacy (Archives, L053/002). Later, at the beginning of 1944, he presented recent advances in physics in a Sunday course at the high school in Troyes. Finally, Langevin could conduct a bit of theoretical research. But instead of continuing on his familiar subjects, he tackled new problems in nuclear physics including neutron capture. He suggested experimental projects to Joliot, and even designed experimental devices (Archives, L073). Thanks to his academic activities, Langevin was not cowed by adversity.

It does not mean that he was always in high spirits. His correspondence with Jeanne Langevin reveals the hardship of his life in Troyes. "Can you send me something to eat? (...) Did you put my slippers in the suitcase?" (Fig. 19.3). Langevin strove to survive in scarcity: he queued to stock up on milk or meat; he cooked for himself in his "kitchen laboratory". But he enjoyed the port wine that was sent for his birthday, remaining a *bon vivant*.

He bravely endured the hassles of life under surveillance: a control visit to the police station every fourth day; continual intimidations, with all his requests for "permission" to go to Paris rejected. He was arrested a second time in October 1941 and spent 3 days in prison. In 1942, he received a proposal from the German authorities for scientific collaboration, which he dismissed.

The correspondence of this period also reveals his family life shared with two women. It seems that the visits of Jeanne, his wife, alternated with those of Éliane Montel, his former mistress and mother of his son Paul-Gilbert Langevin. As for his other children and grandchildren, Langevin flooded them with letters, overflowing with tenderness, signed "your dad and grandpa" (Fig. 19.4). Undeniably, Langevin was something of the patriarch who watched over his tribe. Over the years, when the children got married and the director's apartment of the EPCI became too small, he asked the young couples to settle nearby, in the neighbourhood, or even across the *rue Vauquelin* for Jacques and Hélène Solomon. Langevin was more and more inclined to seek advice from his family, to ask his children and in-laws for their opinions. However, he still ruled over the household, sometimes exercising a bit of authority during family meals. He adopted a protective attitude when he sought to spare his wife bad news about their children.

On 1 March 1942, Jacques Solomon was arrested by the French special brigades and incarcerated at the Cherche-Midi prison. Accused of "a major conspiracy against the security of the State", he was handed over to the Germans and shot on the Mont-Valérien on 23 May 1942, the same day as his friend Politzer. In addition to the pain of losing a son-in-law, who was both esteemed and cherished, Langevin felt responsibility because his arrest had been the origin of Solomon's resistance group (Langevin 1946b). His wife, Hélène Langevin-Solomon was first interned at Romainville, then transferred to Germany in a convoy on 24 January 1943, to Auschwitz. For the next two years, the family lived in sadness, anxiety, hope. Only in December 1944, Langevin heard, from a professor in Geneva, that Hélène had survived the camps (Archives, L053/017). She would be reunited with her parents at the Gare du Nord on 15 May 1945.

The German pressure on Langevin in Troyes increased in 1943 with the confiscation of the furniture from his apartment. Joliot got regular news from Langevin thanks to Eliane Montel's visits, who was working in his laboratory at the *Collège*

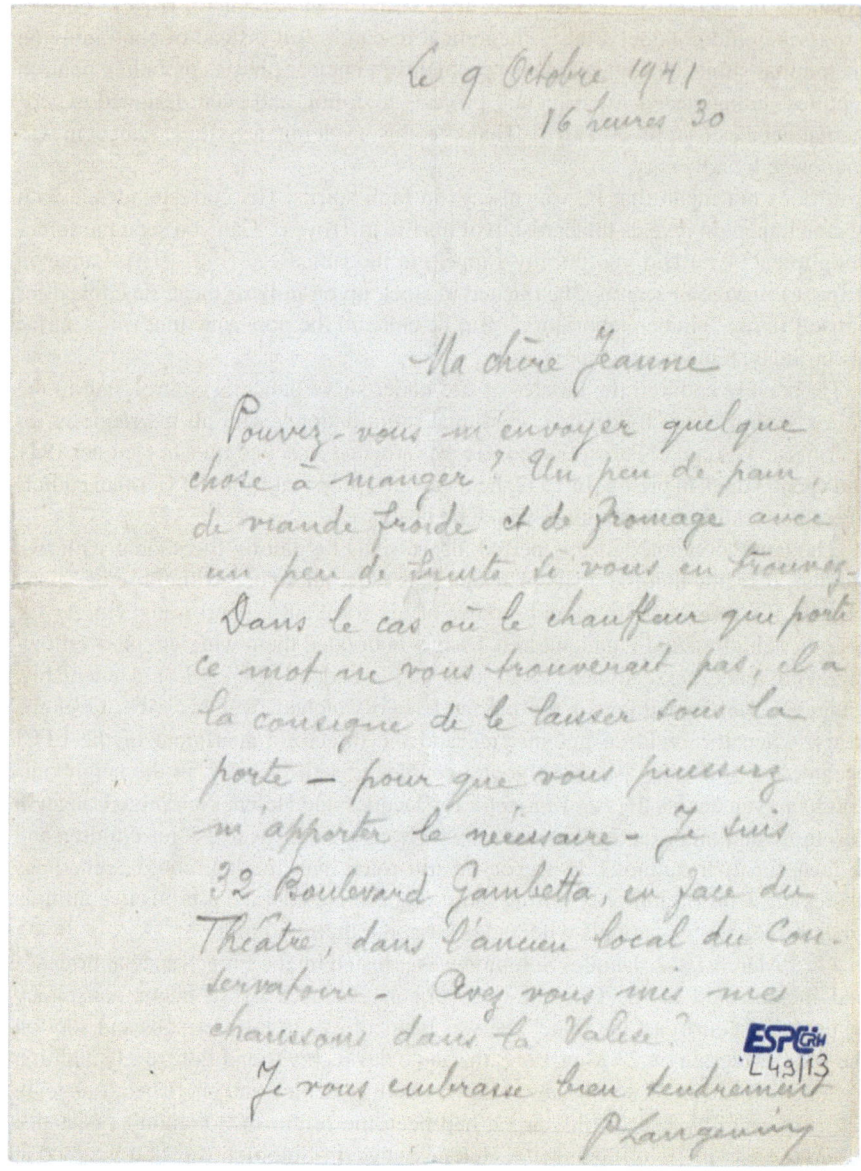

Fig. 19.3 A letter written by Langevin to his wife in Paris on 9 October 1941 while he was under house arrest in Troyes. (ESPCI, PSL University L049/013)

19.2 Mandatory Vacation

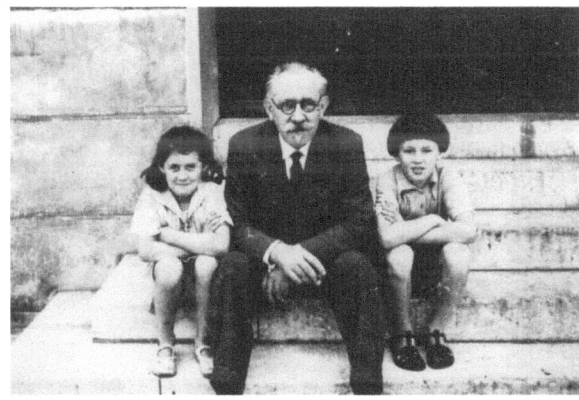

Fig. 19.4 Langevin, grandfather, with two of his grandchildren. (ESPCI)

de France. He organized a daring escape for Langevin through the resistance network. "My escape was a masterpiece of organization. Nothing went wrong. Everything went according to plan, in the shortest possible time", said Langevin when he was safe in Switzerland. Following the plans set up by André Léger and Philippe Alleman, on 2 May 1944 Langevin went to the regular control at the police station then walked to a village nearby, where he waited for a train while trying to hide (Archives, L053/016). He boarded a train at 5 a.m. and arrived in Paris where someone drove him to an apartment. He was given a false identity card and documents for admission in Switzerland.

On 6 May, he arrived in Lyon with a student of the *Paris Ecole des arts et métiers* and was welcome by André Léger. After a quick lunch at a *soupe populaire* with Léger, he left Lyon in a car of the Navigation Service displaying a sign reading "Wasserstrassenant". Inside the car they found a thick file on dam construction in Vautrey, a village near the Swiss border. Their alibi in the event of an inspection was that they were on a field trip around the dam. On their arrival at Chamesol, not far from the dam, they were met by two *Francs-Tireurs-Partisans* (FTP) who helped Langevin across the border (Fig. 19.5). It was a daunting adventure for a 71-year-old because they had to walk across a valley with steep slopes on both sides, especially on the ascent to Switzerland. The two FTPs (loggers by trade) literally carried the professor on their shoulders. When they reached the border post N°455, they met Philippe Alleman who took charge of Langevin, taking him on to meet Irène Joliot-Curie (Fig. 19.6).

In September 1944, when Paris was liberated, Langevin left Neuchâtel and returned to France through freed Haute-Savoie. Still following Joliot's instructions, he was driven to Lyon where he met friends and collaborators, notably Pierre Biquard. He gave a speech on Radio-Lyon, on 24 September: a brief but hopeful speech, calling for the pursuit "without weakness [of] those who by their acts have placed themselves outside the nation" and then to achieve "the economic liberation and spiritual of the country" through deep reforms of work and education (Langevin 1944a). Langevin drove back to Paris on 25 September, with Aragon and Elsa Triolet, his wife (Fig. 19.7).

Fig. 19.5 In May 1944, Langevin left Troyes and travelled secretly to Switzerland with the help of two FTP guides and a with forged identity card that had been obtained by Frédéric Joliot-Curie. (ESPCI)

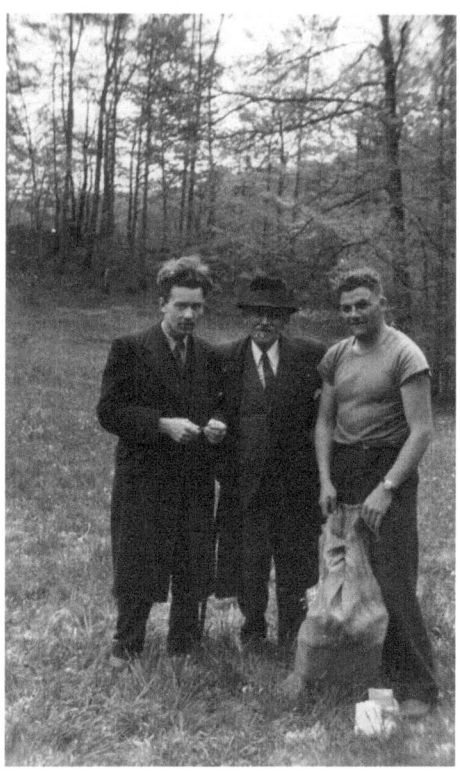

Fig. 19.6 At the end of July 1944, Langevin visited Irène Joliot-Curie, who was also sheltering in Switzerland with her children at *La Chaux-de-Fonds*. (ESPCI)

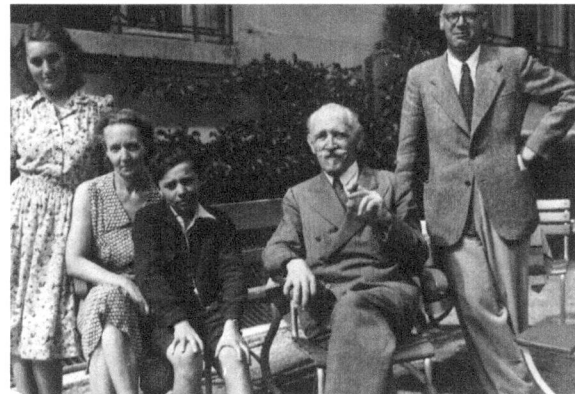

Fig. 19.7 September 1944: Langevin returned from Lyon to Paris with Aragon and Elsa Triolet. (ESPCI)

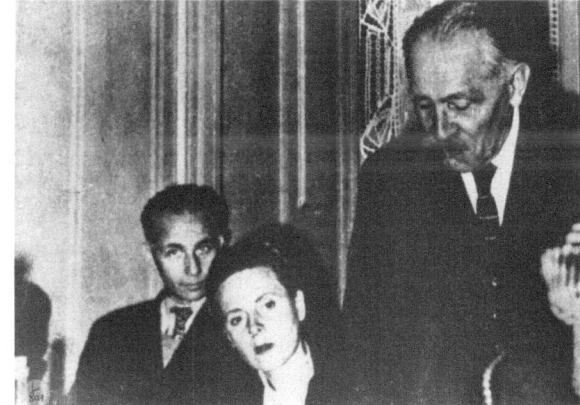

Fig. 19.8 Langevin was celebrated as a hero at a grand reception for his 73rd birthday, at the Sorbonne, on 3 March 1945. To his right, the USSR Ambassador Aleksandr Bogomolov; to his left, the British Ambassador Duff Cooper and Frédéric Joliot. (*Science et Vigilance*)

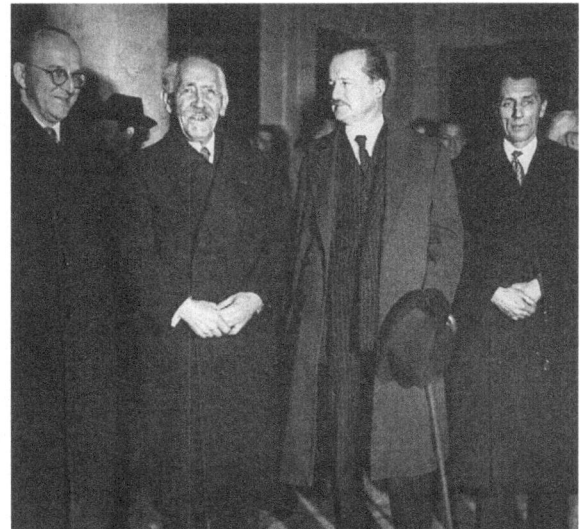

19.3 The Time of Tributes

Better days then began. At the EPCI, where the director's apartment was still occupied by his replacement, Langevin met some of his children. He had to settle in rooms under the eaves, but this was nothing in comparison with the trials of Troyes. Langevin was surrounded, assisted and honoured as a national hero. His 73rd birthday in January 1945 was celebrated with a great fanfare; first by a dinner organized by the Communist Party; then in grand style by a ceremony at the Sorbonne, on 3 March, with ministers and the *Marseillaise* (Fig. 19.8).

Langevin was weak and already drained by illness, but he bravely continued to do his "civic duty". First, he paid tribute to friends who disappeared during the war, Jacques Solomon, Victor Basch, president of the League of Human Rights (Langevin

1945h), Henri Roger, president of the Rationalist Union (Langevin 1946d) and declared that he would continue their work by assuming their tasks as presidents. At 73, Langevin still remained a fervent champion of justice:

> For we all know that the struggle is not over and will require many sacrifices and much effort before, in the current stage of the ongoing revolution, fascism is definitively defeated, a criminal attempt to maintain by brutal force and by stupefaction, an economic and social regime that reason can no longer justify. (Langevin 1945h, p. 11)

The war had enhanced Langevin's aspirations to justice and freedom. Although he shared with his companions of the Liberation the will to see traitors punished, Langevin did not hesitate to help one of his former comrades from the EPCI who was sentenced for collaboration with the Nazis in the development of V2 rockets. He testified at the trial of Georges Claude, member of *Action française*, a notoriously anti-Semitic party (Langevin 1944c). Faithful to his childhood friends, Langevin was less so to his own political habits. For the first time in his life, he accepted direct political responsibilities: he was elected member of the City Council of the fifth arrondissement; member of the General Council of the Seine department. Finally, he was appointed by Charles de Gaulle to be president of the Commission for the Reform of Education (Chap. 20).

19.4 The Flash of Hiroshima

Caught up in the enthusiasm of the tasks of reconstruction, Langevin did not feel the shock of the first atomic bombs with the gravity he had given to the deadly applications of science in World War One. His attitude in the summer of 1945, after the two bombings of Hiroshima on 6 August and Nagasaki on 9 August was in striking contrast with the reactions of French intellectuals who envisaged catastrophic visions of mass-destruction and of a collective suicide. In France, for instance, Albert Camus wrote a famous editorial in the daily newspaper *Combat*:

> The world is what it is—not much. That's what we've all known since yesterday, thanks to the tremendous concert that radio, newspapers and news agencies have just unleashed on the subject of the atomic bomb. […] The mechanical civilization has just reached the ultimate degree of savagery. Within the foreseeable future, we will have to choose between collective suicide or a clever use of scientific conquests. (Camus, *Combat*, 8 August 1945)

On 10 August, the catholic novelist François Mauriac commented in his diary that the bombings of Hiroshima and Nagasaki represented a "planetary suicide" with but a single benefit: to discredit the idea of the progress of humanity [6, p. 340]. Even before the number of victims and the extent of the radiation damage were known, the violence of the explosion created an impression of annihilation, of a global threat, of an end of the world. Jean-Paul Sartre opened the first issue of the monthly *Les temps modernes*:

> Yet here we are, brought back to the year 1000, each morning on the eve of the end of times; on the eve of the day when our honesty, our courage, our good will will no longer have any

19.4 The Flash of Hiroshima

meaning for anyone, and will sink together with wickedness, ill will and fear into a radical indistinction. After the death of God, the death of man is announced. [...] There is no longer a human species. The community that has made itself the guardian of the atomic bomb is above the natural kingdom, because it is responsible for its own life and death: every day, every minute, it must agree to live. This is the anguish we feel today. (Sartre, *Les Temps modernes*, 1 October 1945)

Langevin reacted quickly and vividly, but he had not the slightest feeling of the impact of nuclear bombs. Far from deploring the threat of barbarism or "the prostitution of science" as he had done in the aftermath of World War One, he basked in euphoria. In *La Pensée* of July–August–September 1945, Langevin, one of the journal's editors, published an article entitled *L'Ere des transmutations* ("The Age of Transmutations"), which quietly announced the dawn of a new era, the advent of an unprecedented power:

One cannot exaggerate the importance of the event that represents for the future of humanity, the appearance of the atomic bomb. It is indeed about much more than the invention of a new weapon whose terrible efficiency has just hastened the end of the conflict that, for six years, set the planet ablaze. We are witnessing in reality, in a particularly dramatic form, the beginning of a new era, that of artificial transmutations. This opens up prospects for us that go far beyond the old dream of the alchemists. (Langevin 1945a, p. 3)

The phrase "atomic age" was introduced in Henry Smith's official chronicle of the Manhattan Project. Langevin translated his report on the test on 19 July in New Mexico into French, which begun with the words: "The effective entry of mankind into a new period, the atomic age, took place on 16 July 1945 ...." In September 1945, this report was his main source of information, together with Harry Truman's press release saying: "With the advent of the nuclear age, new dilemmas in the art of warfare arose."

Langevin had no moral dilemma: he was fascinated by the technological prowess, like most of the French daily press. On 7 August 1945, *L'Aurore* announced the atomic bomb on Hiroshima under the title "A Scientific Revolution". The front page of *L'Humanité* included two articles headlined: "The Atomic Bomb Has Its History" and "Freeing Atomic Energy" with a photo of Joliot-Curie (Fig. 19.9). On 9 August, *Le Soir* published the testimony of the pilot of the plane that dropped the bomb, who describes the horrifying impact—"the city rose up and bubbled"—but without reporting the casualties. French people had no factual information about the damage caused by the atomic bombs in Hiroshima and Nagasaki. Because they had access to the official reports of the national press agencies, there was a striking asymmetry between the detailed scientific information about the Manhattan project and the absence of data about the effect of the bombings on the population, the number of casualties and the suffering of the survivors in Hiroshima and Nagasaki [10]. With the US occupation of Japan in September 1945, a strict censorship was imposed by the US administration. The coverage of the event by an official *New York Times* reporter, William Laurence, merely described the awesome beauty of the flash from the bomb dropped on Nagasaki. Even when French officials and journalists were allowed to travel to Japan and wrote reports they insisted on the spectacle of the explosion and the power of the bomb, without showing any empathy for the victims.

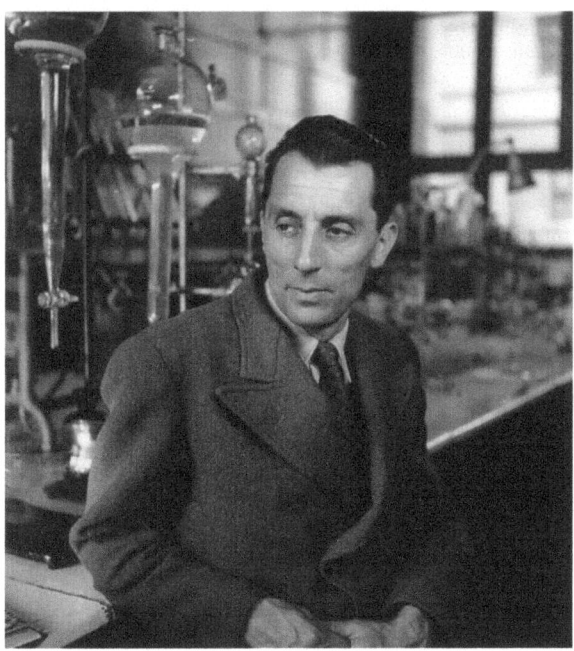

Fig. 19.9 Frédéric Joliot (1900–1958). (ESPCI)

For example, Francis Lacoste, a diplomat who visited Hiroshima in January 1946, wrote on 8 February 1946: "all it took was a single 300 grams projectile to wipe out an entire city and half its population in a flash of lightning". Not until the 1950s would the victims be allowed to a hearing and to talk about the long-term effects of radiation.

Even though Langevin's blindness about the human impact of the first nuclear bombings was shared by most French people in 1945–1946, his insensitivity to the human side of the first nuclear bombings, his lack of concern with the risks of "planetary suicide" never cease to amaze. In our view, his fascination with the perspective of nuclear energy shows the influence that Joliot had on him. In 1945, Joliot, who had rescued him from Troyes, was director of the CNRS, in charge of the organization of the *Commissariat à l'énergie atomique* (Atomic Energy Commission). He was an entrepreneurial scientist who juggled his time between research, ministerial budgets and public projects [8]. As a communist, he wanted to implement the programme outlined by Bernal in "The Social Function of Science". He thus claimed that scientists were responsible for the applications of their science. Still, he was determined to make France into a nuclear power.

In the name of the *Union rationaliste* of which he was the president, Langevin invited Joliot to give a lecture in the Sorbonne in September 1945. In his introduction, he gave a detailed description of the nuclear bomb, presented as a "revolution" in the history of the mastery of energy and a decisive step in the history of the atom. He even claimed that atomic research would change the relationships between genders, "that the future of this new era of transmutations is also that of collaboration

19.4 The Flash of Hiroshima

on all levels, and on the scientific level, in particular, of women and men" (Langevin 1945c, p. 177).

Resolutely triumphalist, Langevin was also reassuring: there is no danger of catastrophe by uncontrolled propagation of nuclear reactions (Langevin 1945a, p. 15). And he ended on the promise of a bright future where each citizen would have "about 50 slaves powered by electricity" to do his work. This "material liberation" would not only enable but make even more necessary the "spiritual liberation" of humans through education and the development of culture (ibid., p. 16). In short, Hiroshima generated a euphoric celebration of nuclear power, occasionally mixed with jokes, for instance when Langevin declared in front of a packed audience in the Sorbonne auditorium:

> Seeing what is happening tonight, we can say that the explosions of two atomic bombs in Japan have had the very distant effect of expanding the Richelieu auditorium where our Rationalist Union usually holds its conferences to the dimensions of the great auditorium of the Sorbonne. (Langevin 1945c, p. 176)

Even though the war slowed the relations with foreign scientists in August 1945, Langevin and Joliot, who both knew John Bernal, could have contacts with England in particular. They were presumably aware of the mobilization of a number of British and American "scientific workers", who acted as whistle blowers. As early as 17 February 1945, a conference on the moral responsibility of scientists was organized by the Association of Scientific Workers in London: Hill, Oliphant, Bernal, Blackett and John A. Simpson, President of Chicago Atomic scientists committee, declared that scientists had the right and duty to question and debate the nature of their own function and its contribution to national and international well-being, and a duty to refuse to cooperate if they have no power of decision and control. Unlike the British community of physics,[2] Langevin and Joliot had no inside knowledge of the Manhattan Project and were not prepared to take a firm position regarding Hiroshima.

This call for responsibility, which could have been signed by Langevin in the prewar period, was totally obscured by his enthusiasm for scientific achievements and his rationalist fervour. In 'La pensée et l'action' he describes the convergence between theoretical physicists and engineers as a model of interactions between thought and action, science and technology (Langevin 1946a, p. 344).

In the first issue of *La Pensée* new series, published a year before Hiroshima, the editorial presented the Resistance and the Liberation as a victory of reason over obscurantism, the triumph of the resilient, infallible French rationalist tradition (*La Pensée* 1944, pp. 1, 3–4). Langevin revived the *Union rationaliste*, because it seemed "more than ever useful to make the voice of reason heard" (Langevin 1946d, p. 61). Far from casting doubt on human civilization, as in 1918, the atrocities of the war consolidated his faith in progress. Science was no longer perceived as a powerful, ambivalent, unpredictable force. He assumed that true science was easily

---

[2] Recruitment of British physicists was prolific, starting with Rudolph Peierls' group from Birmingham, and including Joseph Rotblat, who would become Nobel Peace Prize winner in 1995.

distinguishable from the "pseudo-scientific coatings" that support harmful practices. Science seemed controllable, and its future in our hands. "It depends on us", Langevin argued, to use transmutations for good or evil (Langevin 1945a, p. 15). He thus outlined another figure of science, that of neutral science, that is neither intrinsically good nor bad. Unlike the figure of gentle, maternal science that he invoked in the interwar period, this figure would prevail in the 1950s in the service of the development of nuclear technology. On the assumption that nuclear power was a dual use technology, which can be used for both killing and well-being, the slogan "Atoms for Peace", launched in December 1953 before the United Nations Assembly, rallied politicians, scientists and engineers behind a vast programme to build nuclear power plants. It created a divide between the warlike and peaceful uses of the atom [1].

At the same time, we observe, in Langevin, a kind of transfer of the qualities of science to technology. It is technology that is said to be emancipating both materially and spiritually. It was no longer, as in the 1930s, a side effect that accompanies ("in addition") scientific development. Nuclear science is clearly presented as a promise of technology and comfort for all in a call signed by Langevin, de Broglie and Joliot in the name of the French Academy of Sciences, in December 1945, for the French government to direct the applications of nuclear physics exclusively towards peaceful goals. Science was depicted as a reservoir of "potentials" at "the disposition of the human community", a reservoir fuelled by a world of scientists "fully aware of their responsibilities" and well determined not to let state secrets be imposed on them (Langevin 1945b).

Should we then say that by professing their shared faith in the atomic era, Langevin and Joliot revived the optimism of their elder, Pierre Curie? In his Nobel lecture in 1905, Curie dismissed, as soon as it arose, the concern about criminal uses of the atom by concluding: "I am one of those who think, with Nobel, that humanity will derive more good than harm from new discoveries" [3]. After the shocks of two world wars, was it still possible to express such trust in science and humanity?

Like Curie, 40 years before, Langevin strives to conclude his last papers on an optimistic note. In *La science et la paix*, he revives his hymn to life on a sad note.

> One of the reasons why I'm hoping for the end of wars is that this one has just spread across the whole world and can't go any further, because the earth is round. More than in the fear of the new danger of the atomic bomb, I have confidence, to ward off war, in the general sense of the development of life. (Langevin 1946f, p. 326)

He insists on the immensity of the universe, the slowness of evolution and the youth of the human species. But the evolution of life could hardly dispel the fear of a destruction of mankind, since Langevin acknowledges that the tendency towards mutual aid and solidarity translates, in the immediate, into the formation of enemy blocks and the extension of conflicts to a global scale. He acknowledges that war has long been a remarkable spur of scientific progress and that "the beneficial and harmful possibilities of using nuclear energy are intimately linked" (ibid., p. 324). He cannot help but add a note of regret:

What would not have been the human interest and the fertility of the results if, avoiding immense material destructions and the tragic disappearance of a tenth of the human species, we had shown ourselves wise enough to dedicate directly or exclusively to the works of peace the efforts made in the name of war to supply the feast of death of which only a few crumbs remain for the living! (Ibid., p. 324)

Langevin's reaction to the atomic bomb therefore follows an unexpected evolution: at first, he completely downplayed the human impact of the bombings and blindly advocated nuclear energy. Later in 1946, he tempered his optimism with more alarmist considerations about the dangers of the destruction of humanity and finally resumed his pathetic calls to the responsibility of men of science to face the "madness" that took hold of some political leaders (Langevin 1946a, p. 356, 1946g, p. 205). The Second World War did not diminish Langevin's fervent rationalism, but it seems, on the other hand, to have shaken his beautiful confidence in humans. Perhaps we should link the two and say that Langevin, foreseeing a dark future, found no other way out than the worship of reason? Like Albert Camus in the aftermath of Hiroshima, he would have therefore chosen "between hell and reason" (*Combat*, 8 August 1945).

References

1. Bensaude-Vincent B, Boudia S, Sato K (eds) (2022) Living in a nuclear world. From Fukushima to Hiroshima. Routledge, London
2. Bustamante M-C (in print) Jacques Solomon (1908-1942). Physicien, militant fusillé. Et sa valise de manuscrits dans la clandestinité. Brephols, Brussels
3. Curie P (1905) Radioactive substances, especially radium. Nobel Lecture. https://www.nobelprize.org/uploads/2018/06/pierre-curie-lecture.pdf
4. Fisher D (2004) Les étudiants et la Résistance. Matériaux pour l'histoire de notre temps 74:20–28
5. Langevin A (2022) Paul Langevin my father. EDP Sciences, Paris. English edition: Duck F
6. Mauriac F (2008) Jornal et Mémoires politiques (ed Barré J-L et al). Robert Laffont, Paris
7. Pinault M (1996) Frédéric Joliot, les Allemands et l'université aux premiers mois de l'Occupation. Vingtième Siècle Revue d'histoire 50:67–88
8. Pinault M (2000) Frédéric Joliot-Curie. Odile Jacob, Paris
9. Wallon H (1941) Letter published in "La résistance universitaire devant l'Occupation". Trygée 4, 15 October 1953:11–13
10. Wellerstein A (2021) Restricted data: the history of nuclear secrecy in the United States. The University of Chicago Press, Chicago

Chapter 20
Changing Society Through Educational Reforms

Abstract The government programme of the *Conseil national de la Résistance* (National Council of the Resistance), 15 March 1944, included a vast project to reform education that was entrusted to Langevin and Wallon. This was a huge task for an elderly man weakened by the war years. But this responsibility was the outcome of Langevin's longstanding efforts to change the educational system. Through a survey of his participation in the New Education Movement and contributions to French reform projects in the 1920s and 1930s, this chapter outlines the key ideas that inspired him: developing modern humanities, promoting general culture as a tool to weave the social fabric rather than vocational training and adopting science-based educational methods. Langevin considered such measures to be the only levers in their hands to build up social justice.

The government programme of the *Conseil national de la Résistance* (National Council of the Resistance), 15 March 1944, included a vast project to reform education. In France, the organization and funding of the education system are strictly ruled by the state and the basic principles of education are laid down in the French Constitution. On 8 November, René Capitant, Minister of National Education in the provisional government of the French Republic presided over by Charles de Gaulle, entrusted responsibility for the reform to Langevin and Wallon.[1]

This ambitious project, conceived in a spirit of reconstruction and in the fever of the Liberation, was co-chaired by two professors at the *Collège de France*, an elderly physicist in poor health and a child psychologist who was a bit younger. However, it was the crowning achievement of Langevin's parallel career as an expert in education. It is as an authority in matters of education that he is well known in France, if only because many schools in French towns and villages are named after him.

---

[1] Several other educational projects had been in competition before the end of the war: the project of the Communist Party by Cogniot (30 September 1943); a project by Henri Marrou published in the catholic journal *Esprit*; a project by Stéphane Piobetta, head of the Office of the Baccalaureate published in *Bulletin Officiel de l'Education Nationale* (BOEN) (16 November 1944).

Throughout his life, since his early critical remarks of science teaching in secondary education in 1904, Langevin never ceased working on the reform of educational system, in both international and national commissions. And he was so involved in this milieu that he chaired the *Société française de pédagogie* from 1935 to 1945. His plans for the reorganization of the school system offer the best window on Langevin's worldview for two reasons. First, it is a niche where he could combine thinking and acting (*la pensée et l'action*) a major concern of his. Second, Langevin's educational plans reveal the main lines and nuances of his most intimate political convictions. Unlike the French Communist Party, Langevin never wished to bring about a proletarian revolution in France. Instead, he wanted to rebuild society through the education of its citizens. To remedy injustice and reduce violence, it is necessary to address young people. In order to prevent future conflicts, one has to weave the social fabric. For Langevin, the ultimate goal of education is:

> to enable each being to become part of the great collective that is our species, by receiving the benefits of the efforts and sufferings of previous generations, and by striving, through his or her own work, to enrich these benefits and pass them on to future generations. [4, p. 16]

Inserting everyone into the human cultural heritage is the means towards Langevin's goal: creating a sense of international and intergenerational solidarity. But, what practical measures did he recommend to others in order to achieve this ambitious goal?

This ambition focused Langevin's effort on the primary and secondary educational systems, although he had been also involved in *Les Compagnons de l'université nouvelle*, an association created in 1919 that purposed to reform the French university system. Among its founding members were Edmond Bauer, Langevin's assistant, and Henri Laugier, a physiologist who recruited the psychologist Henri Piéron and Langevin. Most of these "compagnons" were friends from the ENS and l'Arcouest and shared the same ideals of justice and promotion of science. Langevin succeeded Henri Laugier as President of the association but he was not deeply committed in it. The association went bankrupt in 1933 [5].

20.1 Knowledge-Based Methods of Teaching

In the aftermath of World War One, Langevin was not alone in trying to build a fair society through education. He was part of an international movement created by Beatrice Ensor, a theosophical educator, in "a cry of revolt against the war": the International League for New Education (ILNE). The League aimed to promote a "New Era", through the development of new methods of teaching with the purpose of educating the future "citizens of the world". Preventing the periodic return of the horrors of war, this was the objective of its international action, for which it organized large congresses that brought together educators and reformers from all countries. Langevin joined the French section (GFEN) of the International League of New Education in 1921 (Fig. 20.1). By 1932, he had become president of the

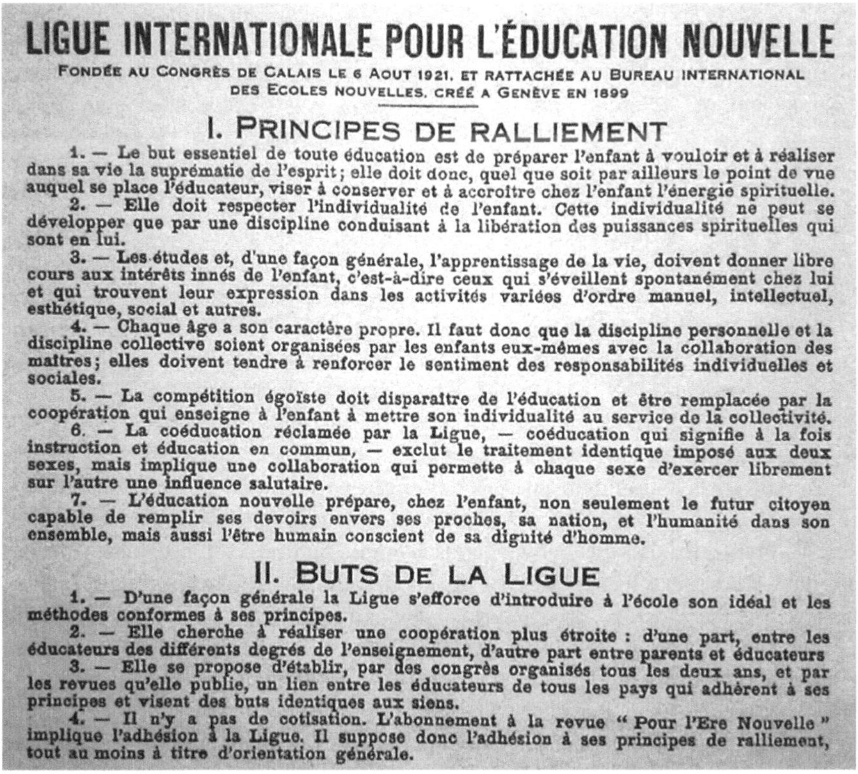

LIGUE INTERNATIONALE POUR L'ÉDUCATION NOUVELLE
FONDÉE AU CONGRÈS DE CALAIS LE 6 AOUT 1921, ET RATTACHÉE AU BUREAU INTERNATIONAL DES ECOLES NOUVELLES, CRÉÉ A GENÈVE EN 1899

I. PRINCIPES DE RALLIEMENT

1. — Le but essentiel de toute éducation est de préparer l'enfant à vouloir et à réaliser dans sa vie la suprématie de l'esprit; elle doit donc, quel que soit par ailleurs le point de vue auquel se place l'éducateur, viser à conserver et à accroître chez l'enfant l'énergie spirituelle.

2. — Elle doit respecter l'individualité de l'enfant. Cette individualité ne peut se développer que par une discipline conduisant à la libération des puissances spirituelles qui sont en lui.

3. — Les études et, d'une façon générale, l'apprentissage de la vie, doivent donner libre cours aux intérêts innés de l'enfant, c'est-à-dire ceux qui s'éveillent spontanément chez lui et qui trouvent leur expression dans les activités variées d'ordre manuel, intellectuel, esthétique, social et autres.

4. — Chaque âge a son caractère propre. Il faut donc que la discipline personnelle et la discipline collective soient organisées par les enfants eux-mêmes avec la collaboration des maîtres; elles doivent tendre à renforcer le sentiment des responsabilités individuelles et sociales.

5. — La compétition égoïste doit disparaître de l'éducation et être remplacée par la coopération qui enseigne à l'enfant à mettre son individualité au service de la collectivité.

6. — La coéducation réclamée par la Ligue, — coéducation qui signifie à la fois instruction et éducation en commun, — exclut le traitement identique imposé aux deux sexes, mais implique une collaboration qui permette à chaque sexe d'exercer librement sur l'autre une influence salutaire.

7. — L'éducation nouvelle prépare, chez l'enfant, non seulement le futur citoyen capable de remplir ses devoirs envers ses proches, sa nation, et l'humanité dans son ensemble, mais aussi l'être humain conscient de sa dignité d'homme.

II. BUTS DE LA LIGUE

1. — D'une façon générale la Ligue s'efforce d'introduire à l'école son idéal et les méthodes conformes à ses principes.

2. — Elle cherche à réaliser une coopération plus étroite : d'une part, entre les éducateurs des différents degrés de l'enseignement, d'autre part entre parents et éducateurs

3. — Elle se propose d'établir, par des congrès organisés tous les deux ans, et par les revues qu'elle publie, un lien entre les éducateurs de tous les pays qui adhèrent à ses principes et visent des buts identiques aux siens.

4. — Il n'y a pas de cotisation. L'abonnement à la revue " Pour l'Ère Nouvelle " implique l'adhésion à la Ligue. Il suppose donc l'adhésion à ses principes de ralliement, tout au moins à titre d'orientation générale.

Fig. 20.1 Principles and rules of the International League for New Education. (B. Bensaude-Vincent)

International League, and chaired the International Congress held in Nice. The theme was "Education in its relationships with social evolution". During just a few days, educators from 57 nations discussed how to lay the foundations of a kind of spiritual League of Nations (Langevin 1932a). Five years later, in 1937, the Cheltenham Congress tried very hard to maintain the ideal of pacification through education at a time of intensified nationalist tensions. The last congress that Langevin attended was the European Congress of August 1946, on "The Reform of Education in Different Countries and Its Relationships with New Education".

In addition to the reconciliation between nations, the League aimed to prevent the increasing mechanization of life that was encouraged by schools aimed at disciplining students. They accordingly promoted alternative teaching methods more concerned with encouraging individual development [6]. Langevin was interested in the new methods of teaching promoted by Rudolf Steiner, Maria Montessori, Ovide Decroly, Célestin Freinet and Maurice Martenot, which stimulate a child's personal initiative. He adopted as a guideline for the reform plan, a principle that had been implemented by Freinet, the opening of the school to the community. He also retained from Decroly the need to balance the intellectual with the emotional. However, Langevin did not subscribe to any particular school of pedagogy, nor did he advocate their formulae. Instead, he retained a holistic spirit, which he quickly integrated into his own reflections on education.

He insisted that school methods must be rooted in a deep understanding of the development of children's capacities. Accordingly, he encouraged educational research and its anchoring in child psychology (Langevin 1932a). He promoted the science of education as early as 1926 when, appointed president of a commission in charge of reorganizing the *Musée pédagogique*, he proposed the creation of an *Institut national de la recherche pédagogique* (National Institute of Pedagogical Research) and a National Centre for Pedagogical Documentation. In this respect, he followed the suggestions of the French physician and psychologist, Ignace Meyerson, nephew of the philosopher Emile Meyerson (Archives, L059/021). He also fully adopted the views of Wallon who had completed his doctoral thesis on *L'enfant turbulent* ('The Troublesome Child') in 1925 and joined the GFEN in the late 1920s [7]. Wallon clearly stated that "to respect children, we must first get to know them, we must have studied them, we must every day gather the information that, in all areas and circumstances of life, can be provided by the behaviour of children" [12] (Fig. 20.2). It does not mean that education is a science-based practice: Wallon added that this knowledge is acquired by parents, physicians, teachers and day-carers rather than by experts in child psychology who rely on rigid categories, such as the division between normal and pathologic.

Langevin adopted the postulate of a strict parallelism between the evolution of the species and the individual development of the child, often invoked by child psychologists, such as Jean Piaget and Wallon. He suggested adapting science teaching to the three stages that he identified both in child development and in the historical evolution of science: experiential observation and experimentation for children from 6 to 12 years old; acquisition of laws and causal series between 12 and 15 years old; finally, initiation to abstract syntheses after 15 years old (Langevin 1931b).

Before describing the measures recommended by the "Plan Langevin-Wallon"—which was presented to parliament in 1947, just after Langevin's death—we should first consider the projects of the inter-war period that shaped his vision of education.

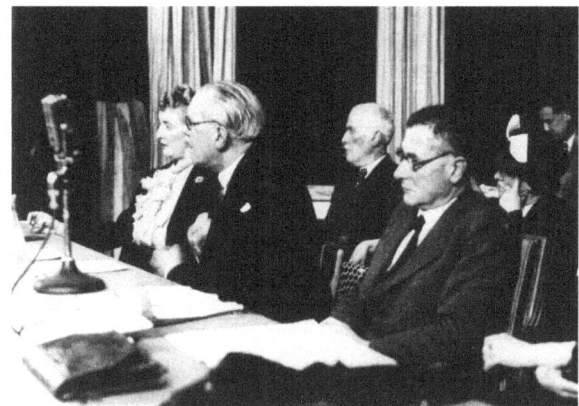

Fig. 20.2 Wallon and Langevin at *la Mutualité* in 1938. Henri Wallon (1879–1962), Professor of Psychology at the *Collège de France* collaborated with Langevin in the *Cercle de la Russie neuve* in the 1930s and was the co-president on Commission for the Reform of Education. (ESPCI)

20.2 L'école unique

The theme of the *L'école unique* did not imply a state monopoly in education. It referred to a simplification and democratization of the educational system with one single curriculum for all children under 15–16. In 1924, this project was an electoral platform and in 1925, the then Prime Minister Edouard Herriot charged de Monzie, Minister of Instruction, to prepare a reform project for submission, without delay, to the Parliament. De Monzie then convened a ministerial commission, subdivided into three sub-commissions corresponding to the objectives set by the minister: control of the private sector, secondary education and tertiary education. Langevin presided over this third sub-commission, which concerned students aged 15–18, and normal schools for teacher training, together with the philosopher Xavier Léon, a founder of the *Revue de métaphysique et de morale* and of the French Society of Philosophy. A Committee for the *école unique* was set up in 1927, which served as a liaison between several partners, Human Rights League, French League of Education, National Union of Teachers, Fraternal Groups of Education to which was added in 1928, as soon as it was created, the General Federation of Education (a trade union). This committee developed a "project for a statute to institute the école unique", which included free education and materials, allowances for students in upper secondary education and tertiary education, with a selection at the entrance of the latter.

The minutes of the meetings show that Langevin's ideas guided the work of the reformers (Archives L059). He advocated the creation of a general core of culture, which was common to all sections. He criticized premature specialization for vocational purposes, on the basis that it feeds ideas of caste or class. Langevin addressed the question: "What should be the general culture common to all tertiary education, i.e. in post high-school curricula?". This was a challenge because the third level is specifically that of specialization. But Langevin asserted that it is possible and desirable to form a culture common to all sections, even in the technological ones, "to avoid the creation of a class or caste spirit; it must also prepare to act in practice".

A confrontation erupted in the Commission over the content of this general core of culture: the supporters of ancient languages and classical humanities opposed Langevin who believed that "the common elements of this culture are manual labour and the arts, experimental and theoretical sciences, the history of ideas and facts, languages, literature, and philosophy". Langevin caused even more indignation by arguing that the same teaching method should be used everywhere.

The text of the resolutions adopted by the sub-commission shows that Langevin ended up imposing his views, in terms of both objectives and methods (Archives, L056): it begins with a critique of premature specialization, followed by Langevin's definition of culture:

> This general culture must represent everything that, independently of vocation, prepares the child for life, that is to say, in contact with things and with men, and allows him to act on things in agreement with men and in accordance with the laws that govern both. (Archives, L056/20)

At the outset, the text specified that history should play a prominent role in general culture. It also proposed the homogenization of male and female teaching

(Archives, L056) and the institution of a competition at the entrance into tertiary education with a system of annual examinations (Archives, L059). While he accepted the principle of selection, Langevin was concerned about the fate of those who would be rejected. He therefore drafted a "bill for mandatory obligatory post-school education" (Archives, L057/027). This should be a secular, free, mandatory course for all teenagers under 18 who had been excluded from the school system. The rationale for its establishment included: "To train the future citizen and the future worker", to avoid wasting intellectual forces, to establish "a bridge between primary school and the barracks" and to "prevent delinquency and maintain the quality of French craftsmanship".

This heterogeneous mix of intentions partly accounts for the unhappy outcome of the reform of the *L'école unique*. It lacked coherence and dispensed measures "in dribs and drabs" such as the creation of a common core in higher primary schools, lower secondary education (French *collèges*) and in high schools.

Such measures stirred up a storm of criticism. Right-wing deputies denounced egalitarianism, monopoly, amalgamation and inefficiency. Left-wing ones argued that free education accentuated selection and social discrimination. The battle dragged on and the reform got bogged down with the end of the *Cartel des gauches*. In 1931, Langevin responded point by point to the objections against the *école unique,* published in a brochure (Archives, L066/016). The project was revived under de Monzie's ministry who extended free education to the secondary level.[2]

However, the ideal of *L'école unique* was never fully implemented. There was no standard timetable and no homogeneity of the contents of sciences in secondary education. Over the years, the project of *l'Ecole unique* revealed its many pitfalls. In particular, the two principles of free education and common teaching to all sections dramatically posed the problem of selection. It was gradually discovered that less than half of the students would be capable of following the ideal training curriculum. Hence there was a need to think differently about a school for all and to invent an alternative to the process of selection.

20.3 Modern Humanities

Another aspect of Langevin's plans for reforming the educational system was the promotion of "modern humanities" to rival the classical humanities, as it was based on the ancient languages Latin and Greek. It consisted of a broader introduction of science, "conceived in its spirit more than in its results" with a broad historical approach (Langevin 1931b, 1932a). For Langevin, it is an essential reform, a question of civilization. Without a satisfactory teaching of modern humanities, the gap

---

[2] Under the *Front Populaire*, Jean Zay, Minister of National Education, passed a number of laws: mandatory school attendance until 14 years (9 August 1936); then a mandatory certificate of primary studies for all; the introduction of classical, modern and technical options from the fifth grade (2 May 1937). Finally, Zay abolished specialized secondary education (3 March 1938).

between science and civilization will continue to grow. To reduce this gap, Langevin suggested that the sciences themselves provide the cement to create the unity of culture (Langevin 1932a, p. 245). However, he did not plan to substitute a new science-based elite for the old one, based on Latin and Greek. He sought to prevent the drama, later named as "the two cultures" by Charles P Snow, by preventing the divide between an increasingly uncultured body of scientists and technicians and a classical elite, ignorant of science and clinging to values of the past. The history of science must, to this end, play an important educational role provided it is connected to general history (Langevin 1926c, 1931b). "We thus return to the necessity of preserving a historic way of teaching: it is necessary to mark the sense of change and teach respect for the past; for it is the past that prepares and guarantees the future" (Langevin 1931b). Langevin suggested delivering the historical teaching of sciences in connection with the teaching of philosophy. In addition, to amplify the educational scope of history, he recommended to use the original memoirs of past scientists, the "sources" of scientific theories, in order to study them before their ossification into a dogmatic system (Langevin 1926c); and to further develop the cultural potential of science, contained in history, he proposed an interdisciplinary course.

It was therefore not a question of sacrificing all other knowledge at the altar of science, but of integrating sciences into general culture. Providing all children with general culture is the central goal of education. For Langevin culture is not an ornament, allowing some beautiful minds to shine among others. It is "an initiation into the various forms of human activity", that forms the cement of society: "We can say that general culture represents what brings people together and unites them, whereas the profession all too often represents what separates them" (Langevin 1932a, p. 232). Langevin insisted that culture is socializing because it weaves a social fabric and it is dynamic, because it drives changes both in the individuals and in the community. Above all, Langevin sought to avoid the compartmentalization of society into socio-professional categories because he viewed this to be a source of conformism and selfishness (Langevin 1934a, p. xv). He tried to promote a general culture, through a dialogue between natural and human sciences, outside vocational practices. These proposals did not remain pious wishes. Langevin did his best to implement them in his ultimate institutional project.

20.4 The Langevin-Wallon Plan

The reconstruction of the education system was considered to be a priority, as many people attributed France's collapse in 1940 to the failure of its elite class, who were seen as notoriously lacking in courage [8]. Both Langevin and Wallon assumed that the Third Republic School carried a heavy responsibility for the recent development of fascism:

> This cancer of fascism, which we observe to be endemic at every moment of our daily life, and particularly so in difficult periods such as those we are still going through, could only develop on our humanity by finding the necessary elements of conformism and selfishness. (Langevin 1946j, p. 37)

The dogmatic, passive, both uniform and competitive methods of teaching "create the bed of selfishness and conformism". Conversely, a new education, with active individual and collective methods, would promote the development of personality and solidarity.

Langevin was appointed to take charge of the project of reform in March 1944. He immediately set up a commission of about 20 members, representing various levels of education as well as scholars "renowned for their scientific work or their corporate activity as specialists in educational issues". To secure the political independence of the Commission, the members were recruited for their responsibilities and their competencies; no nominations were accepted from any party or delegation or to represent any mandate.

The task entrusted to the Commission was: reorganizing the entire structure of education from kindergarten to university, establishing teacher training and also planning the transition between the old and the new systems. This immense task would finally be accomplished two and a half years later, on 17 June 1947, when a reform plan, divided into eight sections was handed to the government [10, 11].[3]

Despite his age and illness, Langevin beat the drum with the rhythm of weekly meetings, every Thursday, in his apartment at EPCI, rue Vauquelin (Fig. 20.3). First of all, on 29 November 1944, he identified the broad outlines of the project, prior to creating subcommittees to work on detailed institutional measures. These outlines were clearly expressed at the end of the tenth session of the commission in March 1945. "The aim is to achieve equality for all children in education and to allow each one to occupy in society the place that corresponds to their own value". A financial effort would ensure free education, allowances, construction and revaluation of the teaching function (BOEN 4 January 1945, 13, 776–778).

On 15 February, the Commission decided to form four subcommittees: (1) general organization, led by Langevin; (2) methods and programs; orientation and selection, led by Piéron; (3) teacher training, led by Wallon; (4) general education led by Lucien Febvre.

The elitism of this organization is worthy of comment. All four chairs of the subcommittees were professors at the *Collège de France*. Two additional subcommittees were created at the ministry which included inspectors, deans, directors and administrators, in order to "fine-tune execution measures involving a start of implementation of the Commission's proposals". However, as important as these

---

[3] The eight sections were: (1) theoretical introduction; (2) structures and organization of education; (3) teacher training; (4) control and improvement bodies; (5) programmes, schedules, methods and sanction of studies; (6) moral and civic education, formation of the man and the citizen; (7) popular education; (8) implementation deadlines; with an appendix: project of organization of education in rural areas.

20.4 The Langevin-Wallon Plan

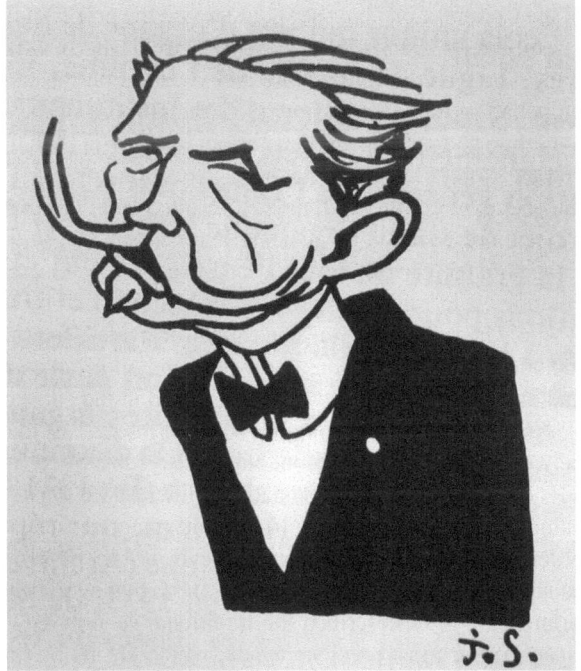

Fig. 20.3 Langevin by Jean Sennep, a famous cartoonist and virulent anti-communist (*Science et Vigilance*)

roles were, the lower categories of teaching staff were strictly subordinated to the guidelines decided by the senior professors of four sub-committees.

It is also worth noticing that humanities had priority over natural sciences, with two psychologists and one historian among the four directors of subcommittees. However, Langevin's emphasis on general culture prevailed in all subcommittees. Culture prevailed over vocation in the subcommittee on general education chaired by Febvre:

> The disciplines included in the framework of General Education (artistic and craft teaching, manual work, physical education and sports, etc.) are intended, outside of any professional training (…) to make closer contact with life, to develop the faculties of expression and action, as well as the qualities of character through the practice of collective actions (Bulletin officiel de l'education nationale, 15 March 1945)

The subcommittee chaired by Piéron also retained Langevin's priorities:

> It is important that a balance is everywhere maintained between general culture and the preparation for a vocation. … The teaching of sciences, essential to most vocational training, should, by constant reference to the history of ideas and the figures of this history, lose its purely utilitarian character, take on a living aspect and be integrated into the general culture. (Ibid.)

After highlighting Langevin's influence on the work of reform, we must also recognize the influence of his collaborators on Langevin. The elderly president was concerned with the expression of the collective opinion of the Commission. In September 1946, Langevin wrote from Geneva to Fernande Seclet-Riou, rapporteur of the Commission, that she should revise the proofs of his last presentation because, "I am not very sure I have described well what *we* think" (Archives, L057/025). Langevin agreed to put culture and vocation on the same level, when he declared, on behalf of the Commission, that "the purpose of the school is twofold: initiation to culture and vocational preparation, to allow in each one the formation of the man and the worker he should become". Vocational training was no longer perceived as the enemy of culture, as long as it resulted from orientation and not from selection. The culture-vocation rebalancing is reflected even in the subcommittee headed by Langevin: the general organization of secondary education provides for a first "orientation cycle", up to 15 years old, duly supervised by child psychology specialists. It would be followed by a "determination cycle", for 15–18 years old, which would include vocational sections and would end with "an examination on general culture and on the vocational knowledge acquired in the chosen group of disciplines".

Not only did Langevin revise some of his dearest ideas, notably on the priorities between culture and vocation, but he also subscribed fully to the orientation policy advocated by Wallon. In the national interest we must "seek the solution that most values the riches, all the spiritual and material riches that France possesses", in order to recover from the war (Langevin 1944b, p. 30). Thus, Langevin married his usual humanist language with a new more managerial style. His last speeches in the summer of 1946 described the traditional school, let's say the class school, as "a waste of our most precious assets, which are human riches" and the reform as a "better management" (Langevin 1946j, p. 37). All in all, Langevin's views significantly changed during these last two years of intensive work on the reform of education. He traded the generous humanistic style of the republican *Dreyfusard* for a more realistic, managerial style. He gradually adopted more political views. A little further and, in his reports, "man" would almost have disappeared behind the "worker" and the "citizen". And it is said that, shortly before his death, Langevin planned to write a book on science and society. Nevertheless, Langevin's last speech, in September 1946, suggests that he was more sceptical than Wallon, who promised to erase professional inequalities and the contempt of manual work by eliminating selection in favour of the orientation of the pupils according to their abilities. Langevin simply considered such measures to be the only lever in their hands, the only way out left to them: either they would make "the necessary effort for the incessant emergence of a new world" or the human species would end tragically (ibid. 39).

20.5 A Dormant Reform?

Despite the synergies between the leaders of the project, there were tensions within the members of the Commission. Fernande Seclet-Riou, the closest collaborator of Langevin in this project, remembered many turbulent sessions of conflicts about Greek and Latin, about the integration of technology into secondary and higher education. But she immediately added that during the 52 plenary sessions presided

20.5 A Dormant Reform?

over by Langevin, his courteous but firm intervention always led to an agreement on the basis of mutual concessions [9, p. 17]. It seems, indeed, that Langevin always imposed himself as a moderator and managed to maintain a consensus within the Commission.

Whatever the inner tensions, the commission's work progressed at a steady pace. Most measures of the reform were already worked out when Langevin ceased his activity, shortly before he passed away in December 1946. And his death barely delayed the project. As early as February 1947, the Commission resumed its regular meetings, under Wallon's presidency. This second phase was much more arid since it involved elaborating the official report, point by point. But nothing slowed it down.

In June 1947, the Langevin-Wallon plan was handed over to the government (Fig. 20.4). It was promptly forgotten, even though officially the reform of education had been considered a top priority in 1944. The work of the Commission was ignored, buried in the filing cabinets of the Ministry of Education [8]. What caused such a failure?

One major cause was the economic situation; the government did not have the means to fulfil its ambitions in the field of education. Rampant inflation led to the reintroduction of rationing in 1947. Rebuilding industry was the priority. The Ministry of Finance rejected all measures that would entail more personnel and most of the budget of the Ministry of National Education was allocated to rebuild schools that had been destroyed in the war.

Even so, economic pressures were insufficient to justify the rejection of some of the measures recommended in the Langevin-Wallon plan, including the common core and a new curriculum for teacher training. The commission encountered resistance from teachers and, above all, it did not benefit from strong political support from the government. The minutes of the meetings of the Commission show that Capitant, who originally instigated the reform project, never attended its meetings, nor did his successors from the Ministry of Education. The Radical-Socialist coalition tried to obstruct the last decisions of the reform plan, complaining about the Communist Party's takeover of the Commission. The socialist group of the Assembly even insinuated that Langevin served the PCF while the orthodoxy of the PCF considered that educational reforms were useless as long as the capitalist system prevailed.

For the French communists, educational reform would never bring about social change; only revolution could build democratic education, with schools at the service of national production, according to the Marxist ideal. Only Cogniot, who was a member of the Commission and also a communist deputy, supported the reform.[4] In August 1947, he presented a bill before the Assembly that held the government accountable for taking up the report of the Commission. To no avail. The communists had lost influence and were increasingly isolated after Prime Minister Paul Ramadier eliminated the communist ministers from his government.

---

[4] It does not mean that Cogniot remained faithful to Langevin's credo in the power of education to change society. On February 1949 he gave a talk *La pédagogie, même nouvelle, est fonction de la société* ("Even New Pedagogy is a Function of Society"), Paris, FEN-CGT, 19.

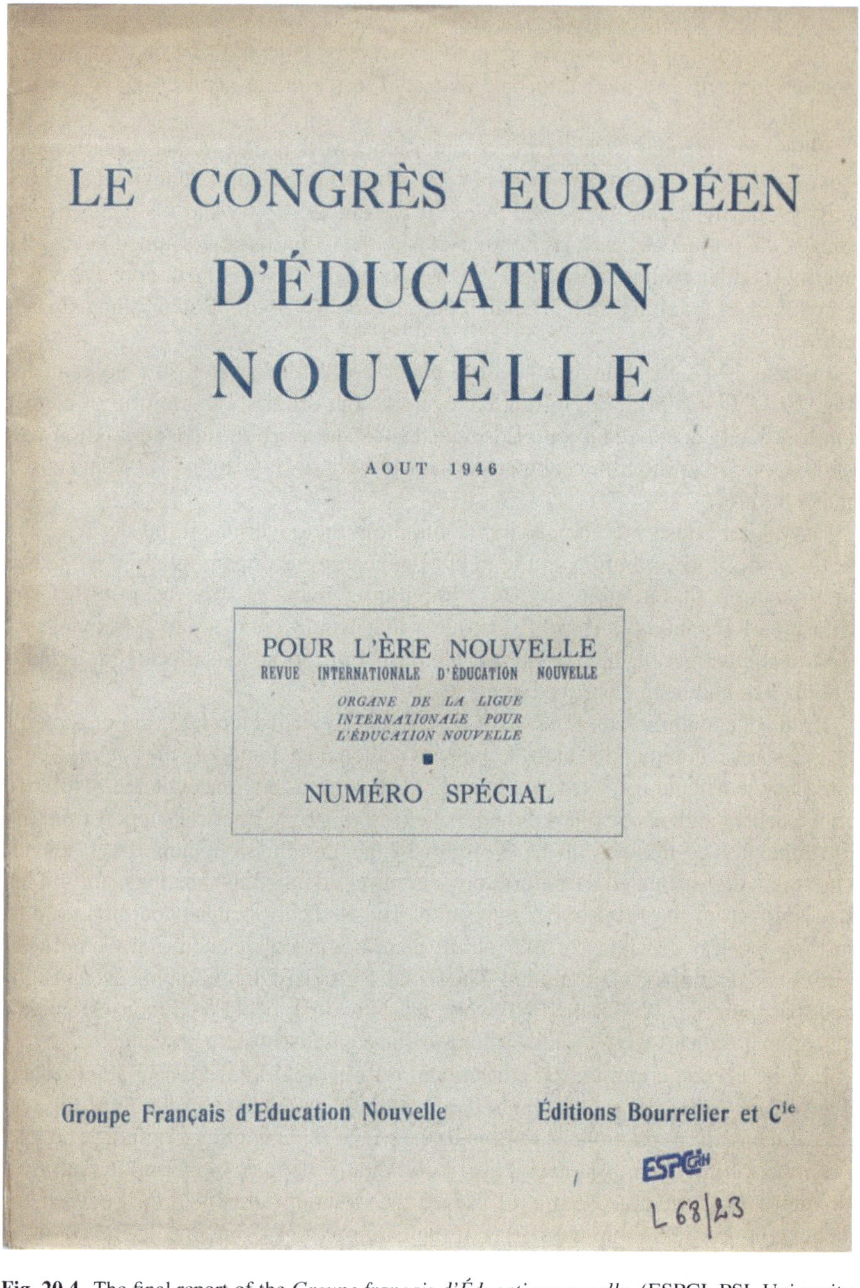

LE CONGRÈS EUROPÉEN
D'ÉDUCATION
NOUVELLE

AOUT 1946

POUR L'ÈRE NOUVELLE
REVUE INTERNATIONALE D'ÉDUCATION NOUVELLE
ORGANE DE LA LIGUE INTERNATIONALE POUR L'ÉDUCATION NOUVELLE
■
NUMÉRO SPÉCIAL

Groupe Français d'Education Nouvelle Éditions Bourrelier et Cie

Fig. 20.4 The final report of the *Groupe français d'Éducation nouvelle*. (ESPCI, PSL University L068/023)

Victim of the economic and political situation at the time of its release, the project of reconstructing the educational system, meant to design the landscape of the new world, has been set aside, archived without even being read. The contrast is striking between the immobility of the file relegated to the archives and the zeal, the speed, of its creation. And yet, the Langevin-Wallon plan is still present in the memory of French educators, especially in trade unions such as the Federation of National Education where it has long served as a reference for democratizing the educational system [2, 3]. It provided the guidelines for future educational reforms. A number of measures put forward at the Liberation have ended up being implemented with political changes of direction. Thus Langevin's convictions and ideals forged in the context of the Third Republic continue to influence educational policy today.

References

1. Bensaude-Vincent B (2010) La place des réflexions sur l'école dans l'oeuvre de Paul Langevin. In: Gutierrez L, Kounelis C (eds) Paul Langevin et la réforme de l'enseignement. Presses universitaires de Grenoble, Paris, pp 15–22
2. Bernardin J (2012) Du Plan Langevin-Wallon à aujourd'hui. Dialogue 144:3–5
3. Boutan P (2017) Le plan Langevin-Wallon. Une ambition pour l'école. Carnets Rouges. https://carnetsrouges.fr/le-plan-langevin-wallon-une-ambition-pour-lecole/
4. Farenc J (1946) Compte-rendu du stage et des journées d'information sur les sixièmes nouvelles. édition L'Education nationale, Paris
5. Garnier B (2010) Paul Langevin et les Compagnons de l'Université Nouvelle. In: Gutierrez L, Kounelis C (eds) Paul Langevin et la réforme de l'enseignement. Presses universitaires de Grenoble, Paris, pp 37–55
6. Gutierrez L (2010) Paul Langevin: le don d'ubiquité. In: Gutierrez L, Kounelis C (eds) Paul Langevin et la réforme de l'enseignement. Presses universitaires de Grenoble, Paris, pp 23–35
7. Gutierrez L, Ohayon A (2010) Henri Wallon, le deuxième homme. In: Gutierrez L, Kounelis C (eds) Paul Langevin et la réforme de l'enseignement. Presses universitaires de Grenoble, Paris, pp 71–86
8. Prost A (2010) Une réforme morte-née: le plan Langevin-Wallon. In: Gutierrez L, Kounelis C (eds) Paul Langevin et la réforme de l'enseignement. Presses universitaires de Grenoble, Paris, pp 55–68
9. Seclet-Riou F (1947) La Commission Langevin. Bref historique des travaux. L'École laïque 1:16–18
10. Sorel E (1997) Une ambition pour l'école. Le Plan Langevin-Wallon (1943–1947). Éditions sociales, Paris
11. Sorel E, Boutan P (eds) (1998) Le plan Langevin-Wallon: une utopie vivante. Actes des rencontres des 6–7 juin 1997. PUF, Paris
12. Wallon H (1927) Allocution d'ouverture. L'Education nouvelle 56:84–85

Chapter 21
Postscript

Abstract The crowd attending the funerals of Langevin suggests that he has achieved the feat of embodying three values that formed the pillars of the French Republic: Science, Education and the People. This postscript highlights the contrasts that make Langevin in the image of his time: sensitive to the dangers of modernity, to the fragility of civilizations but deeply attached to the humanist tradition.

On the morning of 19 December 1946, Langevin passed away, exhausted by too much activity, he who carried a wicker trunk of accumulated "remorse" (André Langevin 2022, p. 203). This son of a worker who became a scholar departs, to be celebrated as a hero of the fatherland with a national funeral at the *Collège de France*, a tricolour flag, with sheaves and wreaths, speeches and the "Marseillaise". In the chilly greyness of a December morning, an immense crowd assembled for a final farewell (Fig. 21.1):

> We saw all the people of Paris file past his coffin, united in brotherhood before his coffin, workers from the suburbs and intellectuals, representatives of the provinces, towns and countryside, Breton sailors followed by miners from the North in working clothes. What could be more moving than to read in the register of signatures deposited at the *Collège de France*, among so many testimonies, the names of the ambassadors of the most diverse foreign powers, next to those of modest artisans of the 5th arrondissement! The workers of the Renault factories signed next to the members of the Academy of Sciences …. (Jacques Nicolle quoted by André Langevin ([1], p. 205))

Around his coffin, inequalities and distinctions were abolished, social classes merged in a single surge of sympathy (Fig. 21.2). By his death, Langevin gave a living image of solidarity.

The procession behind the coffin embodied for a few hours the ideal of society that he has always advocated. In a way, Langevin recomposed the social fabric at the mid-point of a century that had been torn apart by conflicts and wars. "Without

Fig. 21.1 Funeral in front of the *Collège de France*, 21 December 1946 (*Science et Vigilance*)

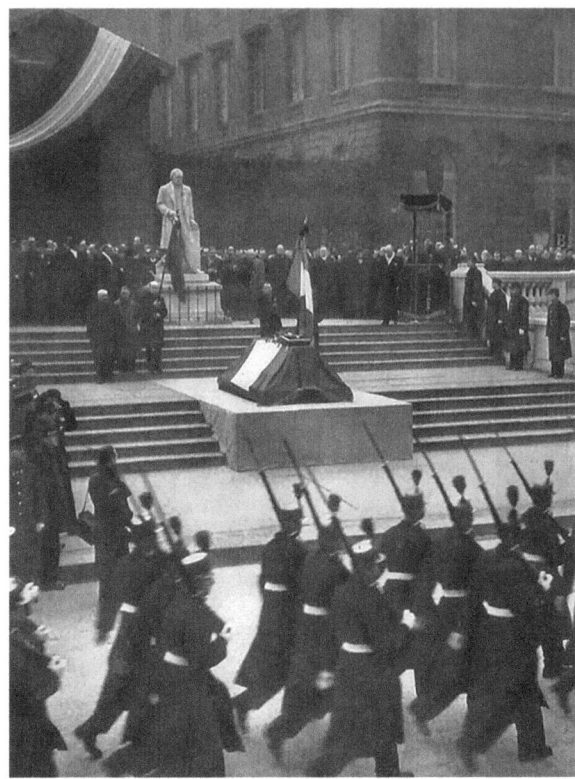

Fig. 21.2 The parade of leftist organizations at Langevin's funeral. (ESPCI)

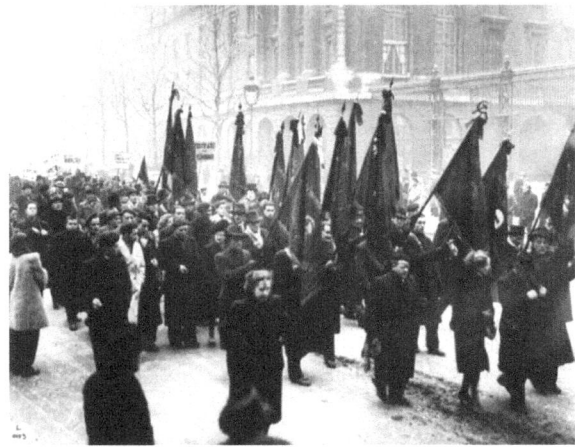

doubt, never has the death of a scholar aroused such widespread popular emotion", wrote E. Kahane a few days later. "In the glorious career of Paul Langevin, each citizen can see a vision of the future we dream of, where society will allow everyone to develop their own faculties (…) It is the role of heroes to provide these stimulating images" (*L'enseignement public*, 15 January 1947).

An exemplary life: Langevin has achieved the feat of embodying three values that formed the pillars of the French Republic: Science, Education and the People.

On 17 November 1948 Langevin's and Perrin's remains were transferred to the Pantheon in a solemn ceremony (Fig. 21.3). Their coffins were placed next to Marcellin Berthelot and Paul Painlevé inside the crypt. Interestingly the speeches and press articles focused exclusively on the scientific achievements of these two French heroes. The miracle alliance of three republican values embodied by Langevin was so fragile and fleeting that it was no longer meaningful in 1948. Today, he is remembered as a scientist more than an activist.

Still, how could we claim that Langevin wasted his talents as an activist? Of course, he never had the aura of a Nobel Prize. But he made discreet and lasting contributions to theoretical, experimental and even applied physics. Through his repeated attacks on the dominance of classical mechanics over physics, through his teaching and influence over an entire generation, Langevin encouraged the rise of a new school of French physics: he not only directed Louis de Broglie in his early days but also guided the career of Frédéric Joliot-Curie; he particularly encouraged theoretical and fundamental research.

Although he shook up traditions and encouraged renewal in physics, Langevin never adopted the professional style of modern scientists. He remained at the limit, closer to the image of the nineteenth-century *savant*, forged in the *Éloges académiques*. A scholar adorned with the noblest virtues, probity, devotion, generosity and selflessness. Langevin nevertheless instantiates a notable variation on this romantic image. To the figure of the genius who devotes himself to the search for truth as to a priesthood, who keeps his eyes fixed on the world of science, without a glance at the troubles of the century, republican mythology has substituted the image of a scholar immersed in the century, in the street, in the forum.

Scholar and worker. Physicist and thinker. Popular and worldly. Lucid and passionate. Incorrigibly scattered, but dreaming of impossible syntheses. Passionate about history and the past, but impatient for new things. Notable and rebellious. Figure of order and progress. So many contrasts that make the man in the image of his time: sensitive to the dangers of modernity, to the fragility of civilizations but deeply attached to the humanist tradition.

Fig. 21.3 In November 1948 Langevin's and Perrin's ashes were solemnly transferred to the Panthéon. (ESPCI)

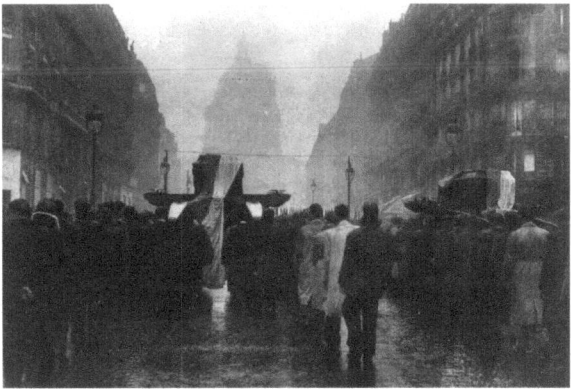

References

1. Langevin A (2022) Paul Langevin, my father. EDP Sciences, Paris. English edition: Duck F

Bibliography

Abbreviations Used in the References

ArchivesLangevin's Archives located in Centre de ressources historiques de l'École supérieure de physique et de chimie industrielles (ESPCI), 10, rue Vauquelin, 75231 Paris, Cedex 05. https://bibnum.explore.psl.eu/s/psl/item-set/249135
BSFP   *Bulletin des séances de la Société française de physique.*
BSIE   *Bulletin des séances de la Société internationale des électriciens.*
CMGF   Comité mondial contre la guerre et le fascisme.
CRAS   *Comptes rendus de l'Académie des sciences.*
CVIA   Comité de vigilance des intellectuels antifascistes.
JP *Journal de Physique théorique et appliquée*; from 1920: *Journal de Physique et Le Radium.*
OS   *Œuvres scientifiques de Paul Langevin*, Paris, CRNS, 1950.
PA*La Pensée et l'action*, textes recueillis et présentés par Paul Labérenne, Paris, Éd. sociales, 1964.
PPE   Bensaude-Vincent, Bernadette ed. *Propos d'un physicien engagé Paul Langevin*. Paris, Vuibert, 2007.
PVA   *La Physique depuis vingt ans*, Paris, Doin, 1923.
PVSFP   Procès-verbaux des communications à la Société française de physique.

Paul Langevin's Publications

1900a: "Sur l'ionisation des gaz", *BSFP*, 3, 39.
1900b: "Les ions dans les gaz", *BSIE*, 17, 203.

1902a: "Recherches sur les gaz ionisés", *CRAS*, 134, 414–417; *OS*, 3–5.
1902b: "Sur la recombinaison des ions dans les gaz", *CRAS*, 134, 533–536; *OS*, 6–8.
1902c: "Sur la mobilité des ions dans les gaz", *CRAS*, 134, 646–649; *OS*, 9–12.
1902d: *Recherches sur les gaz ionisés*, State doctoral thesis, *OS*, 13–150.

1903: "Sur la loi de recombinaison des ions" *CRAS*, 137, 177–179; *OS*, 151–153.

1904a: "L'esprit de l'enseignement scientifique", Conférence at Musée pédagogique 18 February, in *L'enseignement des mathématiques et des sciences physiques*, Paris, Imprimerie nationale, 1904, 73–105; quoted from *PPE* 11–31.

1904b: "La physique des électrons", Rapport au Congrès international des sciences et des arts, Saint-Louis, 22 February 1904; in *Revue générale des sciences*, 1905; quoted from *PPE* 32–60.

1904c: "Sur la conductibilité des gaz issus d'une flame" (with Bloch E.), *CRAS*, 139, 792–794.

1904d: "Sur les ions de l'atmosphère", *BSFP*, 4, 67; *CRAS*, 1905, 140, 232–234; *OS*, 239–241.

1904e: "Notice sur les travaux de Pierre Curie", *Annuaire de l'Association des anciens élèves de l'École de physique et de chimie de la ville de Paris*, 2–36.

1905a: "Recherches récentes sur la théorie de la décharge disruptive", *BSFP*, 4, 25.

1905b: "Recherches récentes sur le mécanisme du courant électrique. Ions et électrons" *BSIE*, 5, 615; in *L'Éclairage électrique*, 1905, 45, 361 and 401.

1905c: "Recombinaison et diffusion des ions gazeux", *JP*, 1905, 4, 322–334; *OS*, 154–163.

1905d: "Interprétation de divers phénomènes par la présence de gros ions dans l'atmosphère", *BSFP*, 4, 79; *OS*, 242–244.

1905e: "Sur un enregistreur des ions de l'atmosphère" (with Moulin M.), *CRAS*, 140, 305–307.

1905f: "Remarques à propos de la communication de M.E. Bloch", *BSFP*, 4, 84.

1905g: "Une formule fondamentale de théorie cinétique" *Annales de Chimie et de Physique*, 1905, 5, 245; *CRAS*, 1905, 140, 35–38; *OS*, 269–300.

1905h: "Sur l'origine des radiations et l'inertie électromagnétique", *JP*, 4, 165; *OS*, 313–328.

1905i: "Sur la théorie du magnétisme", *CRAS*, 139, 1204; *BSFP*, 1905, 4, 13.

1905j: "Magnétisme et théorie des électrons", *Annales de chimie et de physique*, 1905, 5, 70; *OS*, 331–368.

1905k: "Sur la théorie du magnétisme", *JP*, 4, 678.

1905m: "Sur l'impossibilité physique de mettre en évidence le mouvement de translation de la terre", *CRAS*, 140, 1171–1173, *OS*, 395–396.

1905n: *Les quantités élémentaires d'électricité, ions, électrons, corpuscules* (ed. with Abraham, Henri), 2 vol., Paris, Gauthier-Villars.

1906a: "Pierre Curie", *La Revue du mois*, 1906, 2, 5–36.

1906b: "Recherches récentes sur le mécanisme de la décharge disruptive", *BSIE*, 6, 69; *Le Radium*, 1906, 3, 107.

1906c: Preface to the French translation of Oliver Lodge, *Sur les électrons*, Paris.

1907: "Électromètre enregistreur des ions de l'atmosphère" (with Moulin N.), *BSFP*, 3, 264; *Le Radium*, 1907, 4, 218–230; *OS*, 245–265.

1908a: "Sur la théorie du mouvement brownien", *CRAS*, 146, 530–534; *OS*, 301–303.

1908b: "Sur la recombinaison des ions dans les diélectriques", *CRAS*, 146, 1011–1017, *OS*, 164–166.

1909a: "E. Mascart", *Annuaire du Collège de France*, 25. Archives, L088/13.

1909b: "L'œuvre de E. Mascart", *La Revue du mois*, 7, 385–406.

1910a: "Sur les biréfringences électrique et magnétique", *Le Radium*, 7, 249–261; *CRAS*, 151, 475–478; *OS*, 369–391.

1910b: "La théorie électromagnétique et le bleu du ciel", *BSFP*, 4, 80.

1911a: "L'évolution de l'espace et du temps", Lecture at the Fourth International Conference of Philosophy in Bologna, *Scientia*, 1911, 10, 31–54; quoted from *PPE* 61–74.

1911b: "Le temps, l'espace et la causalité dans la physique contemporaine", *Bulletin de la Société française de philosophie*, 1912, 12, 1–46, quoted from *PVA*, 301–344.

1911c: "La théorie cinétique du magnétisme et les magnétons", report to the Solvay Conference, in *La Théorie du rayonnement et les quanta*, Paris, Gauthier-Villars, 1912; *PVA*, 171–198.

1911d: "Remarques au sujet des communications de M. Fouard", *PVSFP*, 1 December 1911, 84: 4 April 1913, 42.

1911e: "Exposé expérimental des phénomènes fondamentaux d'électrostatique au moyen de l'électromètre à quadrants", notes on a conference at the Société Française de Physique written by M. J. Villey, *JP*, 1, 460.

1911f: "Victor Régnault", *La Revue du mois*, 1911, 11, 129.

1911g: Preface to Drude P., *Précis d'optique*, revised and completed by Marcel Boll, Paris, vol I.

1912a: "Sur l'orientation moléculaire", Lettre to M. Voigt, *Gottingen Nachritten*, 1912, 5, 589.

1912b: "Sur la comparaison des molécules gazeuses et dissoutes", *CRAS*, 154, 594–596; *OS*, 475–76.

1912c: "L'interprétation cinétique de la pression osmotique", *Journal de Chimie-Physique*, 10, 524 and 527; *OS*, 477–80.

1912d: "Les grains d'électricité et la dynamique électromagnétique", in *Idées modernes sur la constitution de la matière*, Paris, Gauthier-Villars, 1913.

1912e: "Notions géométriques fondamentales" based on a German text by M. Abraham, *Encyclopédie des sciences mathématiques*, 1912, 4(1), 1–60.

1912f: *La Théorie du rayonnement et les quanta*. Report and discussion of the meeting held at Brussels October–November 1911, under the auspices of M.E. Solvay (with de Broglie M.), Paris, Gauthier-Villars, 1912.

1913a: "Mesure de la valence des ions dans les gaz", *Le Radium*, 1913, 10, 113–119; *OS*, 167–178.

1913b: "Sur les chocs exceptionnels des molécules gazeuses" (with Rey J.J.), *Le Radium*, 10, 142–146; *OS*, 304–310.

1913c: "L'inertie de l'énergie et ses conséquences", lecture at the Société française de physique, 26 March 1913, *JP*, 3, 553–592; *PVA*, p. 345–405; *OS*, 397–426.

1913d: "La physique du discontinu", lecture at the Société française de physique, 27 November 1913, *Les progrès de la physique moléculaire*, Paris, Gauthier-Villars, 1914; *PVA*, 189–264.

1913e: "Remarques au sujet de la communication de M. Wertenstein", *PVSFP*, 34.

1913f: "Henri Poincaré. Le physicien", *Revue de métaphysique et de morale*, 21, 665–718; in Volterra V., Hadamard J., Langevin P., Boutroux P., eds, *Henri Poincaré. L'œuvre scientifique, l'œuvre philosophique*, Paris, Alcan, 1914.

1913g: "Le mécanisme scientifique", lecture 9 December 1913, in *La Valeur de la science*, Archives, L090/006.

1914: "Thermodynamique et statistique (à propos de cinq conférences de M. H. A. Lorentz)", *La Revue du mois*, 97, 29–38.

1916a: "Sur la production des étincelles musicales par courant continu", *Annales des P.T.T.*, 4, 404.

1916b: "Procédés et appareils pour la production de signaux sous-marins dirigés et pour la localisation à distance d'obstacles sous-marins" (with Chilowski C.) French patent 502.913, 29 May 1916; *OS*, 527–36. Also US patent 169,804, German patent 399,723, British patent 125,122.

1917: Note on apparatus for the detection of submerged objects by acoustic waves of high frequency. Board of Invention and Research 3929/17. 12 February 1917. British National Archives, Kew. Archives L194/026.

1918a: "Procédé et appareils d'émission et réception des ondes élastiques sous-marines à l'aide des propriétés piézoélectriques du quartz", French patent, 505.703, 17 September 1918; *OS*, 538–42. Also British patent 145,691.

1918b: "Note sur l'énergie auditive", Publications du Centre d'études de Toulon, 25 September, 1.

1918c: "Interallied conference on submarine detection by means of supersonics". In Compton KT. US Navy. Research Information Committee report 161. Paris. 31 October 1918. Reprinted in Zimmermann, David (2002) "Paul Langevin and the discovery of active sonar or asdic". *The Northern Mariner*, 12, 3–52.

1919a: "Remarques à propos de la communication de M.E. Bauer", *PVSFP*, 21 March 1919, 18.

1919b: *Le Principe de relativité*, Address to the Société française des électriciens 6 December 1919, Paris, Chiron, 1922.

1920a: "Les aspects successifs du principe de relativité", *BSFP*, 138, 5; *PVA*, 406–423; *OS*, 427–435.

1920b: "Utilisation de la détente pour la production des courants d'air de grande vitesse", *BSFP*, 139, 7; *OS*, 607–609.

1920c: "Le théorème de Fermat et la loi du minimum de temps en optique géométrique", *JP*, 1, 188.

1920d: "La structure de l'électricité", Lecture, 20 March at l'École supérieure des postes et télégraphes. Archives L091/001.

1920e: Open letter to *L'Humanité*, 18 May 1920.

1920f: Letter to *L'Humanité*, 6 December 1920, Archives L028/043.

1921a: "Sur les grandeurs champ et induction", *BSFP*, 162, 3; *OS*, 491–92.

1921b: "Sur la théorie de la relativité et l'expérience de M. Sagnac", *CRAS*, 173, 831–834; *OS*, 467–469.
1921c: "Sur la dynamique de la relativité", *PVSFP*, 15 December 1921.
1921d: Introduction to Eddington A., *Espace, temps et gravitation. La théorie de la relativité généralisée dans ses grandes lignes*, Paris. Hermann.
1921e: Meeting at the Salle Wagram about the liberation of A. Marty and the imprisoned sailors, Archives L028/044, extracts in PA, 258–263.

1922a: Note sur la loi de résistance de l'air et sur la correction d'élasticité proposée par M. le Capitaine Darrieus, *Mémorial de l'artillerie française*, 2, 253; *OS*, 610–22.
1922b: "L'aspect général de la théorie de la relativité", *Bulletin scientifique de l'Association des étudiants de Paris*, 2, 2–22. Quoted from *PPE* 75–99:
1922c: "La théorie de la relativité", Session on 6 April 1922, *Bulletin de la Société française de Philosophie*, 17, 349–370. Downloadable version in *Les grandes conférences de la SFP, Philosophie des sciences*: https://www.sofrphilo.fr/activites-scientifiques-de-la-sfp/conferences/grandes-conferences-entelechargement/#I_8211_PHILOSOPHIE_DES_SCIENCES
1922d: Preface to Edmond Bauer, *La Théorie de la relativité*, Paris, Librairie de l'enseignement technique.
1922e: *Le Principe de relativité*, Paris, Chiron, Bibliothèque de synthèse scientifique; *OS*, 436–466.
1922f: "Sur la nature des grandeurs et le choix d'un système d'unités électriques", *BSFP*, 164, 9; *OS*, 493–505.
1922g: Preface to Thomson J.J., *Électricité et matière*, Paris. Science et Civilisation.

1923a: "Note sur les effets balistiques de la détente de la poudre dans une tuyère convergente-divergente", *Mémorial de l'artillerie française*, 1923, 3; *OS*, 623–41.
1923b: "Procédés et appareils pour le sondage et la localisation à distance d'obstacles sous-marins au moyen d'échos ultra-sonores" (with Florisson, C L.) French patent 575,435, 27 December 1923; US patent 1,858,931, 17 May 1932; *OS*, 557–70.
1923c: "Émission d'un faisceau d'ondes ultra-sonores" (with Chilowski C., Tournier M.), JP, 4(Suppl.), 537–539.
1923d: "Utilisation des phénomènes piézo-électriques pour la mesure de l'intensité des sons en valeur absolue" (with Ishimoto M.), *JP*, 4, (Suppl) 539–540; *OS*, 592–93.
1923e: Déclaration au retour de Berlin, 1923, Archives, L028.

1924a: "Procédés et appareils permettant la mesure directe ou l'enregistrement des profondeurs ou des distances en mer par la méthode ultra-sonore", French patent 576.281, 14 January 1924; addition 28–798, 1 March 1924; 2nd addition 29–543, 16 October 1924; *OS*, 571–86. Also British patent 227,801.
1924b: "Procédés et appareils pour la mesure par lecture directe de la distance d'un obstacle dans l'air", French patent 577.055, 11 February 1924; *OS*, 587–91.

1924c: "Sondage et détection sous-marine par les ultrasons", *Bulletin de l'Association technique maritime et aéronautique*, 1924, 28, 407; *Revue hydrographique du Bureau international de Monaco*, 1924, 1, 139; *Recherches et inventions*, 1925, 113, 441,

1924d: Repport on the thesis of Louis de Broglie, reprinted in Wheaton, 1983, 295–97.

1924e: The employment of ultra-sonic waves for echo sounding. *Hydrographic Review*, November 1924 2(1), 53–91.

1926a: "Sondeur ultrasonore", *Recherches et inventions*, 1926, 132, 119.

1926b: "Procédé et disposition améliorant l'efficacité des projecteurs ultrasonores piézoélectriques", French patent 622.035, 27 January 1926; *OS*, 543–56. Also British patents 265,181, 279,878.

1926c: "La valeur éducative de l'histoire des sciences", *Bulletin de la Société française de Pédagogie*, 1926, 22, 692–700; *Revue de Synthèse*, 1933, 6. Quoted from *PPE* 183–194.

1926d: Preface in M. Courtines, *Où en est la Physique?*, Paris, Gauthier-Villars, 1926, i–xi.

1926e: "Fascismus und démocratie", *Frankfurter Zeitung*, 11 April 1926, Archives L028/049.

1927a: "Les étapes de la pensée scientifique", *Comptes rendus du Congrès de l'Association française pour l'Avancement des Sciences*, Constantine, April 1927, 23–32.

1927b: "Procédé et dispositif pour la mesure des variations de pression dans les canalisations d'eau ou autre liquide" (with Rocart, R.) French patent 639,151, 6 August 1927,

1927c: "Procédés et appareils permettant la mesure de la puissance transmise par un arbre", French patent 659,658, 19 December 1927.

1927d: "Banc piézoélectrique pour l'équilibrage des rotors", French patent 659,871, 22 December 1927.

1927e: "L'enregistrement des coups de belier", *Bulletin technique de la Chambre syndicale des entrepreneurs de couverture-plomberie*, 23, 81.

1927f: "A propos des bruits parasites ultrasonores", *Revue hydrographique du Bureau international de Monaco*, 4, 161.

1927g: "Atomes et étoiles", two lectures at the Conservatoire des Arts et métiers, March 1927, Archives L092/006.

1927h: Discours pour l'inauguration du monument aux morts de Levallois-Perret, 3 March 1927. Archives L030/005.

1928a: "Les fonctions sociales de l'investigation scientifique", Lecture in Buenos Aires, 17 August 1928, Spanish version in *La Prensa*, 28 August 1928.

1928b: "Les nouvelles mécaniques et la chimie", (recorded by H. Grandjouan), *Réunion internationale de chimie-physique*, Paris, October 1928, 550–569; *OS*, 509–524.

1928c: "La production et l'utilisation des ondes ultrasonores", *Procès verbal de la Société des ingénieurs civils*, 5, 119; *Revue Générale d'Électricité*, 23, 626–634.

1929a: "La structure des atomes et l'origine de la chaleur solaire", *Bulletin de l'Université de Tiflis*, 22, 10.

1929b: "Les vibrations ultrasonores et leurs applications", *Bulletin de l'Université de Tiflis*, 22, 10.

1929c: "Paul Schutzenberger", in *Centenaire de Paul Schutzenberger, 1829–1897*, Fondation Schutzenberger, Paris, Société des bourses de recherches scientifiques chimiques.

1929d: "Sur le mirage ultrasonore", *Bulletin de l'Association technique maritime et aéronautique*, 1929, 727–733; in *Revue hydrographique du Bureau international de Monaco*, 1931, 8, 140–143.

1929e: *Les Méthodes modernes de guerre et la protection des populations civiles*, Paris, M. Rivière, 1929.

1930a: "L'orientation actuelle de la Physique", in L. Brunschvicg, J. Perrin, P. Langevin, G. Urbain, L. Lapicque, C. Perez, L. Plantefol, L'Orientation actuelle des sciences, Conferences organised in 1929–30 at the ENS. Paris, Alcan, 1930. *PPE* 110–127.

1930b: "En l'honneur de Georges Claude et Paul Boucherot", 15 November 1930, Association des anciens élèves de l'EPCI, 14–15.

1931a: "L'œuvre d'Einstein et l'astronomie", Address to the general assembly of the Société Astronomique de France 10 June 1931, *Bulletin de la société astronomique de France*, 1931, 45, 277–297.

1931b: "La contribution des sciences physiques à la culture générale", *Bulletin de la Société française de Pédagogie*, 1931, 41.

1931c: "Science et laïcité", Groupe fraternel de l'enseignement, Paris, Deshayes, 1931, 7–28.

1931d: "Déduction simplifiée du facteur de Thomas" in Sommerfeld A., *Vereinfachete Ableitung des Thomas faktor*, Convegno di ftsica nucleare, Rome, 1931, 137.

1931e: "Contre la guerre chimique", address to the Fédération Internationale des Instituteurs, July 1931. Archives L029/005.

1931f: "Y a-t-il une crise du déterminisme", *Le mois*, 2, 1931, 273–275.

1931g: "La directivité en acoustique sous-marine", *Bulletin de l'Association technique maritime et aéronautique*, June 1931, 1, 37–47; *OS*, 594–603.

1932a: "Le problème de la culture générale", *Pour l'ère nouvelle*, 81, 1932, 239–245. Quoted from *PPE* 231–246.

1932b: La relativité. Conclusion générale de la deuxième semaine internationale de synthèse, Paris, Hermann.

1932c: "La physique au Collège de France", in Livre jubilaire du quatrième centenaire du Collège de France, Paris, PUF, 61–79.

1932d: *La réorganisation de l'enseignement public en Chine* (with Becker C.H., Falski M., Tawney R.H.), Rapport de la mission d'experts de la Société des

Nations, Paris. Reprinted as *The reorganisation of education in China*. Taipei. Ch'eng Wen. 1974.

1932e: "Ernest Solvay", Discours pour l'inauguration du monument, in *Hommage national à Ernest Solvay*, Bruxelles.

1932f: Preface to M. Haïssinsky, *L'Atomistique moderne et la chimie*, Paris, Doin.

1932g: "La science et la paix", *Cahiers des droits de l'homme*, 28, 651–655.

1933a: *La Notion de corpuscule et d'atome*, Paris, Hermann, 1934. Quoted from *PPE* 253–300.

1933b: "Sur l'évolution de la science électrique depuis cinquante ans", *Cinquantenaire de la Société française des électriciens*, Paris, Gauthier-Villars.

1933c: "Paul Painlevé, le savant", *Les Cahiers rationalistes*, 2, 230–243.

1933d: "Gustave Bémont", discours et notice nécrologique, Nogent-le-Rotrou.

1933e: "De Dimitrov à Thaelmann: échec au fascisme", Paris, no reference.

1934a: "La valeur humaine de la science", Preface to *L'Évolution humaine des origines à nos jours. Étude biologique, psychologique, et sociologique de l'homme*, ed. M. Lahy-Hollebecque, Paris, Quillet, T. I, xi–xv; quoted from *Les Cahiers rationalistes*, 1940, 8, 35–50.

1934b: "L'électron positif", *BSIE*, 4, 1934, 335–379.

1934c: "Sur un problème d'activation par diffusion", *JP*, 5, 57–60; *OS*, 481–87.

1934d: Preface to Maltifano G. and Catoire M., *Les Composés micellaires selon la notion de complexité croissante en chimie*, Paris, Hermann.

1934e: "Allocution de Paul Langevin", given on 5 July 1934 at the EPCI during a ceremony "En l'honneur de P. Langevin", *Association des anciens élèves de l'EPCI*, 1934, 17–24.

1934f: Presentation of S. Erchner, *L'Allemagne, champ de manœuvre. Le fascisme et la guerre* (with Lévy-Bruhl L., Prenant M.), Paris, Éd. Sociales internationales.

1934g: "Le fascisme passera-t-il en France?", Replies to an enquiry 20 December 1934, *Regards*, 3(49).

1934h: "Les prétentions sociales du fascisme" (with Alain, Gérôme P., Prenant M., Rivet P.), Paris, CVIA, June 1934.

1934i: "La jeunesse devant le fascisme "; Paris, CVIA.

1934j: "La notion de corpuscules et d'atomes". Lecture delivered at the opening session of the International meeting of Physical Chemistry, 16 October 1933, *PPE* 139–168.

1935a: Remarques au sujet de la note de M. Prunier "Sur une expérience de Sagnac qui serait faite avec un flux d'électrons", *CRAS*, 200, 48–51.

1935b: "Sur les lois de dégagement d'électricité par torsion dans les corps piézoélectriques", (with Solomon J.) *CRAS*, 200, 1257–1259.

1935c: "Espace et temps dans un univers euclidien", *Livre jubilaire de Marcel Brillouin*, Paris, Gauthier-Villars.

1935d: Lecture: *Jubilé scientifique de M. Brillouin*, Paris, Gauthier-Villars, 1936, 18–26.

1935e: "Statistique et déterminisme", in *La Statistique. Ses applications. Les problèmes qu'elle soulève*, Cinquième Semaine Internationale de synthèse; Paris, PUF, 1944, 245–300.

1935f: Discours d'ouverture à la réunion plénière du 23–24 novembre 1935, *CMGF*, Archives L030/033.

1936a: "La valeur humaine de la science", in "*Entretiens philosophiques*", Broadcast Lectures on the National Channel Radio-Paris (undated), 107–115.

1936b: "La science pure et la technique", in *Ce que la civilisation moderne doit à la recherche scientifique désintéressée*, Broadcast Lectures on the National Channel Radio-Paris (undated), 5–9.

1936c: "Transport et distribution de l'énergie électrique grâce aux découvertes de Faraday," Broadcast Lectures on the National Channel Radio-Paris (undated), 37–41.

1936d: Introduction to Paul Painlevé, *Paroles et écrits*, La Société des amis de Paul Painlevé, 2nd ed., Paris, Rieder, xi–xiii.

1936e: Address for Romain at Rolland's 70th birthday L'Université syndicaliste, February 1936, extracts in *PA*, 274–277.

1936f: "La France en face du problème colonial" (with Alain, Casati M. Rivet P.), Paris, CVIA.

1936g: "Non la guerre n'est pas fatale", (with Alain, Bouché H., Rivet P.) Paris, CVIA.

1936h: "Pas de blocus contre l'Espagne républicaine" (with Duclos J., Zyromsky J., Hénaff E., Branting G.), Press conference, 16 September 1936, *CMGF*.

1937a: "Sur l'expérience de M. Sagnac", *CRAS*, 205, 304–306; *OS*, 470–72.

1937b: Preface to Miss Rathborne, *Français et Britanniques vous parlent de l'Espagne et de la paix*, Paris, 1937.

1937c: "Fascisme et civilisation", *Clarté*, 7, 51–56. PPE 169–174.

1937d: "Tous unis pour défendre la paix" (with Rolland R.), CMGF, June 1937, Archives, L032.

1937e: "L'électricité", in *Le Palais de la Découverte*, Broadcast Lectures on the National Channel Radio-Paris (undated), 22–28.

1937f: "La science et la vie", Lecture at Union rationaliste, summary in *Paix et liberté*, 1937.

1937g: "Fascisme et civilisation", *Clarté*, 7, 51–56.

1938a: "La relativité", *Les Cahiers rationalistes*, 1938, 7, 103.

1938b: "Les courants positiviste et réaliste dans la philosophie de la physique", Report to the meeting of the International Union of Physics, 2 June 1938, in *Les nouvelles théories de la Physique*, Paris, 1939, 231–254.

1938c: "Les actions mutuelles dans le monde physique", Introduction to a lecture by Pierre Auger, *10th Semaine Internationale de Synthèse*, Paris, PUF, 1943, 213–216.

1938d: "Défense de la paix et de la liberté", *Clarté*, July 23, 1938, 827–30; *PA*, 281–287.

1938e: Declaration in the National Conference of the French Communist Party, Gennevilliers, 26 December 1938; extract in *PA*, 291–292.

1938f: Interview in *Femmes*, November 1938. Archives L032/053.

1938g: "Fidélité au serment", Congrès paix et liberté du Front populaire de la Région parisienne, June 1938, *Paix et Liberté*, 11–15.

1939a: "La physique moderne et le déterminisme", *La Pensée*, 1939, 1, 1–14.

1939b: "La science comme facteur d'évolution morale et sociale", *Les Cahiers rationalistes*, 1939, 75, 114–137.

1939c: "Science et liberté, Paix et liberté", undated, special issue for the 150th anniversary of the French Revolution; extracts in *PA*, 288–291.

1939d: "Hommage à Georges Urbain", *La Pensée*, 1, 89–91.

1940a: Preface to Le Boiteux H. et Boussardi R., *Élasticité et photoélasticité*, Paris, Hermann.

1940b: Déposition au procès des députés communistes, draft. Archives L028/056.

1942a: "Sur les chocs entre neutrons rapides et noyaux de masse quelconque", *CRAS*, 214, 517–522; *OS*, 645–50.

1942b: "Sur les chocs entre neutrons et noyaux", *CRAS*, 214, 867–869; *OS*, 651–53.

1942c: "Sur le ralentissement des neutrons", *CRAS*, 214, 889–891; *OS*, 653–56.

1942d: "Sur les chocs entre neutrons rapides et noyaux de masse quelconque", *Annales de physique*, 17, 303; *OS*, 657–70.

1942e: "Résonance et forces de gravitation", *Annales de physique*, 17, 265; *OS*, 673–79.

1942f: Reply to A. Dufour and F. Prunier, "Sur un déplacement de franges enregistré sur une plateforme en rotation uniforme", *JP*, 3, 161–162.

1944a: Radio broadcast at Lyon, 24 September 1944: in Biquard P. *Paul Langevin*, Paris, Seghers, 1969, 100–101.

1944b: "Culture et humanités", *La Pensée*, New Ser. 1, 1944, 25–31.

1944c: Testimony at the trial of Georges Claude, in P. Ribet, *Le procès de G. Claude*, Paris, 1946; extracts in *G. Claude, Ma vie, mes inventions*, Paris, Plon, 1957, 250–253.

1945a: "L'ère des transmutations", *La Pensée*, New Ser. 4, 1944, 3–16; "La era de la energia atomica", *Nueva Cultura*, 89, 6–8; "The era of atomic energy", *Science and Society*, 1946, 10, 3–13.

1945b: "Résolutions de la Commission à l'énergie atomique de l'Académie des Sciences transmises au président du gouvernement provisoire de la République" (with de Broglie M., Joliot F.), *CRAS*, 221, 720.

1945c: "La désintégration atomique", introducing a lecture by F. Joliot-Curie, *Cahiers rationalistes*, 8, 175–177.

1945d: Forward to S. Amiel, *Ce qu'une Française doit savoir*, Paris, Ligue des droits de L'Homme.

1945e: Lecture 3 March 1945, in *Hommage à Paul Langevin*, Union française universitaire, Paris, 1945; extract in *PA*, 308–310. www.ina.fr/ina-eclaire-actu/video/

afe86003016/a-la-sorbonne-le-front-national-universitaire-fete-le-73eme-anniversaire-de-paul-langevin

1945f: "L'Encyclopédie ou la solidarité de l'action et de la pensée", lecture delivered at Palais de Chaillot, 10 June, Inaugural session for *l'Encyclopédie de la Renaissance française*; *Les Lettres françaises*, 60, 16 June. Quoted from the extracts in *PA*, 165–75.

1945g: Translation of Bernal J.D., "La science et le sort des hommes", *La Pensée*, 5, 129–132.

1945h: "Victor Basch. 1863-1944", Memorial lecture, 7 January 1945, Paris, Ligue des droits de l'homme.

1945i: "Les principes de la réforme", Broadcast talk, *Pour l'ère nouvelle*, June 1945, 189–190.

1945j: Christmas message, Radio broadcast recording; Extracts in *PA*, 318–320.

1946a: "La pensée et l'action", lecture 10 May 1946, Paris, *Union française universitaire*, 3–20. Science and Action. *Science and Society* 1947;11(3):209–224. Quoted from *PPE* 180–194.

1946b: "La réforme de l'enseignement". Projet soumis à M. le Ministre de l'Éducation nationale par la Commission ministérielle d'étude présidée par P. Langevin et H. Wallon, Paris, Ministère de l'Éducation nationale, 1947.

1946c: "Hommage à Jacques Solomon", Paris, l'Union française universitaire.

1946d: "Hommage à Henri Roger", *Les Cahiers rationalistes*, 8, 57–61.

1946e: "Pasteur, le savant et l'homme", *La Pensée*, New Ser. 7, 1946, 3–10.

1946f: "La science et la paix", *Quadrige*, February–March 1946, 15–19. *PPE* 321–326.

1946g: "La pensée française au service de la paix", Talk at the Conseil de l'Union nationale des intellectuels, May 1946, *Pour l'ère nouvelle*, 1947, special issue "P. Langevin, écrits philosophiques et pédagogiques", 204–205.

1946h: "La science ne doit pas être une cause de guerre", Talk at the Conseil de l'Union nationale des intellectuels, *Les Étoiles*, 60, 2 July 1946.

1946i: La justice est en retard sur la science, *Les Étoiles*, 65, 6 August 1946.

1946j: "La réforme de l'enseignement dans les différents pays et ses rapports avec l'Éducation nouvelle", *Pour l'ère nouvelle*, August 1946, 36–39.

Compilations of Langevin's Publications

1950: *Œuvres scientifiques de Paul Langevin*, Paris, Éditions CNRS.
1964: *La pensée et l'action*, Paris, Éditions sociales.
2007: *Propos d'un physicien engagé*, edited by Bernadette Bensaude-Vincent, Paris, Vuibert.

Chronology

Year	Paul Langevin's life events	Social and political events	Scientific and cultural events
1871		Paris Commune	
1872	Born 24 January, Paris		
1880			Discovery of piezoelectricity by Pierre and Jacques Curie
1881		J. Ferry law on free primary education	
1882			Creation of the EPCI
1884	Enters l'École primaire supérieure Lavoisier		
1885		Zola: *Germinal*	Pasteur: anti-rabies serum
1888	Student at l'École de physique et de chimie (EPCI)		
1889	Student at EPCI	Bergson, *Essai sur les données immédiates de la conscience*	World Exhibition in Paris
1892	Student at EPCI (Pierre Curie tutor)		Lorentz: theory of electrons Branly invents the radio coherer
1893	Military service		
1894	Student at l'École normale supérieure, rue d'Ulm (ENS)		
1894	Student at ENS	Beginning of Dreyfus Affair (1894–1906)	
1895	Student at ENS	Foundation of the General Labour Confederation (CGT)	Roentgen discovers X-rays HG Wells *Time Machine*

(continued)

Year	Paul Langevin's life events	Social and political events	Scientific and cultural events
1896	Student at ENS		Becquerel discovers radioactivity.
1897	*Agrégé* of Physical Sciences. Scholarship Cavendish Laboratory in Cambridge		JJ Thomson demonstrates electrons
1898	Work on gas ionization Signs a petition in support of Dreyfus Marriage to Jeanne Defosses		Marie and Pierre Curie discover radium
1899	Birth of son Jean		Marconi: first radio link between England and France
1900	*Préparateur* at the Paris Faculty of Sciences		Planck introduces "quantum of action"
1901	Birth of son André		
1902	Defence of doctoral thesis Replacement professor at the *Collège de France*		
1903	Substitute professor at the *Collège de France* Birth of daughter Madeleine		Becquerel, Marie and Pierre Curie receive the Nobel Prize for Physics
1904	Attends International Congress of Arts and Science in St. Louis, USA		
1905	Professor at the EPCI Theory of diamagnetism Theory of Brownian motion Inertia of energy and $e = mc^2$		Einstein: special theory of relativity; interpretation of the photoelectric effect; study of Brownian motion
1906			Boltzmann's suicide Death of Pierre Curie
1907	Prize of the Academy of Sciences		
1909	Full professor at the *Collège de France* (chair of general and experimental physics) Birth of daughter Hélène		Blériot crosses the Channel by air First French radio devices
1910	Electric and magnetic birefringence First of 15 nominations for Nobel Prize for physics (all unsuccessful). Love affair with Marie Curie		

(continued)

Chronology 283

Year	Paul Langevin's life events	Social and political events	Scientific and cultural events
1911	Member of the first Solvay Physics Council Course on the theory of relativity at the *Collège de France*		Relativity thoery discussed at the International Congress of philosophy in Bologna
1912	Lives apart from his wife and children		Death of Henri Poincaré
1913			Bohr-Rutherford, Quantum model of the atom Perrin: *Les Atomes*
1914		Assassination of Jaurès Declaration of war in Europe	H.G. Wells: *The World Set Free* (science fiction of atomic war)
1915	Mobilized in the 30th infantry regiment of Chartres Hughes Medal of the Royal Society of London Starts work on ultrasonic submarine detection	First war-time use of gas by Germany	
1916	Assigned to the Artillery Commission	Battle of Verdun	Einstein, General theory of relativity
1917	Guthrie Lecture at the Physical Society of London First use of piezoelectricity of quartz for ultrasonics	Russian Revolution Entry of the United States into the war Soviet request for armistice	Rutherford demonstrates artificial disintegration of atom
1918	Creates high-speed gas jet for testing military ballistics Sea tests for ultrasonic submarine detector	Nov 11, Armistice at Rethondes First transatlantic flight Civil War in Russia	
1919		Treaty of Versailles Pact of the League of Nations	Eddington, measurement of the deviation of light by the sun, confirming the general theory of relativity Rutherford: induced radioactivity
1920	Scientific director of the *Journal de physique* Supports the sailors of the Black Sea Ultrasonic depth sounding demonstrated	Creation of the League of Nations Congress of Tours: split between the Socialist Party and the Communist Party. General strike in France	
1921	Member of the Scientific Committee of the Solvay Physics Council Member Academy of Lincei, Rome	French sailors' mutiny in Kronstadt in Russia Lenin applies the New Economic Policy	Opening of the Radium Institute (Curie Foundation)

(continued)

Year	Paul Langevin's life events	Social and political events	Scientific and cultural events
1922	Einstein's in Paris at the invitation of Langevin Member of the French Society of Pedagogy Awarded the Order of the British Empire third class (CBE) for services rendered during the war	Mussolini in power Stalin secretary of the Soviet Communist Party Formation of the USSR	
1923	Knight of the Légion d'honneur Member of the Central Committee of the French League of Human Rights Visit to Berlin: meeting of the League of Human Rights Collège de France course on ultrasonics	Occupation of the Ruhr and inflation in Germany	
1924	Member of the PhD jury for Louis de Broglie Member of the Russian Academy of Sciences	Left-wing coalition and financial crisis in France France recognizes the USSR. Death of Lenin Hitler: Mein Kampf	Louis de Broglie thesis: beginning of wave mechanics
1925	Member of the Reform Commission of L'école unique	Locarno Agreements Rif War in Morocco	Millikan: Discovery of cosmic rays
1926	Director of the EPCI Supports imprisoned Romanian democrats. Visits Cambridge Member of Prague Academy of Sciences, Member of Bologna Academy of Sciences	Germany enters the League of Nations	Creation of the Henri Poincaré Institute (Borel, director)
1927	Inaugural speech at the Congress of the French Association for the Advancement of Science, Constantine Vice president of French League for Human Rights Anti-fascist meeting with Rolland, Vaillant-Couturier and Barbusse Honorary doctorate, Bristol University		Fifth Physics Solvay Council "Electrons and photons" Heisenberg indeterminacy principle

(continued)

Chronology 285

Year	Paul Langevin's life events	Social and political events	Scientific and cultural events
1928	Chairman of the Scientific Committee of the Solvay Physics Council Chairman of the French Group for New Education Member of *Amitiés franco-russes* Member of the Royal Society, London Member of Buenos Aires Academy of Sciences Travels to South America and the Soviet Union (lecture tour of Georgia)		Einstein's unitary field theory
1929	Head of the "Natural Sciences" section of the *Centre internal de synthèse* Member of Copenhagen Academy of Sciences Second travel in Soviet Union (Moscow Academy medal)	Beginning of the Great Depression in the United States	
1930	Vice-President of *Union rationaliste* Chair of Sixth Solvay Physics Council "Magnetism"		
1931	League of Nations Mission to China on the reorganization of public education	Japan occupies Manchuria. Economic crisis in Europe	First demonstration of television in France
1932	Officer of *Légion d'honneur* President of the International Congress for New Education in Nice Founding member of *Université ouvrière* Member of the Council of the World Committee against War and Fascism (Amsterdam-Pleyel)	Geneva Conference on arms control Roosevelt becomes president of the United States	Chadwick, discovery of the neutron Lawrence, first cyclotron (California)
1933	President of the French Society of Electricians Participant in *Encyclopédie française* Welcomes German Jewish émigrés to his laboratory. Chair of Seventh Solvay Congress: "Atomic Nucleii"	Hitler Chancellor of the Reich German "Law on the Restoration of Public Services" Japan and Germany withdraw from the League of Nations France: fall of the Daladier ministry Foundation of the *Cercle de la Russie neuve* in Paris	Einstein leaves Germany

(continued)

Year	Paul Langevin's life events	Social and political events	Scientific and cultural events
1934	Election to the French *Académie des sciences* Founding member of the *Comité de vigilance des intellectuels antifascistes*, with Paul Rivet and Alain Member of the Radio Commission for the 1937 International Exhibition	Riots on 6 February in Paris; General strike called by left-wing parties Hitler and Mussolini meet in Venice; "Night of the Long Knives" in Germany Start of the Stalinist purges in the USSR (assassination of Kirov)	Death of Marie Curie Discovery of artificial radioactivity by Frédéric and Irène Joliot-Curie Fermi: production of transuranium elements
1935	Instigator of the Popular Rally Movement Participant on the *Palais de la Découverte* project President of the *Société française de pédagogie*	Formation of the *Front Populaire* Creation of a *Fond national de la recherche scientifique* by merging two previous organizations Germany: exodus of Jews USSR: Stakhanovite movement Italy attacks Ethiopia. "Long March" of the Chinese communists	Iréne and Frédéric Joliot-Curie Nobel Prize for chemistry Synthetic plastics and textiles Development of electro-chemistry and electro-metallurgy in the USA
1936	President of the Board of Directors of Radio-Liberté Joins left-wing delegation to London Campaign to support Spanish Republicans	Popular Front: Blum Prime Minister; social laws Civil War in Spain. Anti-Comintern Pact between Germany and Japan Italy annexes Ethiopia	Alan Turing proposes the "Turing machine"
1937	Leads fund-raising in England for Basque refugees, with Picasso, Matisse, and Virginia Woolf Speaks in Cambridge on the *Front Populaire*	International Exhibition of Arts and Technology in Paris Failure of the Blum ministry Creation of the Under-Secretariat of State for Research Italy and Germany enter the Spanish Civil War; air bombing of Guernica Japanese attack on China, alliance between Tchang Kai-Shek and Mao Tse-Tung	Anderson, discovery of the meson in cosmic rays
1938	President of the *Union rationaliste* Participates in the Conference of the French Communist Party in Gennevilliers	Anschluss: Austria annexed by Germany. Munich Agreement signed by Nazi Germany, the United Kingdom, France and Italy. Withdrawal of the International Brigades in Spain End of the Popular Front and devaluation of the franc	Otto Hahn, L. Meitner, H. Strassmann: discovery of nuclear fission

(continued)

Chronology 287

Year	Paul Langevin's life events	Social and political events	Scientific and cultural events
1939	Founder and director of *La Pensée* Group leader in the *Centre national de la recherche scientifique* (CNRS)	Beginning of the Second World War Germany occupies Czechoslovakia and invades Poland Capture of Madrid by Franco, end of the Spanish Civil War German-Soviet Pact	Joliot, Halban, Kowarski, principles of the chain reaction Creation of the Bourbaki group of mathematicians
1940	Lead for Franco-English scientific co-operation. Awarded Royal Society of London Copley Medal Detained at La Santé prison (30 October–7 December)	Germany invades Europe Franco-German armistice and Pétain government in Vichy. Anti-Semitic laws in France Appeal by General de Gaulle	Development of radar in Great Britain and the United States
1941	Under house arrest in Troyes	Pearl Harbour: the United States and Japan enter the war. Germany attacks the USSR Formation of the National Committee of Free France	G.T. Seaborg produces plutonium by bombarding uranium 238
1942	Under house arrest in Troyes Theory of neutron collisions	Total occupation of France Allied landing in North Africa	Fermi, first atomic pile using uranium and graphite (Chicago): start of the Manhattan Project Death of Jean Perrin and Bergson Death of Jacques Solomon (Langevin's son in law), shot by the Nazis
1943	Under house arrest in Troyes Hélène Solomon-Langevin deported to Auschwitz Reports on the candidacy of F. Joliot to the Academy of Sciences	Victory at Stalingrad Formation of the Free French Forces (de Gaulle), the National Council of the Resistance and the French Committee of National Liberation in Algiers	
1944	Escapes to Switzerland Returns to France with FTP (Francs-tireurs et partisans) escort Joins the French Communist Party	Allied landing and Battle of Normandy Liberation of Paris, provisional government Liberation of the concentration camps German VI and V2 rockets bomb London	

(continued)

Year	Paul Langevin's life events	Social and political events	Scientific and cultural events
1945	President of the Commission for the Reform of Education Member of the Commission for Atomic Energy of the Académie des sciences (with L. de Broglie and F. Joliot-Curie) Co-editor of the *Encyclopédie de la renaissance française* Party for 73rd birthday at the Sorbonne	Germany capitulates Yalta Conference and Potsdam Conference Atomic bombs on Hiroshima and Nagasaki Creation of the UN, end of the League of Nations	
1946	Chairman of the European Congress of New Education (Geneva) Deputy Delegate of France to UNESCO Municipal Councillor of the 2nd Arrondissement of Paris General Councillor of the Seine Died 19 December	Peace Conference in Paris (USSR, United States, Great Britain, France) Beginning of the Indochina War. Nationalization in France Creation of UNESCO United States: atomic bomb tests in Bikini and the Marshall Islands	
1948	19 December: Ashes transferred to the Panthéon, Paris		

Index

A
Abraham, Henri, 99, 155
Académie des sciences, 29, 30, 116, 155, 156
Académie matérialiste, 218
Acceleration wave, 56, 57
Action française, 31, 246
Actualités scientifiques et industrielles, 192, 207
Alain, 155, 160, 161, 187, 227
Albert Hall, 160
Amitiés franco-russes, 105, 226
Ampère, André-Marie, 21, 174
Amsterdam-Pleyel, 159, 161, 218, 227
Andler, Charles, 187, 218
Angell, 159, 160
Appel, Camille, 25
Aragon, 230, 233, 243, 245
Arc transmitter, 81
Arcouest, 26, 76, 107, 254
Argentina, 146
Armengaud, 84, 141
Artillery Commission, 83
Asdic, 99, 103
Association concorde et progrès, 160
Atmospheric ions, 18
Atomism, 41–43, 46, 52
Auger, 27, 164, 169, 188
Auschwitz, 241
Austria, 44, 108
Avogadro's number, 19, 42

B
Bachelard, Gaston, 72, 123, 193, 194, 208
Barbusse, Henri, 106, 159, 161, 187, 227
Bartoli, Adolfo, 15
Basch, Victor, 161, 230, 232, 245
Bateau-lavoir, 10
Bauer, Edmond, 15, 56, 63, 166, 169, 175, 188, 195, 254
Bayet, Albert, 150, 161, 230, 232
Becker, Carl, 109, 110
Becquerel, Jean, 122, 131, 155, 240
Beethoven, 76
Bell, Vanessa, 160
Benda, Julien, 107, 225
Bergery, Gaston, 159
Bergson, Henri, 27, 108, 116, 120, 122, 123, 149, 216
Berlin, 113, 121
Berliner Tageblatt, 32
Bernal, John D., 158, 221, 248, 249
Berr, Henri, 194, 195
Berthelot, Marcellin, 42, 269
Beta (β) particles, 50
Bialobrzeski, Czeslaw, 166
Biological analogies, 67
Biquard, Pierre, 2, 83, 90, 136, 141, 163, 165, 167, 224, 233, 243
Birefringence, 18, 21, 166
Bloch, Jean-Richard, 225, 230, 233
Bloch, Marc, 151, 187
Bloomsbury Group, 160

Blum, Léon, 27, 161, 187
Bogomolov, Aleksandr, 245
Bohr, Niels, 21
Boll, Marcel, 209
Bologna, 19, 65, 66, 68, 72
Boltzmann, Ludwig, 44, 45
Borel, Émile, 25, 31, 42, 83, 107, 116, 150, 165, 197
Born, Max, 179, 201, 212
Bourgeois, Henri, 31
Bournazaud, Louis, 83
Boyle, Robert, 126, 128, 131, 141
Bragg, William Lawrence, 91, 93, 95, 96, 128, 129, 178, 179
Brazil, 114, 160
Breton, Jules, 133, 267
Brillouin, Léon, 83, 131, 141, 165, 168, 179, 192, 216
Brillouin, Marcel, 14, 16, 165, 173, 177, 180, 188
British Board of Inventions and Research, 82, 86, 90–92, 97, 129
British Royal Commission on Awards to Inventors, 140
Brownian motion, 19, 42
Bruhat, Georges, 188
Bruhat, Jean, 230
Brunschvicg, Léon, 70, 119, 193, 194, 201
Brussels, 31, 171, 173, 175, 181, 182, 201
Buber, Martin, 194
Buenos Aires, 19, 146
Buffalo Stadium, 160, 161
Buisson, Ferdinand, 105
Bulletin officiel de l'éducation nationale, 253, 261
Bumstead, Henry, 100

C
Cady, Walter, 140
Cambridge, 12–19, 51, 53, 55, 105, 131, 138, 161
Cambridge Philosophical Society, 19
Cambridge Physical Society, 138
Cambridge Scientists' Anti-War Group, 158
Camus, Albert, 246, 251
Capitant, René, 253, 263
Carco, Franci, 106
Carnot principle, 43, 45
Cathode rays, 13, 15, 16, 50, 52
Cavendish Laboratory, 12, 13, 16, 55, 131
Ce soir, 7

Centre national de la recherche scientifique, 107
Cercle de la Russie neuve, 105, 217, 220, 256
Challaye, Félicien, 158, 217
Chartier, Emile (Alain), 155, 160
Chavannes, Edouard, 26
Chemical weapons, 158
Chilowsky, Constantin, 79–81, 83, 84, 90, 91, 93, 97
Chilowsky, Olga, 79, 80, 140
China, 108–110, 160, 165, 226, 229
Churchill, Winston, 228
Citrine, Sir Walter, 228
Clarté, 106, 158, 159
Claude, Georges, 246
Cogniot, Georges, 1, 2, 211, 218, 220, 224, 225, 230, 233, 253, 263
Colin, Victor, 80, 81, 83, 99, 127
Collège de France
  colleagues at, 26, 56, 71, 79, 133, 151, 187, 217, 253, 256, 260
  courses at, 5, 57, 165
  electrons, 56, 64
  magnetism, 181
  quantum mechanics, 206
  radiation and quanta, 175, 177
  relativity, 64, 115, 198
  ultrasonics, 136, 163
  dismissal from, 235, 239
  Einstein at, 111, 117, 122
  funeral at, 267, 268
  laboratory at, 83, 166, 168, 241–243
  professor at, 4, 12, 14, 23, 34, 239
  students at, 18, 166, 215
Comité d'aide aux victimes du fascisme hitlérien, 159
Comité de vigilance des intellectuels antifascistes, 155, 160
Comité international de coopération intellectuelle (CICI), 108, 109
Comité national de rassemblement populaire, 161, 162
Commissariat à l'énergie atomique, 248
Compagnie générale radiotélégraphique, 81
Complementarity, 216, 219
Comte, Auguste, 41, 117, 147
Congrès de Tours, 225
Conservation of energy, 57
Conservatoire national des arts et métiers, 192
Cooper, Duff, 245
Copenhagen, 19, 177, 213, 216
Copenhagen interpretation, 201, 207, 213
Cot, Pierre, 228

Index

Cotton, 188, 230, 232
Crookes' tube, 17, 50
Crowther, James, 7
Curie, Eugène, 30
Curie, Ève, 29, 78
Curie, Irène ep. Joliot, 26, 107, 181, 243, 244
Curie, Jacques, 89, 90, 92, 126, 133
Curie, Marie, 13, 16, 19, 90, 96, 99, 108, 109, 133, 165, 166, 177, 179, 192, 239
   Académie des sciences, 29
   affair, 30, 31
   encourages Langevin, 78
   health, 35
   laboratory, 35, 137
   Nobel Prize, 31–33, 178
   radium, 32, 90
   at Solvay Congress, 173, 179
   teaching, 23, 26, 29
   wartime x-rays, 77
Curie, Pierre, 5, 13, 14, 16, 20, 45, 127, 129, 166, 250

D
Daladier, Henri, 161
Dale, Sir Henry, 238
Dalton, John, 41
Darwin, Charles, 149
Darwinism, 149
Daudet, Léon, 31, 113
De Broglie, Louis, 7, 15, 166, 177–179, 188, 193, 215, 219, 250, 269
De Broglie, Maurice, 15, 82, 86, 90–93, 128, 164, 173, 175–177, 198
De Gaulle, Charles, 239, 246, 253
De Jouvenel, Henri, 189, 190
De Monzie, Anatole, 187, 257, 258
Debye, Pierre, 179
Decroly, Ovide, 255
Delaisi, F., 161
Democracy, 145
Descartes, René, 151, 230
Desfosses, Jeanne, 23, 24
Determinism, 150, 195, 200–209, 212, 214, 217
Dialectical materialism, 56, 211, 212, 217–220, 222
Diamagnetism, 19–21, 173, 174
Dimitrov, 160
Dirac, Paul, 167, 179, 181, 204, 205, 214, 216
Dominois, F., 161
Dorgelès, Roland, 106
Dos Passos, John, 159

Dreyfus affair, 3
Dreyfus, Alfred, 31
Druault, Jean, 113
Duclaux, Emile, 3
Duclos, Jacques, 229, 232
Duhamel, Georges, 106, 189, 191
Duhem, Pierre, 44–46, 65, 71, 76, 119
Dumas, Jean-Baptiste, 42
Dyson, Frank, 114

E
Ecole municipale de physique et de chimie industrielles (EPCI), 2, 4–6, 10, 11, 13, 16, 23, 34, 78, 81, 104, 105, 166, 168, 217, 235, 239, 241, 260
Ecole normale d'instructrices de l'Aube, 240
Ecole normale supérieure de jeunes filles de Sèvres, 19, 24, 35
Ecole normale supérieure (ENS), 3, 11, 12, 14, 23, 27, 31, 107, 187, 194, 201, 219, 254
Ecole pratique des hautes études, 150, 218, 239
Ecole primaire supérieure Lavoisier, 10
Eddington, Arthur, 114, 205, 208
Education, 37, 38
   children's capacities, 256
   classical, 38
   dogmatism, 40
   higher, 257, 262
   modern humanities, 258
   reform, 38, 253
   in science, 45
   secondary, 37, 38
Eiffel, Gustave, 18
Einstein, Albert, 3, 5, 13, 18, 19, 31, 62, 64, 72, 152, 159, 167, 192, 193, 213, 238
   Bose-Einstein statistics, 206
   Conflict with Bohr, 179, 183, 206
   mass and energy, 58, 64
   methods of thinking, 67, 106
   Paris visit, 113, 114, 116, 117, 122
   photoelectricity, 172, 199
   Solvay, 175
   special relativity, 51
   specific heat, 197
   Witches' Sabbath, 173
   world view, 107, 108
Electromagnetism, 13, 14, 22, 43, 45, 52–55, 62, 63, 66
Emery, L., 161

Encyclopédie française, 149, 151, 187, 191
Energetics, 44
Engels, Friedrich, 211, 218, 220
Ensor, Beatrice, 254
Erhenfest, Paul, 177
Ether, 13, 16, 62, 63, 65, 116
  and spiritualism, 55
Ethiopia, 160
Eve, Arthur S, 128, 133
Exposition de physique et de T.S.F, 136
Exposition nationale des arts et techniques
  dans la vie moderne, 151

F
Fabry, Charles, 126, 141
Falski, Marian, 109
Faraday, Michael, 16, 191
Fascism, 5, 143, 145, 146, 150, 152, 221, 260
Febvre, Lucien, 151, 187, 188, 260, 261
Fermi-Dirac distribution law, 206, 212
Fernandez, R., 161
Ferrié, Gustave, 96
Ferromagnetism, 21, 166
Fitzgerald, George, 13, 55, 63
Flame-tipped shell, 79, 83, 85, 97
Florisson, Charles-Louis, 132–134, 140, 141
Fontenay-aux-Roses, 23, 26, 31
Fournier, G., 161
France nouvelle, 7
France, Anatole, 106
Francs-Tireurs-Partisans (FTP), 243, 244
Frazer, James George, 147
Freinet, Célestin, 255
French Communist Party, 105, 159, 224, 226, 232, 239, 254, 263
  See also Parti communiste française
French Mathematical Society, 14
Fresnel, Henri, 199
Front Populaire, 107, 161, 191, 227, 258

G
Galilean frame of reference, 200
Galileo, Galilei, 39
Gandhi, Mahatma, 159
Gas ionisation, 78, 166, 167
Germany, 44, 55, 76, 79, 104, 108, 111, 126, 131, 133, 134, 150, 158, 160, 194, 230, 235, 241
Gérôme, P., 161
Gestapo, 236
Gide, André, 225, 227

Gide, Charles, 106
Goethe, Johan Wolfgang, 76
Gorki, Maxim, 107, 159
Gouy, Paul, 198
Grains of electricity, 52
Guillaume, Charles-Edouard, 29, 32, 116, 117
Guthrie lecture and medal, 19
Guye, Charles-Eugène, 79, 179, 180

H
Haber, Fritz, 76, 108, 169
Hadamard, Jacques, 79, 117, 119, 165
Hahn, Otto, 181
Hall, Albert, 160
Haller, Albin, 34
Hamilton, 199, 200
Hardy, Thomas, 106
Harwich, 93, 99
Hauser, Fernand, 31
Hegel, Friedrich, 216, 219, 221
Heisenberg, Werner, 172, 179, 213, 214
Hermann, 192
Herriot, Edouard, 27, 187, 257
Hertz, Heinrich, 55
Hiroshima, 144
Holweck, Fernand, 96, 98, 127, 131, 132
Hughes Medal, 19
Hugo, Victor, 3, 10
Huyghens, Christiaan, 199

I
Illustrated London News, 7
Inertia of energy, 6, 18, 57, 59
Institut de France, 156
Institut national de la recherche
  pédagogique, 256
International Congress in St Louis, 18
International League for New Education
  (ILNE), 143, 187, 254, 255
International Research Council, 108
Ionization of gases, 18
Ishimoto, Mishio, 136

J
Japan, 108, 131, 134, 136, 160, 247, 249
Jaurès, Jean, 27, 76
Jeance, Maurice, 80
Jeans, James, 173, 175
Jewish refugees, 160
Joffe, Abraham, 178

Index

Joliot-Curie Hélène, 27
Joliot-Curie, Frédéric, 61, 81, 83, 90, 93,
    163, 166, 181, 188, 222, 230,
    232, 244, 247, 269
Jourdain, Francis, 159, 213
Journal de physique, 35, 104, 110,
    166, 168
Justice, 145

K
Kabbale, 147
Kamerlingh Onnes, Heike, 173, 177, 179
Kant, Imanuel, 76, 120, 208
Kapitza, Piotr, 105, 238
Karlsruhe Chemistry International Conference
    (1860), 42
Kinetic theory, 6, 14, 16, 18, 21, 42
Kirchoff, August, 14
Koyré, Alexandre, 194, 209
Kropotkin, Piotr, 149

L
Labérenne, Paul, 233
Laboratoire du centre d'études de Toulon
    (LCET), 131
Lacaze, Admiral, 128
L'Action française, 31, 113
Lahy, Jean-Maurice, 218
La Libre pensée, 150
Lamarck, Jean Baptiste, 149
Landau, Lev, 105
Langevin, André, 10, 23, 26, 30, 131, 169,
    178, 224, 233
Langevin, Jean, 23, 165, 169, 217
Langevin, Jeanne, 26, 30, 31, 35, 51,
    236, 241
Langevin Hélène ep. Solomon, 23, 34, 169,
    215, 224, 227, 236, 241
Langevin, Luce, 169, 224
Langevin, Madeleine, 23, 34, 169
Langevin, Michel, 27
Langevin, Paul-Gilbert, 35, 241
Langevin's noise, 19
Langevin stack, 138
Langevin, Victor, 9
Langevin-Chilowsky Mission, 83
Langevin-Colin Mission, 85
Langevin's traveller, 116, 122
Langevin-Wallon plan, 4, 256, 259–263, 265
la Pasionaria, 229
La Pensée, 90, 209, 231, 247, 249

La pensée et l'action, 254
Lapierre, G., 161
Laplace, 212, 214
Larmor, Joseph, 16, 55
La Santé prison, 236, 240
L'Aube, 7
Laugier, Henri, 150, 254
L'Avant-garde, 7
Lavoisier, Antoine, 39
Lawrence, Ernest, 166
League of Human Rights, 105, 121, 143–145,
    150, 159, 226, 230, 245
League of Nations, 108, 109, 145, 158, 159,
    165, 255
Le Chatelier, Henry, 39
L'école unique, 257, 258
Le Corbusier, Henri, 225
Lefebvre, Raymond, 106
Le Figaro, 12
Léger, André, 243
Légion d'honneur, 103
Le Mois, 204, 207
Lenard, Philipp, 76
Lenin, Vladimir Ilitch, 56, 211, 218
L'Entente féminine, 159
Léon, Xavier, 118, 257
Le Roy, Édouard, 70
Les Cahiers rationalistes, 151
Les Compagnons de l'université
    nouvelle, 254
Les Lettres françaises, 2
Le Temps, 31
Lévy–Bruhl, Lucien, 147
L'Humanité, 105, 158, 220, 226, 247
Li Lin Yu, 110
Li Yu Ying, 110
Liard, Louis, 38
Liberation, 4, 105, 109, 146, 149, 228, 243,
    246, 249, 253, 265
Lippmann, Gabriel, 45
Littré, Emile, 3
Lodge, Oliver, 55, 56
Loomis, Alfred, 97, 141
Lorentz, Hendrik, 52, 53, 55, 62, 63, 108, 111,
    168, 177, 179, 180, 183
    contraction, 63
    group, 63
    transformation, 58, 62, 64, 66
Louisiana Purchase Exposition, 19, 49, 51
Lucas, René, 165, 166
l'Université libre, 239
Lupesco, Stephan, 209
Luquet, G.H., 161

M

Mach, Ernst, 43, 44, 119, 121
Magnetism, 5–7, 14, 18, 20, 21, 98, 165, 167, 178, 180, 181, 185
Malfitano, Giovanni, 83
Manhattan Project, 247
Mann, Heinrich, 107, 159
Marbo, Camille, 25, 27
Margueritte, Victor, 158
Mariotte's law, 42
Marrou, Henri-Irénée, 253
Marti, Pierre, 132
Marty, André, 105
Marx, Karl, 187, 211, 216–218, 220
Marxism, 216–221
Mascart, Eleuthère, 12, 14, 65
Matisse, Henri, 160
Maublanc, René, 217, 230, 233
Maxwell, James Clerk, 16, 52, 54, 55, 58, 62, 67, 197
Mechanics, 13, 14, 16, 18, 22, 41–43, 46, 121, 149, 188
   classical, 44, 52, 54, 63, 68, 118, 213, 214, 217
   quantum, 21, 168, 179, 193, 194, 201, 204, 205, 212, 240
   statistical, 15, 201
   wave, 198, 201, 205
Meitner, Lisa, 181
Ménard-Dorian, Aline, 27, 149
Metaphysics, 43
Metz, André, 122, 167
Meyerson, Emile, 72, 120, 123, 167, 193, 207–209, 216, 256
Meyerson, Ignace, 256
Michelson, Albert, 13
Michelson-Morley experiments, 18, 53, 62
Milhaud, Edgard, 79
Mineur, Henri, 209
Minister of Public Education and Inventions, 82
Moch, Jules, 155, 156
Montel, Eliane, 35, 241
Montessori, Maria, 255
Montmartre, 9
Morin, Charles, 133
Morley, Edward W., 13
Moscow, 19, 79, 225, 226, 230, 238
Moulin, Alfred, 156
Moulin, Marcel, 15, 18
Mourgues (Miss), 42
Mouton, Henri, 26
Murray, Gilbert, 108

Musée national d'histoire naturelle, 239
Musée pédagogique, 38, 42, 256
Mussolini, Benito, 187

N

Nagasaki, 246, 247
Nawa, Takeshi, 137
Néel, Louis, 21
Nernst, Walther, 171–173, 175, 177
Neutron, 181, 241
Newcomb, Simon, 50, 51
Newton, Isaac, 53, 146, 147, 220
Nicolson, Alexander McLean, 127, 140
Nie wieder krieg movement, 121
Nizan, Paul, 232
Nobel Prize, 5, 21, 31, 166, 167, 178, 179, 192, 198, 203, 239, 269
Nordmann, Charles, 113, 115–117, 122
Nuclear energy, 18, 248, 250, 251
Nuclear mass deficit, 18
Nuclear physics, 192

O

Odessa, 105
Ostwald, Wilhelm, 43, 55, 76

P

Painlevé, Paul, 27, 34, 79, 80, 82, 83, 107, 116, 117, 119, 122, 133, 269
Palais de la découverte, 151, 186, 189–191
Palladino, Eusapia, 24
Pantheon, 3, 103, 269
Paramagnetism, 21, 61, 174
Paris Commune, 9
Parkeston Quay, 93, 99
Parti communiste français (PCF), 105, 159, 216–218, 224, 225, 232, 239
Pascal, 42
Pasteur Institute, 26
Pasteur, Louis, 3, 46, 152
Patent, 83, 84, 92, 126–133, 138, 140, 191, 192
   capacitive transducer, 84
   claims, 140, 141
   conflicts concerning, 125, 126
   echo sounding, 134
   quartz sandwich, 128, 129, 132
   Richardson, 80
   ultrasonic transducers, 137
   USA, 127, 140, 141

Pauli, Wolfgang, 179, 204, 212, 216
Peace activist, 145
Peierls, Rudolph, 249
Perrin, Francis, 188
Perrin, Henriette, 29, 30
Perrin, Jean, 52, 119, 131, 151, 165, 204,
    235, 269
  activism, 107, 150, 226, 230, 232
  cathode rays, 15
  encyclopedie français, 188
  friendship, 3, 19, 25, 26, 28, 76, 78
  Solvay, 173, 178, 180
  WWI, 83
Philosophy, 68, 205
  concepts of time, 70
  French influence on, 123
Photoelectricity, 199
Physical Society of London, 19
Piaget, Jean, 256
Picard, Emile, 39, 76, 240
Picasso, Pablo, 160
Piéron, Henri, 209, 254, 260, 261
Piezoelectricity, 5, 90, 91, 97, 136, 138, 140,
    141, 166
Pinel, Marie-Adèle, 9
Piobetta, Stéphane, 253
Pivert, M., 220
Planck, Max, 13, 15, 44, 76, 172, 173, 175,
    179, 197, 199, 200, 205, 207,
    208, 213
Plato, 151
Poincaré, Henri, 13, 14, 16, 18,
    53, 58, 62–64, 67, 71,
    173, 175, 193
Poincaré, Raymond, 32
Politzer, Georges, 216, 218, 230, 239, 241
Prague, 19
Prenant, Marcel, 161, 218
Prout's Law, 59
Pupin, Michael, 97, 127
Pyroelectricity, 166

Q
Quanta, 13, 165, 175, 179, 180, 188,
    195, 197–200, 204, 208,
    212, 220
Quartz, 80, 90, 96, 97, 103, 166
  Curies', 92
  hydrophone, 138
  x-cut, 92, 141
Quartz piézo-électrique, 89–92, 133

R
Radiation force, 81
Radio, 80
Radioactivity, 13, 15, 16, 30, 50, 59, 91, 166,
    181, 192, 239
Radio-Liberté, 186
Radium, 13, 14, 18, 32
Ramadier, Paul, 263
Raman effect, 166
Ramette, Arthur, 232
Rathenau, Walter, 111
Rayleigh, Lord, 136, 198
Réforme, 2
Relativity, 13, 15, 18, 35, 104, 111,
    136, 185, 186, 192–195, 198,
    208, 219
  frames of reference, 66, 70, 117
  general, 113, 115, 116, 118
  and gravitation, 114, 115
  history of, 62, 64, 67
  and philosophy, 71, 72, 121
  principle of, 53, 56, 62–66, 69, 113
  special, 52, 62, 63, 117, 118, 201, 213
  theory of, 62, 67, 119, 122, 165,
      200, 212, 216
Renan, Ernest, 150, 152
Renard, E., 161
Renoult, Daniel, 105
Renseignements généraux, 157, 232, 233
Resonance, 129, 219
Revue du mois, 27
Rey, Abel, 44, 194, 209
Richardson, Lewis Fry, 80
Righi, Augusto, 56, 178
Rivet, Paul, 155, 158, 160, 161,
    227, 228, 239
Roger, Henri, 150, 246
Rolland, Romain, 7, 107, 158, 159, 163, 187,
    226, 228, 233
Romains, Jules, 106
Rome, 19
Röntgen, Wilhelm, 16, 97
Rosny, J.H., 27, 106, 186
Rostand, Jean, 149
Rotblat, Joseph, 249
Roussy, Gustave, 239
Royal Institution, 19
Royal Society of London, 19, 61, 238
Russell, Bertrand, 106, 107, 159
Rutherford, Ernest, 15, 16, 31, 49–51,
    59, 90–92, 126–128, 138,
    140, 173, 177

S

Sagnac, Georges, 65, 116
Sartre, Jean-Paul, 106, 246, 247
Saville Lt., R, 93
Schrödinger, Erwin, 179, 201, 203
Schuster, Arthur, 15
Schutzenberger, Paul, 10
Seclet-Riou, Fernande, 261, 262
Secours rouge international, 160
Seignobos, Charles, 26
Semard, Pierre, 232
Sennep, Jean, 261
Séverine, 106
Simpson, John A., 249
Sinclair, Upton, 107, 159
Snow, Charles P, 259
Société de condensation et d'applications mécaniques (SCAM), 133–135, 137, 141
Société française de pédagogie, 143, 156, 163, 254
Société française de philosophie, 65, 70, 71, 116, 118, 119
Société française de physique, 57, 111, 173, 197, 198
Solomon, Hélène Langevin, 169, 215, 224, 227, 236, 241
Solomon, Jacques, 138, 169, 188, 192, 195, 209, 215–217, 219, 224, 227, 230, 232, 239, 241, 245
Solvay Council, 163, 169, 206
    1911, 172, 173, 176
    1913, 177
    1923, 111
    1927, 194, 197, 200–202, 204
    1933, 182
    1936, 183
    chairman, 180
    chemistry, 180
    president, 168
    scientific committee, 179
Solvay, Ernest, 171–173, 175, 177, 178, 180
Sommerfeld, Arnold, 66, 173, 198, 199
SONAR, 7, 99, 103, 129
Sondeur Ultra-sonore Langevin-Florisson-Marti, 134
Spain, 160, 228, 229
Speed of light, 13, 58, 59, 65
Sp. Kamerlingh Onnes, Heike, 177
Stalin, Joseph, 226
Steiner, Rudolf, 255
St. Louis, 49–51, 53, 56, 65

Stokes, George, 13
Stoney, George J, 52
Surrealism, 225

T

Tawney, Robert, 109
Téry, Gustave, 31, 34
Thaelmann, 160
Thinking in ether, 54–57
Thomson, John J., 13, 15, 16, 51, 131, 178, 199
Thorez, Maurice, 161, 227, 232
Thorndike, Sybil, 160
Time, 70
The Times, 7
Tonnelat, Ernest, 236
Torsion balance, 81, 136
Toulon, 83–86, 93, 96, 97, 99, 100, 126–128, 131, 132
Tournier, Marcel, 81, 83, 85, 89, 90, 93, 95–99, 126, 127, 131–133
Townsend, John, 15, 166, 180
Triolet, Elsa, 243
Trotsky, 225
Trouton-Nobel experiment, 63
Troyes, 240–242, 244, 245, 248

U

Ultrasonics, 89, 90, 97, 164–167
    British work in, 91, 93
    capacitive transducer, 80, 84, 86, 97
    carbon microphone, 81, 85
    CMUT, 86
    diffraction, 192
    echo sounding, 133, 134, 137
    first echoes, 85
    laboratory, 82
    layered quartz transducer, 98, 138
    medical, 103, 133, 141
    non-linear loss, 141
    non-resonant transducer, 128
    patent, 84, 109, 141
    power, 81
    quartz receiver, 95
    quartz transducer, 89, 92, 93, 95, 99, 126, 128, 129
    radiation pressure, 81
    sea trials, 86, 132
    submarine detection, 94, 99, 100, 125
    supersonics, 138

Union des intellectuels pour la justice, la liberté et la paix (UDIF), 230
Union rationaliste, 143, 150, 151, 216, 248, 249
Union sacrée, 104
Université ouvrière, 187, 216
Urbain, Georges, 32, 188
USSR, 105, 159, 217, 226, 227, 238, 245

V
Vaillant-Couturier, Paul, 106, 186, 225
Valéry, Paul, 27, 108, 189, 191
Velocity waves, 56
Vichy government, 161, 165, 239, 240
Vienna Circle, 207, 209, 213, 215

W
Wallon, Henri, 161, 163, 217, 221, 226, 233, 236, 240, 253, 256, 259, 260, 262, 263
Walther Nernst, 76
Wave mechanics, 188
Weiss magneton, 166
Weiss, Pierre, 21, 166, 173, 177, 181

Wells, H.G., 68, 69, 106, 228
Werlein, Ivan, 93
Wien, Wilhelm, 15
Wilson, Charles, 15, 179
Wood, Robert, 97, 98, 127, 141, 166
Woolf, Virginia, 160
World Committee against War and Fascism, 143
Wurmser, André, 161

X
X-ray, 13, 15, 16, 77, 78, 91, 97, 166, 178, 221

Y
Yan Jici, 110

Z
Zangwill, Israel, 106
Zay, Jean, 258
Zeeman effect, 16
Zola, Emile, 3, 152
Zweig, Stefan, 106

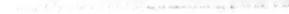

The manufacturer's authorised representative in the EU is Springer Nature Customer Service Centre GmbH, Europaplatz 3, 69115 Heidelberg, Germany. If you have any concerns regarding our products, please contact ProductSafety@springernature.com

Printed and bound by CPI Group (UK) Ltd, Croydon, CR0 4YY

23/03/2026

02076380-0006